Making Medical Progress

Answers to the question "what is medical progress?" have always been contested, and any one response is always bound up with contextual ideas of personhood, society, and health. However, the widely held enthusiasm for medical progress escapes more general critiques of progress as a conceptual category. From the intersection of intellectual history, philosophy, and the medical humanities, Vanessa Rampton sheds light on the politics of medical progress and how they have downplayed the tensions between individual and social goods. She examines how a shared consensus about its value gives medical progress vast political and economic capital, revealing who benefits, who is left out, and who is harmed by narratives of progress. From ancient Greece to artificial intelligence, exploring the origins and ethics of different visions of progress offers valuable insights into how we can make them more meaningful in future. This title is also available as open access on Cambridge Core.

VANESSA RAMPTON is an intellectual historian and senior researcher at Assisted Lab in the University of St. Gallen's Medical Humanities Chair.

Making Medical Progress

History of a Contested Idea

VANESSA RAMPTON
University of St. Gallen

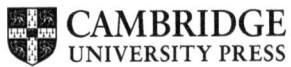

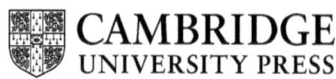

Shaftesbury Road, Cambridge CB2 8EA, United Kingdom

One Liberty Plaza, 20th Floor, New York, NY 10006, USA

477 Williamstown Road, Port Melbourne, VIC 3207, Australia

314–321, 3rd Floor, Plot 3, Splendor Forum, Jasola District Centre, New Delhi – 110025, India

103 Penang Road, #05–06/07, Visioncrest Commercial, Singapore 238467

Cambridge University Press is part of Cambridge University Press & Assessment, a department of the University of Cambridge.

We share the University's mission to contribute to society through the pursuit of education, learning and research at the highest international levels of excellence.

www.cambridge.org
Information on this title: www.cambridge.org/9781009602631

DOI: 10.1017/9781009602662

© Vanessa Rampton 2026

This publication is in copyright. Subject to statutory exception and to the provisions of relevant collective licensing agreements, with the exception of the Creative Commons version the link for which is provided below, no reproduction of any part may take place without the written permission of Cambridge University Press & Assessment.

An online version of this work is published at doi.org/10.1017/9781009602662 under a Creative Commons Open Access license CC-BYNC 4.0 which permits re-use, distribution and reproduction in any medium for non-commercial purposes providing appropriate credit to the original work is given and any changes made are indicated. To view a copy of this license visit https://creativecommons.org/licenses/by-nc/4.0

When citing this work, please include a reference to the DOI 10.1017/9781009602662

First published 2026

Cover credit: Philadelphia Museum of Art: The Louise and Walter Arensberg Collection, 1950 (1950-134-104)

A catalogue record for this publication is available from the British Library

Library of Congress Cataloging-in-Publication Data
Names: Rampton, Vanessa, 1980– author
Title: Making medical progress : history of a contested idea / Vanessa Rampton.
Description: Cambridge, United Kingdom ; New York, NY : Cambridge University Press, 2026. | Includes bibliographical references and index.
Identifiers: LCCN 2025007707 | ISBN 9781009602631 paperback | ISBN 9781009602655 hardback | ISBN 9781009602662 ebook
Subjects: MESH: Biomedical Research – history | Philosophy, Medical – history | Bioethics – history | Personal Autonomy | Health Equity – history | History 20th Century | History, 21st Century
Classification: LCC R852 .R27 2026 | NLM W 20.5 | DDC 610.72/4–dc23/eng/20250703
LC record available at https://lccn.loc.gov/2025007707

ISBN 978-1-009-60265-5 Hardback
ISBN 978-1-009-60263-1 Paperback

Cambridge University Press & Assessment has no responsibility for the persistence or accuracy of URLs for external or third-party internet websites referred to in this publication and does not guarantee that any content on such websites is, or will remain, accurate or appropriate.

For EU product safety concerns, contact us at Calle de José Abascal, 56, 1°, 28003 Madrid, Spain, or email eugpsr@cambridge.org

The open access publication of this book has been published with the support of the Swiss National Science Foundation.

Contents

Acknowledgments	*page* vii
Introduction	1
I.1 Spotlight on Medical Progress	3
I.2 Scope and Aims	6
I.3 Dimensions of Personhood and Patienthood	10
I.4 Health and Values	13
I.5 Problematizing Medical Progress	16
I.6 Historiography of Progress	22
I.7 Historiography of Medicine and Progress	25
I.8 Medical Progress: A Multidimensional View	30
1 History: Medical Progress in Context	34
1.1 Notions of Selfhood and Progress in Antiquity	36
1.2 Health in Christianity and the Middle Ages	40
1.3 Progress and the Person in the Renaissance	46
1.4 Medical Progress, Self, and Enlightenment	49
1.5 Nineteenth Century: Medical Progress and Civilization	56
1.6 Early Twentieth-Century Visions of Progress	61
1.7 Conclusion	64
2 Medical Progress as Biomedical Knowledge Gains	66
2.1 The Importance of (Biomedical) Scientific Knowledge after War	67
2.2 Challenges to Scientific Knowledge Progress from Medicine and the Social Sciences	71
2.3 Challenges to Scientific Knowledge Progress from the Philosophy of Science	76
2.4 No Progress in Medicine: Questioning Cumulative, Progressive Knowledge	78
2.5 Pluralism, Information, and Knowledge	82

	2.6	Defending Progress in Medicine	86
	2.7	Conclusion	101
3	Medical Progress as Becoming Free	104
	3.1	From Technical Knowledge Gains to "Moral Knowing"	106
	3.2	The New Bioethics: Progress as Patient Autonomy	110
	3.3	Challenges to Negative Freedom	114
	3.4	Taking Autonomy Seriously: Freedom versus (Technological) Progress	121
	3.5	Reclaiming Progress as Freedom	131
	3.6	Conclusion	140
4	"Health for All": Medical Progress as Justice	142
	4.1	Progress as Medical Access: Origins	144
	4.2	Progress on Health Equity I: Primary Care and "Health for All"	147
	4.3	Progress on Health Equity II: Upstream Determinants of Health	152
	4.4	Progress, the Social Determinants of Health, and Health Justice	154
	4.5	Progress as Justice: Critiques	161
	4.6	Medical Progress and COVID-19	165
	4.7	Conclusion	170

Epilogue: Medical Progress as Achieving Sustainability   171

Bibliography   188

Index   230

Acknowledgments

This book is a product of the Branco Weiss Fellowship that provided the impetus, funding, and protected time necessary to complete it. I am deeply grateful for many kinds of help I received along the way.

This book greatly benefited from the erudition, questions, and unwavering support of Professor Lutz Wingert, who gave the project a home at his Chair for Philosophy at Eidgenössische Technische Hochschule (ETH) Zürich. I am grateful to Johann Steurer for numerous valuable observations and for his interest in the study from the very beginning. Profound thanks to Victoria Laszlo for all manners of administrative help and support. For encouragement and generous insights, I thank Martin Beckstein, Cornelius Borck, Rachele Delucchi, Fabienne Forster, Jörg Goldhahn, Michael Hagner, Michael Hampe, Martin Hurni, Oskar Jenni, Matthias Kettner, Christine Kuhn, Jérôme Léchot, Nadia Mazouz, Raphael Meyer, Michael Mittelman, Silvan Moser, Tobias Rees, Edith Schmid, Lisa Schurrer, Kaj Späth, Romila Storjohann, Dieter Sturma, Effy Vayena, Sophie Witt, and Monika Wulz. In Zürich, I feel particularly lucky for the feedback and friendship of Maria Böhmer, Nadja El Kassar, Janina Kehr, Anita Winkler, and Vera Wolff.

In a second phase, the project profited enormously from the knowledge and enthusiasm of Daniel Weinstock, who enabled it to find a home at McGill, first at the Institute for Health and Social Policy and then at the Department of Equity, Ethics, and Politics. In Montréal, I learnt from the work of wonderful interns, particularly Esther Kim, Sarah Kim, Alua Kulenova, and Kristin Vanderwee. I am particularly lucky to have collaborated with Athena Ko. Grateful thanks to Anaik Fortier and Sonia Bichler for their long-standing support and perfect administrative work. I am profoundly grateful to Mary Bartram, Michael Da Silva, Hazar Haidar, Jonathan Kimmelman, Nicholas King, Arijit Nandi, Thomas Schlich, and David Wright for their insights into aspects of this project and organizational help. Warmest thanks to Phoebe Friesen for the comradeship.

Every time I presented elements of this work at the Branco Weiss Symposium, I came away seeing it differently. I am very grateful to Peter Chen, Detlef Günther, Angelika Steger, Heidi Wunderli-Allenspach, and Josef Zeyer for accepting me into the fellowship and supporting my project. Thank you to Sonja Isliker, Alessandro Monachesi, Kathrin Ringger, George Slavich, Martine Vernooij, and Eberhard Zangger for all manners of administrative and personal support. The solidarity of different fellows meant so much to me; I am particularly thankful to Kelly Clancy, Lea Haller, Laura Hendriks, Stephanie King, Rain Liivoja, Hannah Mumby, Carolin Schurr, Aurore Schwab, Tetyana Vasylyeva, Anna-Sophia Wahl, Karim Bschir, Klaus Eyer, and Matthieu Galvez. I feel very lucky that Marie Kolkenbrock and Simone Schürle were there during the fellowship and beyond. Lara Keuck illuminated and inspired me in this project, and our meetings during long COVID weeks kept it afloat.

I am grateful to organizers and audiences at workshops and conferences where I discussed this work, among others at Ludwig Maximilian University (LMU) Munich, ETH Zurich, University of Zurich, Vrije Universiteit (VU) Amsterdam, University of St. Gallen, University of Twente, Leibniz University Hannover, Humboldt University Berlin, and McGill University. Ideas I develop here are related to research funded by the ETH Postdoctoral Fellowship program, the support of which I gratefully acknowledge. In the project's last stages, I profited from being surrounded by wonderful colleagues at Assisted Lab, including Charlotte Frank, Marc Keller, Jordan McCullough, Alexander Meienberger, Robyn Otto, Carlos Pittella, and Joe Wood.

At Cambridge University Press, I am very grateful to Rosa Martin and Lucy Rhymer, the editing team, and to anonymous reviewers whose suggestions and references improved this book. I gratefully acknowledge the Swiss National Science Foundation for providing open access funding for this project. I also thank the Philadelphia Museum of Art for supplying the cover image.

Academic research relies on a huge amount of behind the scenes support. I thank the personnel at institutions where I worked in both Zürich and Montréal, as well as educators at institutions ranging from Kinderkrippe to école secondaire. I am grateful to friends, in particular Penelope Bruha, Elgin Brunner, Noah Cannon, Rocío Carvajo, Jérome Ebiner, Mayssun El-Attar, Manon Fantini, Nazlie Faridi, Muriel Gschwend, Florin Ivan, Aleksandra Kucharczyk, Cara

MacMillan, Fabienne Müller, Lorraine Price, Christine Rösch, Stefan Rösch, Louisa Sage, Maude Théoret, Susan Turcot, Sonia Vedrunes, Chris Wilbert, and Milena Zulczyk for helping me with aspects of this project and acting as sources of inspiration. Isabelle Cornaz has thought through my projects with me for decades and improved the book with her suggestions. I am so lucky for the friendship and colleagueship of Anna Elsner, who has been a source of solidarity and support for this project since its inception.

A special kind of gratitude to my extended and immediate family, particularly to my mother and father, and to Alexis, Adrian, and Nicholas. I am most grateful to Nour, Maya, Anouk, and Roman for being with me throughout.

Introduction

In today's era of modern Western medicine, organ transplants are routine, and daily headlines about the mysteries of DNA and the human genome promise that the secrets of life itself are tantalizingly within our reach. Yet to reach this point took thousands of years. One step at a time [...] humanity's medical knowledge has moved forward from a time when even the slightest cut held the threat of infection and death[.]

These words, taken from a popular history of medicine course, have been cited to illustrate the "amazing progress humankind has made from the Stone Age until today."[1] They also bear witness to a widespread contemporary belief, namely, the tendency to associate medicine with the idea of progress. Today, the term "progress" is used by a wide range of people – including politicians, scientists, physicians, and patients – to speak of past medical developments and desired future changes. The notion that impressive progress is being made, and occurring in such a step-by-step fashion that it has the potential to "stall" or be "set back," is a common way of making sense of the developments in medicine.[2]

Despite its popularity in the medical field, the idea of progress is out of fashion as a concept with explanatory power. The notion of

---

[1] See Sherwin B. Nuland, "Doctors: The History of Scientific Medicine Revealed through Biography," *The Great Courses*, The Teaching Company, www.thegreatcourses.com/courses/doctors-the-history-of-scientific-medicine-revealed-through-biography and Clifford A. Pickover, *The Medical Book: From Witch Doctors to Robot Surgeons* (New York: Union Square, 2012), p. 5.

[2] See, for example, the statement by the CEO of the American Medical Association (AMA) in "America Speaks: Polling Data Reflecting the Views of Americans on Medical, Health and Scientific Research," *Research!America: An Alliance for Discoveries in Health*, 14 (2022), p. ii and "AMA President Applauds Members Moving Medicine Forward," *AMA Press Release*, June 8, 2019, www.ama-assn.org/press-center/press-releases/ama-president-applauds-members-moving-medicine-forward.

progress as a cumulative process that enables an individual or a society to attain something, and then go on to achieve something better, is largely seen as a naïve and misleading way of presenting historical change. The English historian Herbert Butterfield, in his famous work *The Whig Interpretation of History* (1931), drew attention to the flaws inherent in seeing the present as an improvement on the past.[3] In Butterfield's account, and the generations of students who absorbed it, "Whig history," or presenting history as a tale of progress, was exactly what not to do as a historian.[4] Numerous critics have pointed to the ways in which the idea presupposes a Eurocentric sense of civilizational and moral superiority and how narratives of progress are bound up with practices of domination, oppression, and violence. Genocide, the nuclear era, wars, and the persistent threat of war, global inequalities, and climate change; it is possible to argue that empirical claims for progress are undermined by reality. "How does it happen that serious people continue to believe in progress in the face of massive evidence that might have been expected to refute the idea of progress once and for all?"[5] With this rhetorical question, social critic Christopher Lasch sums up the widely held disdain for the notion of progress in history.

This book scrutinizes progress rhetoric in the post-World War II period by focusing on medicine, a field that is arguably the paradigm case for an intense belief in progress. Using the tools of intellectual history, it traces the rise and proliferation of the concept of medical progress, which is influenced in complex ways by changing definitions of health, technological capabilities, and politics. Uncovering and cataloging the multiple meanings of medical progress is important because of the concept's impressive emotional power. The commitment to it is remarkably widespread and that commitment – regardless of its precise meaning – influences scientific and political agendas, as well as shared beliefs about the goals of medicine. Clarifying what people mean when they talk about medical progress shows what gets

---

[3] Herbert Butterfield, *The Whig Interpretation of History* (London: G. Bell and Sons, 1931).

[4] Among the voluminous literature on Butterfield's impact on historians, see Naomi Oreskes, "Why I Am a Presentist?," *Science in Context*, 26 (4) (2013), 595–609.

[5] This is the first line of his book *The True and Only Heaven: A History of Progress and Its Critics* (New York: W. W. Norton & Company, 1991).

left out when it is associated with particular kinds of knowledge, as well as who benefits from a specific narrative of progress, and who is harmed by it. In particular, I argue that the most optimistic advocates of medical progress endorse simplified, static views of health and downplay the tensions between individual and social goods. Starting from the normative premise that health is a complex biopsychosocial state and that illness is not fixed, but rather influenced by norms and values, this study shows how progress in medicine is necessarily multidimensional.

I.1 Spotlight on Medical Progress

Why focus on medical progress in particular? Let me start by saying that it is certainly true that the term and the concept of progress have substantial rhetorical and political power in a number of fields. The commitment to measuring and facilitating progress is a fundamental part of the mandate of various international organizations, including the Organisation for Economic Cooperation and Development (OECD), the World Health Organization (WHO), and the United Nations (UN), which reflects the fact that discussions of progress often have explicitly global aspirations. Making progress is a fundamental motivation for both mainstream and alternative economic approaches.[6] It is also a notion able to transcend traditional political boundaries, as the same term "progress" is used by otherwise antagonistic politicians.[7] International science, meanwhile, generally considers the aspiration for progress to be its driving force; there is a virtually unanimous agreement that science is a progress discipline.[8]

---

[6] See, for example, "Our Founding Mission," *The Economist*, www.economistgroup.com/businesses/the-economist, and Abhijit Banerjee and Esther Duflo, *Poor Economics: A Radical Rethinking of the Way to Fight Global Poverty* (New York: PublicAffairs, 2012), p. viii.

[7] See, for example, The White House, "Highlighting a Year of Progress: The Biden-Harris Cancer Cabinet Takes Action to End Cancer as We Know It," March 8, 2024, https://bidenwhitehouse.archives.gov/ostp/news-updates/2024/03/08/highlighting-a-year-of-progress-the-biden-harris-cancer-cabinet-takes-action-to-end-cancer-as-we-know-it/ and "President Donald J. Trump's State of the Union Address," The White House, January 30, 2018, www.whitehouse.gov/briefings-statements/president-donald-j-trumps-state-union-address/.

[8] John Losee, *Theories of Scientific Progress: An Introduction* (London: Psychology Press, 2004), p. 1.

The interest in medical progress, however, is particularly diffuse; whenever I have looked for the term "progress" – and related notions of "better," "improve," and "advance" – with reference to medical practices and their effectiveness, I have found it. An interdisciplinary project devoted to understanding the goals of medicine highlighted precisely the commitment to "unbounded progress" as the main belief that has inordinately shaped modern medicine.[9] Today, the term progress is regularly used to characterize, among other things, health artificial intelligence (AI), brain imaging technologies, datasets of cancer genomes, and bionic limbs. For example, entrepreneur and philanthropist Mark Zuckerberg connects medical progress with the natural and engineering sciences and praises the AI software, chips, and monitoring devices his organization funds for that reason.[10]

As I argue throughout this study, the myriad of criticisms of the idea of progress as a conceptual category have not had the same impact in medicine that they have had in other fields. It is well known that scientific and technological progress can be used for harm as well as for good, while economic progress, for example, has been roundly criticized for its association with environmental destruction. But medicine is regularly cited as the field in which the benefits of progress outweigh potential harms. Amid a new awareness of the ambivalent effects of progress, dedication to the idea of specifically medical progress in advertising, media, political rhetoric, and societal expectations grew steadily in the past decades. At times, progress in medicine became the answer to the question of "What, if anything, constitutes progress?" Medical progress is, I suspect, one field in which the hope for progress and the belief in technological power and its ability to be harnessed for human well-being are particularly intertwined. Even academics in the humanities, who have long been wary of using normative concepts to assess historical changes, agree that progress in medicine has occurred.[11] I am not a relativist, and I believe that medical knowledge

---

[9] *The Goals of Medicine: The Forgotten Issues in Health Care Reform*, eds. Mark J. Hanson and Daniel Callahan (Washington, DC: Georgetown University Press, 1999), p. 5.

[10] Mark Zuckerberg, "Can We Cure All Diseases in Our Children's Lifetime?," September 21, 2016, Chan Zuckerberg Initiative, https://chanzuckerberg.com/newsroom/can-we-cure-all-diseases-in-our-childrens-lifetime/.

[11] See the following exemplary material: a medical anthropologist colleague told me – "Clearly, progress *has* happened: Life expectancies are longer and

and practice can improve, but I also show that medicine is not immune to the multiple epistemological and ethical critiques of progress developed in the past century.

In his comprehensive study of the history of the idea of progress, sociologist Robert Nisbet acknowledges the impossibility of empirically or logically verifying the concept of progress per se, while noting that medicine is an exception to this rule:

> One may say, precisely and verifiably enough, that the art of medicine [...] has advanced, given our perfectly objective ways of noting the means toward the long-held end or purpose in each art: saving or healing life [...]. Plainly, penicillin is, and can be proved to be, superior to old-fashioned remedies – blood-letting or leeching, for example.[12]

Yet as I show in what follows, assessments of medical progress occur in the context of much broader beliefs about human health and well-being than simply "saving or healing life." In particular, largely justified claims about first-order medical progress – the superiority of penicillin to blood-letting to treat a bacterial infection, for example – become bound up with second-order thinking, that is, normative visions of medical historical progress.[13] As a rule, this masks how progress in one dimension – for example, the development of an antibiotic – is entangled with its existence and distribution in complex social circumstances and power structures. What is at stake is the extent to which progress in different aspects of life relates to and interacts with each other.

---

medical procedures did get better. I also don't want to deny the possibility of future progress in science or medicine. Why would I? I actually hope for progress." This was also the upshot of a conversation I had with Amy Allen, author of *The End of Progress: Decolonizing the Normative Foundations of Critical Theory* (New York: Columbia University Press, 2016) on the sidelines of the Summer School "Progress, Regression and Social Change," in Berlin in 2017. See also her "How Not to Critique the Critique of Progress: A Reply to Payrow Shabani," *Journal of Value Inquiry*, 51 (2017), 681–87. Conversations with medical historian Maria Böhmer and philosophers Lutz Wingert and Nadia Mazouz have furthered my thinking on this issue.

[12] Robert A. Nisbet, *History of the Idea of Progress* (New Brunswick & London: Transaction Publishers, 1980), p. 6.

[13] Second-order thinking can be roughly summarized as thinking about thinking. See Yehuda Elkana, "The Emergence of Second-Order Thinking in Classical Greece," in *The Origins and Diversity of Axial Age Civilizations*, ed. S.N. Eisenstadt (Albany, NY: State University of Albany Press, 1986), p. 40.

A disjunction that philosopher Ruth Macklin highlights between "wholly uncontroversial" technological progress, on the one hand, and "highly controversial" moral progress on the other is at the heart of this study.[14] This is because medicine is an art that, while it relies on an extensive body of scientific knowledge and treatment possibilities, remains a humanistic practice. Medicine still requires that the doctor recognize the patient as a full human being with their own preferences, values, and uncertainties, which can change rapidly. Moreover, some medical goals – to save life, for example – do not fit together easily with others – such as the goal to provide equitable care to all. These humanistic and social dimensions of medicine sit uneasily with simplistic conceptions of medicine-as-technological-progress.

I.2 Scope and Aims

This book examines the recent focus on medical progress with reference to North America and Western Europe. I have chosen to focus on the Global North for both practical reasons – this study was composed in Switzerland and Canada – and conceptual ones. OECD countries are at the forefront of technological developments in medicine, and this has influenced their sense of embodying progress. For example, Geneva University Hospitals, one of the largest hospitals in Europe, presents itself as ensuring privileged access for its patients to the latest technological developments and medical progress.[15] At the same time, the use of medical technologies in these countries has significantly influenced rising healthcare costs, which has, in turn, intensified discussions about whether technology-driven medical progress can continue indefinitely. Contributing to these discussions are aging populations, as well as the fact that health inequalities within high-income countries persist and are sometimes glaring, even as they coexist alongside sophisticated medical facilities. In many respects, the rising popularity of complementary and alternative medicine in these regions can be understood as a reaction against traditional (biomedical) approaches to progress. The successes and limitations of scientific-technological medicine, then, have led to backlash and rethinking commonly held

---

[14] Ruth Macklin, "Moral Progress," *Ethics*, 87 (4) (1977), 370.
[15] Hôpitaux Universitaires Genève, Recherche & Innovation, www.hug.ch/recherche-innovation-0.

views of progress in medicine. The idea of simple, straight-line progress in medicine has encountered both theoretical and practical obstacles in the Global North.

In this book, I write about "modern," "contemporary," and "Western" medicine. These terms are not unproblematic, but I think that there are, nevertheless, justified reasons for employing them here. Current debates about medical progress are bound up with transnational scientific achievements, but they are also informed by developments occurring in what used to be designated "the West." Chinese medicine, for example, at times acts as a counterpoint for the focus on progress I describe here.[16] To be sure, it would be a mistake to consider contemporary Western medicine a monolithic entity that contrasts with other medical systems; it is certainly possible to argue that the term "Western" subsumes substantial differences and can therefore be misleading. That said, I do want to argue for thinking about attitudes toward progress in medicine in light of a set of traditions in which individuals and societies participate and share to different degrees. Valuable philosophical work has shown that we participate in shared social practices founded on assumptions that we have difficulty perceiving because they appear to be self-evident.[17] With this approach to Western/globalized medicine, we can see that even as biomedicine is grounded in specific, localized cultural assumptions and practices, it nevertheless claims neutrality and universality.[18] Furthermore, we can conceive of the commitment to the idea of progress as a tenacious assumption of Western medicine.[19] Indeed, the notion of progress in medicine is rarely made explicit and problematized, but rather accepted as something inherently good.

That shared ideas about progress influence how we perceive the goals of medicine has not gone unnoticed. Research by bioethicists,[20]

---

[16] See Paul U. Unschuld, *Medicine in China: A History of Ideas* (Oakland: University of California Press, 1985).

[17] See, for example, Charles Taylor, *Modern Social Imaginaries* (Durham, NC: Duke University Press, 2004).

[18] See Deborah Lupton, *Medicine as Culture: Illness, Disease and the Body* (Los Angeles: Sage, 2012 [1994]).

[19] See Deborah R. Gordon, "Tenacious Assumptions in Western Medicine," in *Biomedicine Examined*, eds. M. Lock and D. R. Gordon (Kluwer Academic Publishers, 1988), pp. 19–56.

[20] Daniel Callahan, *What Kind of Life? The Limits of Medical Progress* (Washington, DC: Georgetown University Press, 1990) and Claudio Sartea, "Il

historians of medicine,[21] philosophers,[22] physicians, and public health workers[23] has used medicine as a case study for ideas about progress in a way that resonates with my approach. Studies of progress have, in their own right, sometimes mentioned medicine as a field in which the theoretical concept could benefit from further empirical inquiry but have not undertaken this task themselves.[24] Thus, it is possible to conclude that the idea of progress in medicine, while crucial, has only ever been studied in a limited way, or discussed briefly, for example, in an article or as the topic of a chapter in an edited volume. At present, there is a lack of academic studies that attempt to bridge the divide between philosophical–historical engagements with progress and the use of the term and concept of progress in the medical context. To my knowledge, there are no full-length studies devoted to the topic, and that is the gap that this work attempts to fill.

passato dell'idea di progresso ed il futuro della bioetica," *Medicina e Morale*, 69 (3) (2020), 293–310; Jean-Paul Thomas, "La médecine progresse-t-elle?," *Raison présente*, 189 (2014), 31–41.

[21] Brigitte Lohff, "Fortschritt mit der Wissenschaft: Wissenschaft ist Fortschritt. Der Wandel der Fortschrittsidee in der deutschen Medizin im 19. Jahrhundert," *Wissenschaftstheorien in der Medizin*, eds. Wolfgang Deppert, Hartmut Kliemt, Brigitte Lohff and Jochen Schäfer (Berlin and Boston: De Gruyter, 2015), pp. 327–54 and Bert Hansen, *Picturing Medical Progress from Pasteur to Polio: A History of Mass Media Images and Popular Attitudes in America* (Newark, NJ: Rutgers University Press, 2009).

[22] Mark J. Hanson, "The Idea of Progress and the Goals of Medicine," in *The Goals of Medicine*, pp. 137–51, Lucien Sève, "La querelle du progrès," in *Pour une critique de la raison bioéthique* (Paris: Editions Odile Jacob, 1994), pp. 209–82, and Anetta Breczko, "'Interest of the Individual' versus 'Common Good' and 'Public Interest' in the Context of Technological Progress in Medicine," *Journal of the Polish Section of IVR*, 3 (2020), 41–52.

[23] Leon Eisenberg, "Medicine and the Idea of Progress," in Leo Marx and Bruce Mazlish, eds., *Progress: Fact or Illusion* (Ann Arbor: University of Michigan Press, 1998 [1996]), pp. 45–64, Didier Sicard, "Réflexions sur le progrès en médecine," *Médecine & Hygiène*, 2491 (2004), 1535–38, Ståle Fredriksen, "Tragedy, Utopia and Medical Progress," *Journal of Medical Ethics*, 32 (2006), 450–53, and Philippe Lazar, "The Idea of Progress and Human Health," in *The Idea of Progress*, eds. Jürgen Mittelstrass, Peter McLaughlin, and Arnold S. V. Burgen (New York: W. de Gruyter, 1997), pp. 219–29.

[24] See, for example, Philip Kitcher, "On Progress," in *Performance and Progress: Essays on Capitalism, Business, and Society*, ed. Subramanian Rangan (Oxford: Oxford University Press, 2015), pp. 115–33, and "Pragmatism and Progress," *Transactions of the Charles S. Peirce Society: A Quarterly Journal in American Philosophy*, 51 (4) (2015), 475–94. See also Stuart Firestein, *Failure* (Oxford: Oxford University Press, 2015), Chapter 9: "Failure in the Clinic."

In this book, I show, first, that the shared agreement about the value of medical progress rests on the assumption that no one wants to be sick or to die.[25] But this purported agreement does not translate into any one conception of progress; health is a complex biopsychosocial state, and illness is not fixed, but rather influenced by norms and values. This poses problems for simplistic definitions of progress such as, for example, eliminating pathogens. While narrowly scientific conceptions of medical progress have captured the public imagination, the possibilities of meaningful medical progress are much more chastened than the claims of techno-optimists. But inclusive visions of medical progress as better health for the largest number of citizens are also political appeals that entail trade-offs, for example, with regard to expensive procedures or rare disease research. It is for this reason that multidimensional approaches to persons and to health are less likely to channel reductionist and potentially harmful views of medical progress.

Second, I demonstrate that answers to the question "What is medical progress?" have always been contested; the answer that predominates in any particular context is bound up with a specific approach to health and is also a question of power. In what follows I document how medicine – an art that deals with existential questions about human finitude – experiences firsthand the tensions between different kinds of progress and resolves them differently in particular circumstances. Current ways of thinking about medical progress are, therefore, historically contingent. As detailed in subsequent chapters, progress rhetoric in medicine has been associated with a range of ideas about personhood, knowledge, freedom, and justice in the post-Cold War Global North. As I illustrate, these ideas depend on historical and geographical contexts, as well as on personal experiences of illness and therapy, and there are certainly further iterations of medical progress to come. The title of this book *Making Medical Progress* – also a nod to Miriam Solomon's study *Making Medical Knowledge*[26] – reflects the fluidity

---

[25] On how this assumption is linked to ableism, sanism, and suicidism, see Alexandre Baril, *Undoing Suicidism: A Trans, Queer, Crip Approach to Rethinking (Assisted) Suicide* (Philadelphia: Temple University Press, 2023).

[26] Miriam Solomon, *Making Medical Knowledge* (Oxford: Oxford University Press, 2015). See also Paul Rabinow, *Making PCR: A Story of Biotechnology* (Chicago: University of Chicago Press, 1996).

with which progress can be associated with different dimensions of selfhood and health.

Finally, this book fits with recent attempts to blend intellectual and cultural history by paying attention to the significance of an idea for its own sake, as well as tracking its broad diffusion and circulation. Medical progress is, I think, particularly able to illustrate the porosity between cultural and intellectual divides and to illuminate how an idea is absorbed into broader patterns of cultural beliefs and expectations. It is arguably in medicine that the agreement about progress is the greatest, it is with reference to medicine that "progress" is popularly used, and it is in medicine that the search for progress acts as an agenda that drives research and shapes the aims of those applying for funding.[27] Moreover, a study of the idea of progress in medicine cannot be separated from medical practices and the varieties of experiences of healthcare recipients. With this in mind, this book adopts a research agenda that breaks down traditional distinctions between the professional and popular. More specifically, my analysis draws on a variety of sources, often academic engagements with the history and philosophy of progress, but also the insights of physicians, patients, and tech actors. Combining these perspectives provides the resources for an in-depth analysis of the idea of progress outlined above.

I.3 Dimensions of Personhood and Patienthood

Any theory of progress in medicine rests on or defends some vision of individual persons and what it means to live together. Indeed, the problems of what it means to be a healthy person or an ill person in a given social context are foundational for coming to grips with medical progress. Historian Jerrold Seigel describes three interconnected aspects of the self that are helpful for understanding how these underpin different views of progress.[28] The first way of approaching the self is bodily or

---

[27] See, for example, the Swiss National Science Foundation, *The SNSF's Model of Excellence*, www.snf.ch/en/theSNSF/research-policies/model-of-excellence/Pages/default.aspx#Question, or the National Institutes of Health and National Human Genome Research Institute, Advancing Genomic Medicine Research Exploratory/Developmental Grant, https://grants.nih.gov/grants/guide/rfa-files/RFA-HG-20-037.html.

[28] Jerrold Seigel, *The Idea of the Self: Thought and Experience in Western Europe since the Seventeenth Century* (New York: Cambridge University Press, 2005).

material, involving the corporeal existence of individuals, our physical needs, and the conditions that, for example, make us more or less susceptible to experiencing pain. This facet of the self considers that our health and wellness are determined primarily by our physiological demands and that progress is evaluated in relation to its ability to meet those needs. The second dimension is the self as a reflexive being, able to take distance from bodies, physical limits, impairments, and social relations, and examine them critically, thereby actively participating in its own self-realization. On this level, the self is able to judge its feelings and symptoms, make choices, and pursue self-knowledge; this is the dimension most likely to be associated with self-determination or autonomy. Progress in such an account takes into account the capacity of human beings to give meaning to their lives, their illnesses, and their suffering. Third, the self can be understood as relational, with collective identities, orientations, and values that are shaped within particular social and cultural contexts. Health is relational, to the extent that people consider their own health in relation to the health of others, their environment, their capacity to perform their work or occupation, and so on. In relational views of medical progress, the health of one cannot be detached from the health of others.

These categories help demonstrate how approaches to selfhood and to progress are inextricably bound up with context. For example, ideas about the physical self are very different if one links bodily functions to certain temperaments, as Greek thinkers did, if the body is seen as the means by which genes can achieve their end, as some evolutionary biologists have argued, or if the body is perceived as matter governed by the rules of physics and chemistry, as Director of the Massachusetts Institute of Technology (MIT) Artificial Intelligence Laboratory Rodney Brooks describes it.[29] In the specific case of medical progress, the three dimensions of the self have played different roles at different times. Recently, relational approaches to the self have become fundamental in narrative accounts of illness, in care ethics, and in nursing philosophy. Such approaches also underpin increased attention to the social determinants of health. But the bodily dimension continues to be exalted in optimistic visions of medical progress, and the reduction of the person to the body and its mechanisms is a

---

[29] See his *Flesh and Machines: How Robots Will Change Us* (New York: Pantheon, 2002), pp. 173–75.

recurring theme underpinning contemporary visions of medical progress. Brooks, cited above, argues that since humans are composed of biological mechanisms, albeit complex ones, they are mere machines. If a self is reducible to the fundamental science behind basic body functions, medical progress is virtually identical to technological progress. "More medical research, more medical technology, more progress," is how Mark Hanson has characterized this way of thinking.[30]

In addition to acknowledging different dimensions of the self, it is important to recognize the dangers of reductionism when thinking about persons. Philosophical theories that hold that human beings are not merely highly complex organisms but that they are persons do not fit neatly into any one category. Yet what joins them is their interest in the multifaceted realities associated with personhood.[31] Sociologist Christian Smith, for example, shows that human persons are "emergent," in that they cannot be reduced to their component parts, and that the capacity for free will, the ability to create meaning and an identity, relationships, and a sense of virtuous action all contribute to how persons understand themselves and each other.[32] Physician and bioethicist Eric J. Cassell argues in a similar fashion that a person is a composite entity made up of its body, its history, its beliefs, its imagined future, and its subconscious life.[33] A great deal of medical literature has drawn attention to the importance of person-centered care, which involves knowledge of social relationships and normativity.[34] Healing illness requires more than healing specific body parts; it requires acknowledging persons as complex entities, with hopes and needs that go beyond purely physical ones. Such an approach to

---

[30] Mark J. Hanson, "The Idea of Progress and the Goals of Medicine," in *The Goals of Medicine: The Forgotten Issues in Health Care Reform*, ed. by Mark J. Hanson and Daniel Callahan (Washington, DC: Georgetown University Press, 1999), p. 143.

[31] See Randall Poole, "Conceptions of Humanity in Health Humanities," presentation at the International Health Humanities Conference, McGovern Center for Humanities and Ethics, University of Texas Health Sciences Center at Houston, March 2017.

[32] See Christian Smith, *What Is a Person?: Rethinking Humanity, Social Life, and the Moral Good from the Person Up* (Chicago: University of Chicago Press, 2010), p. 25 e passim.

[33] Eric Cassell, *The Nature of Healing: The Modern Practice of Medicine* (Oxford: Oxford University Press, 2012), p. 25.

[34] A seminal text in this regard is Francis Peabody, "The Care of the Patient," *The Journal of the American Medical Association*, 88 (12) (1927), 877–82.

persons means that reducing a person to any one dimension of the self, for example, the body, is a misguided, reductionistic exercise that flattens what is ultimately a stratified reality.

As I argue throughout this study, views of personhood that emphasize the integrated nature of and inner tensions within persons – for example, that a person is a complex, thinking, feeling, relational entity – are less likely to develop one-dimensional views of medical progress. Multidimensionality resists these tendencies because it accepts that the knowledge of any one aspect of a person is fundamentally incomplete. It also illustrates how the demands of different dimensions of the self are sometimes in tension. This multiform approach is necessary to develop a more nuanced and realistic approach to medical progress.

I.4 Health and Values

In addition to endorsing some vision of personhood, any theory of medical progress rests on a conception of human health, that is, a set of ideas about what we need to sustain health and its connection to life. The fact that health is linked to maintaining life, and is important – though not sufficient – for a good life is, I contend, the basis of a sturdy societal consensus that promoting health is a worthy social and medical goal. If a person's arm is bleeding profusely, there is a robust, shared agreement that medical intervention and treatment are necessary and that a person in a difficult, life-threatening situation should be helped. This is analogous to the notion that basic physiological requirements are primary goods, normally regarded as such by all human beings, who similarly desire to be protected from primary evils, including avoidable ill-health.[35]

The shared commitment to health as a valuable social good appears more robust than other areas of political life; health has been described as one of those rare goods that benefits from continuous public support.[36] At the descriptive level, healing or attempting to heal the sick has been identified as a "human universal" because it occurs in all societies across time.[37] But what exactly is the health that so many

---

[35] On primary goods, see John Kekes, *The Morality of Pluralism* (Princeton, NJ: Princeton University Press, 1993).
[36] For a discussion, see Shlomi Segall, "Is Health Care (Still) Special?," *The Journal of Political Philosophy*, 15 (3) (2007), 342–61.
[37] See Donald Brown, *Human Universals* (New York: McGraw Hill, 1991).

people seek? At times, the question of what is health is approached less through the lens of what it means to be a person who is ill and seeks to be healthy and more often reduced to the bodily dimension of the self. This approach to health underlies medical education, which teaches students that healthcare interventions are designed to restore biological functioning. The biomedical sciences, meanwhile, have appropriated the task of defining what a normally functioning organism – and therefore what health – is. The use of technologies in the medical encounter also tends to rely on a somatic view of health that diminishes the significance of the mind or other factors. It is possible to argue that the entire biomedical model of disease is predicated on the idea that the body and the mind are two distinct substances and that the body is the locus of health.[38]

Physicalist models of health have been associated with ambitious aims for medical progress and significant achievements. But other approaches to health have illuminated various shortcomings with a narrow, somatic definition. Numerous examples – from a nervous stomach and tension headaches to the effects of racism on stress and mental health – attest to how emotional reactions or social life affect bodily systems. In 1977, George L. Engel presented a classic paper on the biopsychosocial model of illness, which sought to address the lacunae of reductionist and mechanistic conceptions of health by adding psychological and social factors.[39] Indeed, health has a reflexive aspect: Being healthy involves feeling healthy, which integrates a necessarily subjective element into the idea of normal functioning. Mental suffering is as real as physical suffering, yet more difficult to grasp and treat; a recent study notes that blurred boundaries between the normal and the pathological are a persistent theme in research attempting to classify mental disorders.[40] Meanwhile, in Western countries, neuropsychiatric conditions such as depression and anxiety are the diseases that cause the most sickness overall. Moreover, health

---

[38] Neeta Mehta, "Mind-Body Dualism: A Critique from a Health Perspective," *Mens Sana Monographs*, 9 (1) (2011), 202–9.

[39] George Engel, "The Need for a New Medical Model: A Challenge for Biomedicine," *Science*, 196 (4286), 129–36. See also Derek Bolton and Grant Gillett, *The Biopsychosocial Model of Health and Disease: New Philosophical and Scientific Developments* (Cham, Switzerland: Palgrave Pivot, 2020).

[40] *Vagueness in Psychiatry*, eds. Geert Keil, Lara Keuck, and Rico Hauswald (Oxford: Oxford University Press, 2017), p. 3.

has an inherently relational dimension; French philosopher Georges Canguilhem famously has shown that disease is a deviation from societally defined norms.[41] The social aspects of health are in view, for example, in the World Health Organization's definition of health as "a state of complete physical, mental *and social* well-being" (my emphasis).[42] They also inform the social model of disability, which depicts how society is constructed around a particular idea of normal and thus creates barriers for people with disabilities that would not exist in other circumstances.[43] Much recent work in epidemiology and public health has revealed to what extent health depends on background social and cultural factors that occur beyond the boundaries of classical disease notions.

The conceptual flaws in refusing to consider factors beyond the body are significant: Symptoms with no identifiable physiological cause are a common reason that patients visit doctors.[44] Medicine that reduces persons to their bodies, without taking into account their personal and social contexts, can be dehumanizing as well as misguided because it misses possible causes of illness. This is linked to how patients experience illness. Questions like "Why me?" and "Why now?" matter to patients: Contributions from narrative ethics show that patients benefit when physicians understand the importance patients attribute to their health in relation to different aspects of their lives.[45] Another failure of a reductionist attitude to health concerns its ability to provide comfort. In an interventionist medical system, if the disease is

---

[41] Georges Canguilhem, *On the Normal and the Pathological*, trans. Carolyn R. Fawcett, intro. Michel Foucault (Dordrecht: D. Reidel Publishing Co., 1978).

[42] "Constitution of the World Health Organization," in *Basic Documents*, 49th ed. (Geneva: World Health Organization, 2020), https://apps.who.int/gb/bd/PDF/bd47/EN/constitution-en.pdf?ua=1.

[43] For an overview, see Mike Oliver, "The Social Model of Disability: Thirty Years On," *Disability & Society*, 28 (2013), 1024–26.

[44] *Medically Unexplained Symptoms, Somatisation and Bodily Distress: Developing Better Clinical Services*, eds. Francis Creed, Peter Henningsen, Per Fink (Cambridge: Cambridge University Press, 2011), p. vi. See also Anne Harrington, *The Cure Within: A History of Mind-Body Medicine* (New York: W. W. Norton, 2008).

[45] See *Narrative Ethics: The Role of Stories in Bioethics*, special report, ed. Martha Montello, *Hastings Center Report*, 44 (1) (2014), 2–44 and Chiara Fioretti, et al., "Research Studies on Patients' Illness Experience Using the Narrative Medicine Approach: A Systematic Review," *BMJ Open*, 6 (2016), e011220.

real but little or nothing can be done, patients tend to experience this negatively. That is, if patients have unrealistic expectations of medical progress, they experience their illness situation as a failure of medical actors, rather than an aspect of the human condition with which they must cope.

Views of personhood that emphasize the complexity and contradictions of life as a person tend to align with conceptions of health that refer to a complex state of affairs that includes individual experience and social context. But recognizing that physical, mental, and social health are not cleanly divided challenges definitive claims for medical progress. Engel, the "father" of the biopsychosocial model of health, flagged progress toward bridging the biological and psychosocial aspects of health as "slow and halting," both because of the complexities inherent to the endeavor and due to unremitting pressures to favor the more tangible, physical aspect of health.[46] And in a reflective article considering his tenure as a prominent WHO employee, Kenneth Newell argued that there are so many facets of health that have to be seen together, "There is no objective way of judging whether one mix is better or worse than another."[47] By these accounts, medical progress is a complicated process with multiple dimensions, and the goal is an ephemeral, constantly changing one.

I.5 Problematizing Medical Progress

In light of these reflections regarding health and persons, what do people referring to progress in medicine in the media, in politics, in scholarly interventions, and in conversations mean when they use the term? There is no easy answer to that question. The wide range of ways in which health and persons can be understood, and how the term progress is used, makes it difficult to grasp; progress is a popularly used but fundamentally vague concept.[48] "Progress" is a noun, but sometimes a verb or the root of the adjective "progressing," a variety that enables it to carry different amounts of political baggage. In its most common

---

[46] George Engel, "The Need for a New Medical Model," p. 134.
[47] Kenneth W. Newell, "Selective Primary Health Care: The Counter Revolution," *Social Science and Medicine* 26 (9) (1988), 903.
[48] Anat Itay, "Conceptions of Progress: How Is Progress Perceived? Mainstream versus Alternative Conceptions of Progress," *Social Indicators Research*, 92 (2009), 530.

use, "progress" refers to advancement to a better state or condition. But etymologically, "progress" has not always implied betterment; the notion that a disease is "progressing" is one of the few contemporary uses of progress in its negative valence.

I have been using the word progress freely up until now, but in the main, I am interested in a specific idea of progress that has been accepted for centuries in Western culture, whereby progress refers to a cumulative process that enables an individual or a society to obtain something and then go on to attain something better.[49] This kind of progress has a normative component in that it evaluates change according to a broadly shared framework or a goal. Such progress also involves an epistemological claim, in that it valorizes certain kinds of knowledge – biomedical knowledge, for example – and posits specific relationships between knowledge gains and other spheres of life. Thus conceived, progress is also an ontological phenomenon, linked to an understanding of how historical change occurs. Examples of such assumptions about reality can be found in statements such as "you can't stand in the way of progress" made by enthusiastic engineers or in the well-known definition of progress as "*irreversible* meliorative change" (my emphasis).[50]

In the medical case, there is a persistent tendency to associate medical progress with the above cumulative-historical view, even as progress in medicine is often best described in a much more limited fashion. Speaking to broader cultural desires that associate medicine with notions of progress, surgeon and writer Atul Gawande observes that Western medicine is singularly focused on the idea of machinelike perfection.[51] The high stakes involved in healthcare mean that there is an urgent and intense need to believe that medical intervention can be constructive for patients. The very notion of progress is associated with the benefits of intervention, as opposed to resignation, or

---

[49] To paraphrase one of the foremost commentators of the idea, British philosopher John Gray. See his "Cats Can Teach Us about the Meaning of Life," *JSTOR Daily*, December 6, 2020, https://daily.jstor.org/john-gray-cats-can-teach-us-about-the-meaning-of-life/.
[50] Conversation with the author on the sidelines of the Moral Machines Workshop, Zurich, Switzerland, February 23, 2017. The definition comes from Charles Lincoln Van Doren, *The Idea of Progress* (New York: F. A. Praeger, 1967).
[51] Atul Gawande, *Complications: A Surgeon's Notes on an Imperfect Science* (London: Profile Books, 2002), pp. 37–38.

being with the patient, as in the conceptual framework of palliative care. Hope, an emotional attitude that desires an outcome, implies the possibility – if not the certainty – of progress.[52] Given the importance of hope when confronted with one's own vulnerability and finitude, Adrienne Martin describes it as the watchword for the medical research industry as a whole.[53]

This study does not attempt to provide a comprehensive answer to the question of whether a given intervention or development "genuinely" constitutes progress, in the sense of improvement over time. It makes no attempt to conclusively prove that any specific practice or technique can be unambiguously designated as medical progress or not. What interests me rather is the belief in the existence of progress, what can be called progress as a second-order concept, and the variety of forms this belief takes on. This contrasts with various existing engagements with medical progress, which often are evaluative, and seek to demonstrate that a particular change constitutes a first-order advance.[54] What I am particularly concerned with is the widespread rejection of the idea of progress as a valid conceptual category for describing historical change – a tendency that became particularly pronounced in the post-war period – and the insights that these debates offer into the widely held attachments to the idea of medical progress today. Therefore, I focus on the medical story where the term and concept of progress have been especially widely used, but the medical case is important to me as part of the larger, transdisciplinary story of the vagaries of progress as a conceptual category.

I want to acknowledge the more questionable assumptions inherent in its Enlightenment heritage but also to contend that progress need not be teleological nor linear, as well as to show that I do think there are justified reasons for believing in it. With regard to the epistemological dimension of progress, we must consider how every statement about progress is a statement about change in relation to a contested time slice. Depending on the time reference chosen, statements about

---

[52] See Jakob Huber, "Looking Back, Looking Forward: Progress, Hope, and History," *Constellations*, 28 (2021), 126–39.
[53] Adrienne Martin, *How We Hope: A Moral Psychology* (Princeton, NJ: Princeton University Press, 2013), p. 3.
[54] See, for example, Jeremy R. Simon, "How to Make Real Constructive Progress in Medicine," *Journal of Evaluation in Clinical Practice*, 17 (5) (2011), 845–51.

progress will look very different; it is harder to describe the industrial revolution as "progress" in light of climate change. Particularly in the medical case, factors such as side effects – a necessary part of intervening in the human body – and unintended consequences are likely to gain or to lose prominence.[55] For instance, the achievements of "frontier" fields like neonatal medicine and their ability to allow very premature babies to survive are often cited as exemplary medical progress.[56] But depending on when we take stock of the effects thereof – on the date babies are released from the neonatal intensive care unit or later in life with reference to their overall health – there is a very different sense of the progress involved; while more babies survive, a premature birth means higher risks of chronic health problems and disability.[57] Other examples abound; while penicillin has been widely recognized as a "perfectly objective" example of progress – as per Robert Nisbet above – no full account of the antibiotic era can be given without reference to the antibiotic resistance challenges of the present day. Or consider, for example, how the drive to have pain taken seriously as a medical condition and to provide relief is bound up with the current opioid crisis, which itself has been described as caused by modern medicine. In short, claims of medical progress are valid with reference to a particular time frame.

Furthermore, the knowledge we require to grasp the health of a holistic entity such as a person is complex. Gaining knowledge of a particular dimension of health, biophysical for example, remains fundamentally incomplete. A biophysical model of health presumes that health problems are measurable and therefore can be solved by well-defined interventions, procedures, and technologies, something that needs to be considered alongside insights from health's other dimensions. In general, knowledge gains raise the standards for justification and require that related interventions be evaluated by more

---

[55] See Diana B. Dutton, *Worse than the Disease: Pitfalls of Medical Progress* (Cambridge: Cambridge University Press, 1992).

[56] See Linda L. Layne, "How's the Baby Doing?' Struggling with Narratives of Progress in a Neonatal Intensive Care Unit," *Medical Anthropology Quarterly*, 10 (4) (1996), 624–56.

[57] See Amber Dance, "Survival of the Littlest: The Long-Term Impacts of Being Born Extremely Early," *Nature*, 582 (2020), 20–23. Tracy McVeigh, "Interview: Nathan was born at 23 weeks. If I'd known then what I do now, I'd have wanted him to die in my arms," *The Guardian*, March 20, 2011, www.theguardian.com/society/2011/mar/20/nathan-born-premature-life-death.

demanding criteria. Increased knowledge also uncovers new uncertainties and new sources of potential error. Such gains also increase the responsibility to act on them, actions that, in turn, have secondary and unintended consequences.

The normative framework we might use to evaluate medical progress is similarly contested. The fact that health has multiple dimensions, and the ways that different dimensions may be in tension with each other, means that there is no objective measure of health nor standard for measuring progress. Medicine has multiple fundamental goals, the way these goals fit together cannot be determined in advance, and there are conflicts among them. The mandate of medicine to save and extend life, for example, may be in tension with the relief of suffering and the pursuit of a peaceful death. Privileging resource-intensive techniques is not reconcilable with the goals of an equitable medicine accessible to all. Medicine is constantly performing a balancing act between the pursuit of individual health and well-being and the common good. Indeed, for a single goal of medicine against which progress can be measured, local solutions generate new difficulties. In essence, this provides that there are only limiting cases in which progress could be judged. We can claim that medical progress exists in relation to the shared commitment to a vital minimum of health needed to sustain life since we know that there are health conditions that we are morally compelled to treat given available material resources. But any further progress in medicine will remain relative to mitigating what we consider shared evils with regard to health.

Moreover, we have to take into account the fact that rather than having a stable ontological status, the confines and scope of medicine and health are the subject of ongoing disputes and are constantly renegotiated. Far from having a unified, consistent mandate, medicine can be defined as a diverse set of ideas, methods, procedures, and practices that have constantly varied depending on time and place.[58] There now exist entire categories of disease that doctors did not use to treat, including attention-deficit hyperactivity disorder, obsessive-compulsive disorder, phobias, chronic fatigue, social anxiety disorder, post-traumatic stress disorder, and various kinds of depression. In a

---

[58] Diego Gracia, "What Kind of Values? A Historical Perspective on the Ends of Medicine," in *The Goals of Medicine*, p. 88.

similar vein, there are multiple examples of behaviors that were previously labeled as diseases, such as drapetomania, a disease that caused slaves to run away, masturbation, or hysteria.[59] Concepts of diseases emerge from specific cultural and scientific priorities, while diagnostic innovation goes hand in hand with both treatment innovation and the experience of both illness and therapy.

Taken together, these remarks show that there is no stable standard for measuring progress, nor any stable goal toward which medical progress could orient itself. The criteria we can apply to compare and judge medicine, health, and disease in different contexts are complex and ultimately value based.[60] Determining what progress is necessary to overcome disease and to achieve health is always a social and political act. In sum, the standards by which we might evaluate progress change over time, progress consists in confronting a new set of problems in each historical moment and trying to overcome them, and this means that we can only determine progress in hindsight.[61] Progress might consist in improved epistemic or moral assumptions, but human learning also implies forgetting; progress comes with pauses and regressions. Therefore, rather than seeing progress as a unified process proceeding lawfully across societies, it is better described as localized and circumscribed. Crucially, if progress is nonlinear, but rather multidimensional, progress in one domain – such as one aspect of health – may coexist alongside losses in another.[62] Part of making progress that is neither metaphysical nor deterministic therefore involves facing up to the difficulties involved in weighing the relative importance of problems. Such progress is necessarily a chastened idea of progress.

---

[59] On disease concepts, see Jacalyn Duffin, *Lovers and Livers: Disease Concepts in History* (Toronto: University of Toronto Press, 2005) and Brandon Conley and Shane Glackin, "How to Be a Naturalist and a Social Constructivist about Diseases," *Philosophy of Medicine*, 2 (2021), 1–21.

[60] For related discussions, see Steven Shapin, "Possessed by the Idols," *London Review of Books*, 28 (3) (2006), 31–33.

[61] See Amanda Roth, "Ethical Progress as Problem-Resolving," *The Journal of Political Philosophy*, 20 (4) (2012), 385.

[62] Andy Stirling argues that ideas of progress are thus best represented, "not as a single-track 'race,' but as palimpsests of branching counterfactual paths." "Pluralising Progress: From Integrative Transitions to Transformative Diversity," *Environmental Innovation and Societal Transitions*, 1 (1) (2011), 82–88.

I.6 Historiography of Progress

Given the wide range of contexts in which progress-talk occurs, it will come as no surprise that the academic literature on the concept is vast. As we shall see in Chapter 1, the eighteenth century is usually considered the heyday of the concept of progress, while it continues to be referred to as the guiding idea (*Leitbegriff*) of the nineteenth century.[63] At the time, the idea was bound up with the optimistic hope that human reason can and will construct a better, more enlightened society. It was also the term of choice to describe new knowledge, improved material conditions, and better societal institutions and to understand them as part of an overarching scheme of improvement.

The theme of progress fundamentally changed the character of history writing by introducing a developmental structure to global history, and it merged with a simultaneous interest in universal histories of the world. Implicit in this idea of progress was the notion of the superior state and civilizing mission of European nations; with the idea of progress, the history of humankind as told in the West became identical with the history of civilization.[64] Documenting the enlightened and reasoned developments that count as progress was bound up with history writing, which aimed at documenting the errors of the past and the present inferiority of non-Western nations.

And yet, tales of progress have always had their skeptics.[65] By the end of the nineteenth century, the widespread fascination with progress in the West was matched by a significant revolt against the view that the future development of human societies was moving in any discernible direction or whether there were common standards or objective truths achievable by reason. In the twentieth century, different families of theories, including critical theory, moral relativism, postmodernism, and postcolonialism, further questioned and undermined the notion. When I told a medical historian colleague that I was working on the idea of progress in medicine, she asked me, "haven't you read Foucault?" Today, prominent critics of progress and the

---

[63] Thomas Nemeth, "Positivism in Late Tsarist Russia: Its Introduction, Penetration and Diffusion," *The Worlds of Positivism: A Global Intellectual History, 1770–1930*, eds. Johannes Feichtinger, Franz L. Fillafer, and Jan Surman (Cham, Switzerland: Springer, 2018), p. 274.

[64] See *Versions of History from Antiquity to the Enlightenment*, ed. Donald R. Kelley (New Haven, CT: Yale University Press, 2008), p. 440.

[65] See, for example, Henry Vyverberg, *Historical Pessimism in the French Enlightenment* (Cambridge, MA: Harvard University Press, 1958).

violence that has been conducted in its name abound.⁶⁶ A global crisis in the ideology of progress has been linked to phenomena ranging from the enthusiasm for "post" words to the resurgence of popularity of analog objects. Historian and philosopher of science Naomi Oreskes writes that history has come to be seen, no longer as a linear story of progress, but as a story in which the notion of progress can only be considered in relation to the question: progress for whom?⁶⁷

Given its charged history, progress is by no means a neglected topic in academia.⁶⁸ The concept has recently benefited from increased scholarly attention across a range of fields including in philosophy of science,⁶⁹ law,⁷⁰ anthropology,⁷¹ sociology,⁷² and

---

⁶⁶ For an overview, see Joshua Foa Dienstag, *Pessimism: Philosophy, Spirit, Ethic* (Princeton, NJ: Princeton University Press, 2009). See also the multiple writings of John Gray, particularly *The Silence of Animals: On Progress and Other Modern Myths* (London: Penguin, 2013), and *Heresies: Against Progress and Other Illusions* (London: Granata Books, 2015), Eileen B. Leonard, *Women, Technology, and the Myth of Progress* (Upper Saddle River, NJ: Prentice Hall, 2003), and Joseph R. Winters, *Hope Draped in Black: Race, Melancholy and the Agony of Progress* (Durham, NC: Duke University Press, 2016).

⁶⁷ Oreskes, "Why I Am a Presentist," p. 602.

⁶⁸ Older studies include J. B. Bury, *The Idea of Progress: An Inquiry into Its Origin and Growth* (London: Macmillan & co., 1920), Charles Frankel, *The Faith of Reason: The Idea of Progress in the French Enlightenment* (New York: Columbia University Press, 1948), Ernest Lee Tuveson, *Millennium and Utopia: A Study in the Background of the Idea of Progress* (Berkeley and Los Angeles: University of California Press, 1949), John Baillie, *The Belief in Progress* (London: Oxford University Press, 1950), W. Warren Wagar, *Good Tidings: The Belief in Progress from Darwin to Marcuse* (Bloomington: Indiana University Press, 1972), Sidney Pollard, *The Idea of Progress* (London: C. A. Watts, 1986), and Friedrich Rapp, *Fortschritt: Entwicklung und Sinngehalt einer philosophischen Idee* (Darmstadt: Wissenschaftliche Buchgesellschaft, 1992).

⁶⁹ Yafeng Shan, "A New Functional Approach to Scientific Progress," *Philosophy of Science*, 86 (2019), 739–58 and Juha Saatsi, "What Is Theoretical Progress in Science," *Synthese*, 196 (2019), 611–31.

⁷⁰ Tilmann Altwicker and Olivier Diggelmann, "How Is Progress Constructed in International Legal Theory," *The European Journal of International Law*, 25 (2) (2014), 425–44 and Thomas Skouteris, *The Notion of Progress in International Law Discourse* (The Hague: TMC Asser Press, 2010).

⁷¹ See Maximilian C. Forte, "Progress, Progressivism, and Progressives," *Zero Anthropology*, February 28, 2018, https://zeroanthropology.net/2018/02/28/progress-progressivism-and-progressives/.

⁷² Angelos Mouzakitis, "Modernity and the Idea of Progress," *Frontiers in Sociology*, 2 (3) (2017), 1–11 and Nancy Folbre et al., *Rethinking Society for the 21st Century: Report of the International Panel on Social Progress*, vol. 3 (Cambridge: Cambridge University Press, 2018).

intellectual history.[73] Attention has also been paid to how the idea of progress has been shaped by and itself influenced different historical periods.[74]

The popularity of the concept is further reflected in the number of recent international events and related publications devoted to progress.[75] Some of the most sustained supporters of the idea of progress are a cluster of academics and thinktank operatives – sometimes called "New Optimists," the most prominent of whom is psychologist Steven Pinker – who argue that humanity should be much more sanguine about the genuine progress it has made.[76] Such commentators point to different measures – first and foremost modern medicine – to show that the world is becoming a better place. As a rule, such interventions have a stabilizing function in that they validate current systems, namely, capitalism and democracy. They assume that whatever political and economic arrangements we currently have are working well and therefore ought to be maintained.[77]

---

[73] Carlo Altini, *Le maschere del progresso: Ascesa e caduto di un'idea moderna* (Bologna: Marietti, 2018), Matthew Slaboch, *A Road to Nowhere: The Idea of Progress and Its Critics* (Philadelphia: University of Pennsylvania Press, 2017), and Yohan Ariffin, *Généalogie de l'idée de progrès. Histoire d'une philosophie cruelle sous un nom consolant* (Paris: Editions du Félin, 2012).

[74] *Tradition, Innovation, Invention: Fortschrittsverweigerung und Fortschrittsbewusstsein im Mittelalter*, ed. Hans-Joachim Schmidt (Berlin: Walter de Gruyter, 2005), Wolfram Kinzig, *Novitas Christiana. Die Idee des Fortschritts in der Alten Kirche bis Eusebius* (Göttingen: Vandenhoeck & Ruprecht, 1994), David Spadafora, *The Idea of Progress in Eighteenth-Century Britain* (New Haven, CT: Yale University Press, 1995).

[75] See, for example, *After Progress*, eds. Martin Savransky and Craig Lundy (Thousand Oaks, CA: Sage, 2022), the *After Progress Digital Exhibition*, www.after-progress.com/, and related symposium series at the University of London in 2019, the *Human Progress and Social Enhancement* workshop at LMU Münich in 2020, organized by Jason Branford and Jan-Christoph Heilinger, "Moral Progress: Special Issue," *Ethical Theory and Moral Practice*, eds. A. W. Musschenga and G. Meynen, 20 (1) (2017), 1–183 and related conference, and "Progress, Change, Development: Special Issue," *International Journal of Postcolonial Studies*, 19 (5) (2017), 599–705.

[76] See, for example, Johan Norberg, *Progress: Ten Reasons to Look Forward to the Future* (New York City: Simon and Schuster, 2016), Michael Shermer, *The Moral Arc: How Science Leads Humanity toward Truth, Justice, and Freedom* (New York: Henry Holt and Co., 2015), and Steven Pinker, *The Better Angels of Our Nature* (London: Penguin, 2011).

[77] See Oliver Burkeman, "Is the World Really Better than Ever?," *The Guardian*, the Long Read, July 28, 2017, www.theguardian.com/news/2017/jul/28/is-the-world-really-better-than-ever-the-new-optimists.

Other engagements with progress seek to reclaim the concept's emancipatory potential and link it to a more disruptive politics. Philosopher Axel Honneth observes that "'progress' is a necessary and unavoidable perspective for all those of us today who aim at revitalizing emancipatory action."[78] The notion that progress is essential but problematic, and requires new, reconstructed conceptual foundations, runs through a number of works in contemporary philosophy and political theory. Thus, scholars have probed the different meanings of progress in history and the need for a reformulation of the idea today,[79] the potential tensions between scientific and technological progress and other more humanistic forms of progress,[80] the links between progress, normativity, and social change,[81] the extent of moral progress in history,[82] as well as the question of what it means to make political progress.[83] Among other things, representatives of "neoprogressivism,"[84] as Jakob Huber terms contemporary philosophical reappraisals of progress, have sought to reconceive progress in a nondogmatic way, which relies on the notion of learning processes in which human agency plays an important but unstable role.

I.7 Historiography of Medicine and Progress

Given the ubiquitous use of the term progress in professional medical contexts and popular ideas about medicine, it may come as a surprise

---

[78] Axel Honneth and Felix Koch, "The Normativity of Ethical Life," *Philosophy and Social Criticism*, 40 (8) (2014), 824.
[79] Peter Wagner, *Progress: A Reconstruction* (Cambridge: Polity Press, 2016).
[80] Nicholas Agar, *The Sceptical Optimist* (Oxford: Oxford University Press, 2015).
[81] Amy Allen, *The End of Progress: Decolonizing the Normative Foundations of Critical Theory* (New York: Columbia University Press, 2016) and Rahel Jaeggi, *Fortschritt und Regression* (Berlin: Suhrkamp, 2023).
[82] Allen Buchanan and Russell Powell, *The Evolution of Moral Progress: A Biocultural Theory* (Oxford: Oxford University Press, 2018), *Philip Kitcher: Moral Progress*, ed. and intro. Jan-Christoph Heilinger (Oxford: Oxford University Press, 2021) and Hanno Sauer et al., "Moral Progress: Recent Developments," *Philosophy Compass*, 16 (10) (2021), e12769.
[83] Christopher F. Zurn, "Political Progress: Piecemeal, Pragmatic, and Processual," in *Debating Critical Theory: Engagements with Axel Honneth*, eds. Julia Christ et al. (Rowman & Littlefield: Lanham, 2020), pp. 269–86 and Catherine Lu, "Progress, Decolonization and Global Justice: A Tragic View," *International Affairs*, 99 (1) (2023), 141–59.
[84] Jakob Huber, "Looking Back, Looking Forward: Progress, Hope, and History," *Constellations*, 28 (2021), 126–39.

that the topic has not been more investigated in academia. Historians of medicine have a particular relationship with and perhaps a particular aversion to the idea of progress. One reason is that the history of medicine was originally told by doctors and from a heroic perspective. The first specialized historians of medicine in the nineteenth and early twentieth centuries were themselves practitioners, and they characterized medicine as a continuous tale of progress. In the English-speaking world, the best-known spokesperson for this model was Canadian physician and educator William Osler (1849–1919), who saw medicine as a fundamentally progressive science and sought in his history lectures to provide a bird's eye view of medical progress.[85] It was only in the 1970s and 1980s that trained historians began to engage substantially with the history of medicine, something that occasioned new historiographic controversies about whether nonphysicians could sufficiently grasp medical practices.[86] At stake was also the question of whether the history of medicine should be embedded in a narrative of progress, which both confirmed the superiority of science-based medicine to what came before and perpetuated that view of history.

"Unilinear scientific progress,"[87] a "linear march of progress,"[88] "the march of medical progress,"[89] as a rule, such depictions of medical history were seen as the worst kind of presentism by academic historians. Today, historians of medicine are uniquely aware of the pitfalls of seeing the development of history as a straightforward path to current truths. Rather, history is perceived as uniquely able to raise inconvenient perspectives and an antidote to perpetuating the "dangerous illusion" that medicine is on a progress track from religion

---

[85] "Preface," *The Evolution of Modern Medicine: A Series of Lectures Delivered at Yale University on the Silliman Foundation in April* (Champagne, IL: Project Gutenberg, 1998 [1913]), p. 3.

[86] See Leonard Wilson's editorial, "Medical History without Medicine," *Journal of the History of Medicine*, 35 (1) (1980), 5–7, and David Rosner's response, "Tempest in a Test Tube: Medical History and the Historian," *Radical History Review*, 26 (1982), 166–71.

[87] Frank Huisman, "Shaping the Medical Market: On the Construction of Quackery and Folk Medicine in Dutch Historiography," *Medical History*, 43 (1999), 359.

[88] Mark S. Pernick, "Bioethics and History," in *The Cambridge World History of Medical Ethics*, eds. R. Baker & L. B. McCullough (New York: Cambridge University Press, 2009), pp. 16–20.

[89] Jonathan Sadowsky, *Electroconvulsive Therapy in America: The Anatomy of a Medical Controversy* (New York and London: Routledge, 2017), p. 6

Introduction 27

to science.⁹⁰ In addition to history, insights from science and technology studies highlight how medical innovations and their application are bound up with social contexts and constraints. Medicine, increasingly, has come to be seen as part of an intricate network, involving market forces, institutions, power hierarchies, and ideologies, and one in which lawful, inevitable progress has little meaning.

The interest of the medical humanities, then, has largely been to move away from triumphalist narratives by recapturing the complexities, roads not taken, and undocumented effects of simplistic accounts of medical progress. The notion of linearity that clings to progress implies that the acceptance of new, more refined techniques is nearly inevitable and therefore inherently oversimplifies what are often complex and circuitous adoption procedures.⁹¹ In many cases, there is no clear move from theory to practice, as shown, for example, by the introduction of antisepsis and asepsis or the adoption of surgical gloves.⁹² Moreover, many therapeutics initially perceived as cutting-edge and desirable are ineffective or end up harming patients.⁹³ Other studies meticulously document how views of disease – for example, diagnostic judgments based on "objective," laboratory evidence rather than "subjective" evidence such as patients' sensations – are inherently partial, with losses as well as gains.⁹⁴ This has led some historians to argue that the technological orientation of modern medicine is a contingent development.⁹⁵

---

⁹⁰ Gerald N. Grob, *Aging Bones: A Short History of Osteoporosis* (Baltimore: Johns Hopkins University Press, 2014), p. xvii.
⁹¹ On this point, see Sally Frampton, *Belly-Rippers, Surgical Innovation and the Ovariotomy Controversy* (Cham: Palgrave Macmillan, 2018).
⁹² See Thomas Schlich, "Introduction," *Palgrave Companion to the History of Surgery*, ed. Thomas Schlich (New York: Palgrave Macmillan, 2018).
⁹³ See Gerald N. Grob and Allan V. Horwitz, "Rhetoric and Reality in Modern American Medicine," *Diagnosis, Therapy, and Evidence: Conundrums in Modern American Medicine* (New Brunswick, NJ: Rutgers University Press, 2010), pp. 1–32.
⁹⁴ Mary Fissell, "The Disappearance of the Patient's Narrative and the Invention of Hospital Medicine," *British Medicine in an Age of Reform*, eds. A. Wear and R. French (London: Routledge, 1991), pp. 92–109.
⁹⁵ I am grateful to historian Thomas Schlich for discussing this issue with me. See also John V. Pickstone, "Introduction," in ibid (ed.), *Medical Innovations in Historical Perspective* (Houndsmills: Macmillan, 1992), pp. 1–16 and Ilana Löwy, "Medicine and Change," in ibid (ed.), *Innovations in Health and Medicine. Diffusion and Resistance in the Twentieth Century* (London: Routledge, 2002), pp. 1–15.

The critique of progress by medical historians also means reflecting on the relativistic implications thereof. In a well-known intervention on nineteenth-century therapeutics, historian Charles Rosenberg sought to break with past scholars who presented change as equating progress.[96] In doing so, he tried to move the study of past medicine away from questions of physiological efficacy and to connect it to broader contexts of explanation and meaning-making. Once historical context was taken into account, he argued, medical therapies of the past "worked" in the sense that they produced physiological effects that were predictable for physicians and experienced by patients as relief. Reflecting on the wider import of Rosenberg's conclusions for medical progress, John Harley Warner argues that relativism is an important tool for historical understanding because it forces us to acknowledge that the very claim about whether a treatment "works" is context dependent.[97] Ultimately, this methodological premise implies that techniques such as blood-letting "worked" for those physicians and patients who used them, and antibiotics "works" in a later era.[98] But if each system of therapeutics works according to its own criteria, determining progress becomes more complex. The upshot of this line of reasoning is that while we are invested in the therapeutic regimes of our own time and can prefer them on that basis, broader claims of progress are difficult.

Progress-oriented stories of medicine often focused on a series of breakthroughs in medical science, accompanied by "heroic" acts of a small number of affluent, influential white men, who were ideally positioned to reap the fruits of progress. In 1985, Roy Porter published a seminal article, "The Patient's View," that questioned writing the history of medicine as a story of scientific progress and called for

---

[96] Charles E. Rosenberg, "The Therapeutic Revolution: Medicine, Meaning, and Social Change in Nineteenth-Century America," in *The Therapeutic Revolution: Essays in the Social History of American Medicine*, eds. Morris J. Voegel and Charles E. Rosenberg (Philadelphia: University of Pennsylvania Press, 1979), pp. 3–23.

[97] John Harley Warner, *The Therapeutic Perspective: Medical Practice, Knowledge, and Identity in America, 1820–1885* (Princeton, NJ: Princeton University Press, preface to 1997 edition [1986]). For Warner's reflections on methodological relativism, see his "Preface to the Paperback Edition," p. ix.

[98] See Ian Kerridge and Michael Lowe, "Bloodletting: The Story of a Therapeutic Technique," *Medical Journal of Australia*, 163 (4) (1995), 631–33.

taking into account the views of patients, and linked medical events to social rituals, in which families and communities play a part.[99] New historical sensibilities to the voices of patients, including the stories of women, minorities, and communities facing barriers, have drawn attention to the fact that social positions associated with age, abilities, class, gender, and race intersect to determine who benefits from specific kinds of medical progress and who suffers from it.[100] This insight exists alongside the awareness of the difficulty inherent in recovering such voices when few of them recorded their views on illness and treatment. But it also draws attention to the fact that historical narratives of progress are necessarily selective, and these are precisely the viewpoints that have been omitted to allow a relatively uncomplicated story of progress to emerge.

It would, however, be an exaggeration to say that historians of medicine have not at times been very clear about what constitutes progress. Historian David Wootton, for example, set 1865, the date that Joseph Lister used antiseptic surgery, as the moment marking the beginning of the first real progress in medical therapy.[101] He argues that historians of medicine have a simple choice: either understanding the past on its own terms, in which case Hippocrates' and Galen's cures saved lives, or in light of modern science, in which case these cures were often deadly.[102] Wootton, however, remains the exception; as historian of science Steven Shapin observes, in the past few decades, academic historians of medicine "didn't – with rare exceptions – criticize the idea of medical progress so much as fall silent about it, seeing their job as something other than its documentation and celebration."[103] And if academic historians did not so much talk about progress as avoid it, popular accounts have filled the gap. Given medicine's extraordinary technical prowess, triumphant histories of medicine remain remarkably popular today.

---

[99] "The Patient's View: Doing Medical History from Below," *Theory and Society*, 14 (2) (1985), 175.

[100] See, for example, Deirdre Cooper Owens, *Medical Bondage: Race, Gender and the Origins of American Gynecology* (Atlanta: University of Georgia Press, 2017) and Elinor Cleghorn, *Unwell Women: Misdiagnosis and Myth in a Man-Made World* (London: Penguin, 2022).

[101] David Wootton, *Bad Medicine: Doctors Doing Harm since Hippocrates* (Oxford: Oxford University Press, 2007).

[102] David Wootton, "Understanding the History of Medicine," *BMJ*, 334 (7597) (2007), 762.

[103] Shapin, "Possessed by the Idols," *London Review of Books*.

Widely read books aimed at a general public, in the genre of *Physicians, Plagues and Progress: The History of Western Medicine from Antiquity to Antibiotics* and *The Medical Book: From Witch Doctors to Robot Surgeons*, contribute to our understanding of medicine as the locus of progress in contemporary society.[104] Often, they use evolutionary metaphors to portray modern medicine as an inevitable history of progress, emphasizing cumulative achievements and minimizing the ways in which these are entangled with significant failures and rejections.

I.8 Medical Progress: A Multidimensional View

This book is about the politics of medical progress and the real-world implications of conceptual choices. For example, we might describe a specific medical technology as progress, we may associate progress with the ability of individuals to determine what happens to them in healthcare, or we might see progress in a given procedure being made available to all. These differing visions are better understood not as more or less accurate reflections of what medical progress "really" is – arguably they are all justified first-order instances of progress – but rather as normative positions underpinned by specific ideas of personhood, of society, and of health.

In the chapters that follow, I unpack and historically contextualize ideas of progress that hold currency in particular circumstances. I do so with a special interest in the terms "medicine" and "progress." To avoid overuse, I alternate the usage of progress with other words such as advance, improvement, or even development. I am, of course, aware that these terms are not entirely synonymous with progress; in particular, they do not link back to the larger tradition of progress rhetoric that I am particularly interested in. In the case of medicine, I do at times refer to health progress, as do the actors who are interested in minimizing the role of biomedicine and who favor broader conceptions of health. That said, rather than focusing on a wider thematic cluster of terms, I look specifically at medical progress to offer a *Begriffsgeschichte* – a conceptual, semantic history – of the term "progress" and its recent incarnations in medicine.

---

[104] Allan Chapman, *Physicians, Plagues and Progress: The History of Western Medicine from Antiquity to Antibiotics* (Oxford: Lion Books, 2018) and Pickover, *The Medical Book* (2012).

Chapter 1 offers a historical overview of progress rhetoric up to 1945, and specifically how the interest – or disinterest – in progress is entangled with contemporary understandings of what it means to be a healthy/ill person, and the medical priorities of the time. While present-day ideas about medical progress rest on very different understandings of the human person from other cultural and historical contexts, their emergence from a combination of scientific knowledge and ethical preoccupations recurs throughout history. Indeed, both utopian and modest visions of medical progress have historical antecedents. This rough historical guide, therefore, explores the roots of contemporary statements about progress and explains how they relate to current epistemological and ethical priorities.

Subsequent chapters offer a more or less chronological survey from 1945 to the present day, each of them focusing on different operative concepts for medical progress – knowledge, freedom, and justice – before concluding with an epilogue on sustainability. Chapter 2 describes the heady excitement surrounding scientific medical progress in the post-war period and subsequent theoretical challenges culminating in the idea that progress claims are only valid in relation to context. It also scrutinizes how, in light of relativistic questions about to what extent knowledge can be progressive, medicine continues to be portrayed as uniquely immune to these uncertainties. It concludes by analyzing two recent examples, evidence-based medicine and health AI, both of which have been praised as objective examples of a particular kind of medical knowledge progress.

Chapter 3, on freedom, begins by showing how awareness of the insufficiencies of medical progress as "merely" scientific knowledge gains led to a new interest in knowledge with the ability to empower patients. This chapter also details how, in some cases, taking individual freedom seriously meant challenging traditional (technological) forms of medical progress because they were not patients' preferred methods of intervention. It concludes with a detailed examination of the most recent instances in which technological progress is presented as being highly compatible with personal freedom. To that end, I discuss the way in which genomic medicine promises to make "empowered patients in the twenty-first century" – to paraphrase the title of a recent book.[105]

---

[105] Barbara Prainsack, *Personalized Medicine: Empowered Patients in the 21st Century?* (New York: New York University Press, 2017).

The final chapter traces debates on progress and social justice focusing on the late 1980s onward. The critique of a medical marketplace, the perceived need to challenge an autonomy-based notion of progress, and a certain sociopolitical optimism all contributed to reimagining medical progress by placing left-wing sensibilities front and center. Effectively, the idea of progress lost its narrower "medical" focus, in favor of the idea of health progress and became associated with ambitious projects for achieving social equality. Part of the story told in this chapter is the extent to which increased knowledge of health inequalities has come to embody progress. But here too, a single-minded commitment to the notion of progress as health justice comes replete with trade-offs and unresolved tensions.

The book concludes by considering one possible future incarnation of the idea of medical progress, progress as achieving sustainability. Visions of sustainable medical progress enlarge the concept of human health to include the health of nature, call for expanding the time frame in which medical progress is assessed, and posit environmental limits as a constraint on open-ended progress. At the same time, few of these visions engage with the pluralistic nature of medical progress, preferring to understand measures that support a robust natural environment as intrinsically good for the health of individuals and societies.

In structuring my chapters this way, I am not arguing that these incarnations of medical progress are somehow exclusive to a particular time or were ever hegemonic; I rather think they occur simultaneously and all have deep historical roots. Nevertheless, there are moments in which specific ideas gain a particular resonance. My research shows that the notion of medical progress grafts particularly well onto the normative high ground of a particular historical moment. Within the chapters, I do two main things. First, I show the way in which the progress of knowledge, freedom, and justice has been both justified and contested and the implications for specifically medical progress of these debates. This task is epistemological, that is related to investigating the methods, validity, and scope of different kinds of medical knowledge.

The second aim is ethical and related to ideas about what is a person and what constitutes health. Throughout the book, I contend that the most vocal proponents of medical progress have tended to believe one of two things. Either they have focused on one particular element of health (biological or psychological or social) or they have argued that the three elements (biopsychosocial) are mutually reinforcing and progress in one aspect leads to progress in the other two. I, therefore, show that when thinking about medical progress, not only do we have to consider the epistemological aspects of how progress in any one dimension of health is not uncomplicated but also that health has multiple dimensions and that progress in one dimension does not necessarily mean progress in another.

1 History
Medical Progress in Context

We may believe in the doctrine of Progress or we may not, but in either case it is a matter of interest to examine the origins and trace the history of what is now, even should it ultimately prove to be no more than an *idolum saeculi*, the animating and controlling idea of western civilisation.

J. B. Bury, *The Idea of Progress*, p. 6

In his seminal study of the idea of progress published in 1920, J. B. Bury emphasizes the concept's deep rootedness in Western culture. Others who have traced the idea's transformations over time agree on its crucial importance for the self-definition of the West: Robert Nisbet calls it the single most important idea for Western modernity, and conceptual historian Reinhart Koselleck associates it with a historical change whereby the future came to be seen as open-ended.[1] Current scholarship on progress notes the peculiarity and contingency of modern versions of this belief. "Normally," writes historian Charles Frankel, "people have believed that the future would repeat the past."[2] In addition to its importance, recent contributions remark on the inherent neutrality and elasticity of the concept. This variety creates significant challenges for attempting an overview of the history of progress: Charles van Doren, the author of a multiyear collaborative study on the topic, differentiates between fifteen types of theories of progress and nine primary forms of progress denial.[3]

---

[1] Robert Nisbet, *History of the Idea of Progress* (New Brunswick & London: Transaction Publishers, 1980), p. 4 and Reinhart Koselleck and Christian Meier, "Fortschritt," in *Geschichtliche Grundbegriffe*, Historisches Lexikon zur politisch-sozialen Sprache in Deutschland, ed. Otto Brunner, Wilhelm Conze, and Reinhart Koselleck (Stuttgart: Klett-Cotta, 1977), vol. 2, pp. 352, 371.

[2] Charles Frankel, "Progress, Idea of," in *Encyclopedia of Philosophy*, 2nd ed., ed. Donald M. Borchert (Detroit: Thomson Gale, 2006), p. 45.

[3] van Doren, *The Idea of Progress*, pp. 26–32.

1 History: Medical Progress in Context

This chapter does not attempt to retell the rich history of the idea of progress in the West. The aim, rather, is to describe and to analyze the specific role that the art of medicine has historically played in relation to broader cultural attachments to, or rejections of, the idea of progress. In this chapter, I link historical–philosophical engagements with the concept of progress with contemporary understandings of what it means to be a healthy/ill person and the aim and remit of medicine. Daniel Callahan observes that "modern people love progress, *particularly* medical progress" (my emphasis).[4] That progress is important for how contemporary Western societies conceive of the history of medicine is undisputed; in what follows I scrutinize the status of medicine for a survey history of the idea of progress itself.

Inevitably, the following historical sketch provides only partial answers. I rely on recent research into progress rhetoric and draw attention to historical transitions and caesurae in the intellectual history of progress that help illuminate how we got to where we are today. I shift rapidly between periods and contexts, and I refer primarily to philosophical engagements with the idea of progress, material in line with my academic interests. In addition, looking for a modern notion of progress in the past runs into both linguistic and conceptual obstacles. The term progress does not appear in all historical periods discussed in this chapter; in that case, what I examine are equivalents, namely alternative terms and notions that reflect a substantial agreement that significant improvements in the human situation have occurred. As we shall see, both the reduction of the word "progress" to betterment and the idea that there are necessary linkages between advances in different spheres of human life are present only toward the end of the period discussed here.

These limitations notwithstanding, the historical overview that follows is crucial for considering how answers to the question "what is medical progress?" have always been contested and historically contingent. As I show in what follows, improved medical care had very different meanings depending on the respective value ascribed to individual and societal well-being, attitudes toward death, and the role

---

[4] Daniel Callahan, "Finite Lives and Unlimited Medical Aspirations," in *The Contingent Nature of Life: Bioethics and the Limits of Human Existence*, ed. Marcus Düwell, Christoph Rehmann-Sutter, and Dietmar Mieth (New York: Springer, 2008), p. 164.

of physicians. And within these shifting ideas of medical progress are numerous longer running threads that return in the post-World War II focus of Chapters 2–4.

1.1 Notions of Selfhood and Progress in Antiquity

To grasp what is distinctive about contemporary views of medical progress, we must put them in context, and ideas of progress dating back to classical times are an obvious point of reference. It is widely accepted in academic scholarship that various worldviews developed in ancient Greece are crucial for the history of the idea of progress itself. Classicist Ludwig Edelstein observes that ancient Greeks formulated most of the thoughts and sentiments that later generations went on to associate with progress.[5] There is no direct translation of the term progress in ancient Greece, though possible equivalents, such as ability awareness or consciousness of human capacity, have been proposed.[6] Already this etymological hurdle requires acknowledging that a modern idea of progress is an unfamiliar category in the ancient world. Greek thinkers had an entirely different horizon for considering historical change, one in which the future is not open-ended, but rather connected back to the present in a cyclical way. And yet a sense of novelty and progress did exist in ancient Greece; fifth-century Greeks were concerned not so much with continuous advances through time to a far-off future but rather with increases in knowledge and technical capabilities. Moreover, the Latin analog, *progressus*, of the Greek words most commonly used to describe progress, has entered all modern European languages.[7]

---

[5] Ludwig Edelstein, *The Idea of Progress in Classical Antiquity* (Baltimore: Johns Hopkins Press, 1967), p. xxxiii. See also W. Burkert, "Impact and Limits of the Idea of Progress in Antiquity," in *The Idea of Progress*, ed. Arnold Burgen, Peter McLaughlin, and Jürgen Mittelstrass (Berlin, New York: De Gruyter, 1997), pp. 19–46 and Armand d'Angour, *The Greeks and the New: Novelty in Ancient Greek Imagination and Experience* (Cambridge: Cambridge University Press, 2011).

[6] See Christian Meier, "Ein antikes Äquivalent des Fortschrittsgedankens: das 'Könnens-Bewusstsein' des 5. Jahrhunderts v. Chr.," *Historische Zeitschrift*, 226 (1) (1978), 265–316.

[7] Leonid Zhmud, *The Origin of the History of Science in Classical Antiquity*, trans. Alexander Chernoglazov (New York: De Gruyter, 2006), pp. 17–18.

1 History: Medical Progress in Context

Greek thinkers viewed history as having both a mythical point of origin and being subject to recurrent cycles. But they drew attention to the ability of citizens to alter and improve their lives through individual will and actions. Historian F. J. Teggart argues that the poet Hesiod (c. 700 BCE) first articulated an idea of human progress, namely that a good life is attainable and that humans have the power to achieve such a life.[8] These views resounded in the works of philosopher Xenophanes (570–475 BCE) who portrayed the various steps by which humans acquired the knowledge and skills to make their life more comfortable: "Indeed not from the beginning did gods intimate all things to mortals, but as they search in time they discover better."[9] Edelstein, who also cites these words, refers to them as the first statement of the idea of progress in Western history.[10]

The Greek interest in progress was stimulated by what has been referred to as the triumphant experience of progress in the fifth and fourth centuries BCE.[11] Various contemporary accounts of these improvements consider *technê* – arts or skills including medicine – central for enabling human beings to overcome the tribulations of their natural situation. Medicine in the tradition associated with Hippocrates of Cos (c. 460–370 BCE) envisaged illness as having natural causes as opposed to being a result of, for example, religious sin or superstition, which is also the reason that Greek medicine has been described as closer to modern medicine than any other historical form.[12] But ancient notions of discovery and the idea of gradual, cumulative progress also influenced the aspirations of medicine at the time. Hippocratic physicians believed that their observations built on what was already known to add to a continually growing body of medical knowledge. The author of the Hippocratic Treatise, "Ancient Medicine," wrote as follows:

---

[8] Frederick J. Teggart, "The Argument of Hesiod's Works and Days," *Journal of the History of Ideas*, 8 (1) (1947), 77.
[9] Xenophanes, Fragment 18 in James H. Lesher, *Xenophanes of Colophon: Fragments* (Toronto: University of Toronto Press, 1992), p. 150.
[10] Edelstein, *The Idea of Progress*, p. 4. On various relevant points of translation, see Alexander Tulin, "Xenophanes Fr. 18 D.-K. and the Origins of the Idea of Progress," *Hermes*, 121 (2) (1993), 129–38.
[11] E. R. Dodds, *The Ancient Concept of Progress and Other Essays on Greek Literature and Belief* (Oxford: Clarendon Press, 1973), p. 6.
[12] Erwin H. Ackerknecht, *A Short History of Medicine* (Baltimore: Johns Hopkins University Press, 2016 [1955]), p. 36.

[M]any and excellent discoveries [in medicine] have been made over a long period of time; and what remains will also be discovered, if an inquirer is competent and, being cognizant of the discoveries already made, conducts his researches beginning from these. [...] [And since medicine] has been able by reasoning to rise from deep ignorance very close to perfect accuracy, I think we should admire its discoveries as the work, not of chance, but of scientific inquiry honestly and correctly conducted.[13]

Thus presented, knowledge growth is a cumulative process rooted in systematic observation, with the potential to uncover the mysteries of health in their entirety.[14] This worldview is evident in another Hippocratic essay on the art of medicine, which states that "to discover something among things unknown, which would be better if it were discovered rather than left undiscovered," is the proper ambition and task of intelligence.[15]

But this interest in discovery and the steady growth of knowledge occurred in the context of a broader worldview in which physicians approached health in relation to a structured, predetermined natural order influencing human life.[16] The humoral medicine practiced at the time considered disease the result of an imbalance in vital bodily fluids (e.g., blood/phlegm/yellow bile/black bile) that had different properties (hot–cold/moist–dry) and were themselves identified with natural forces (air/water/fire/earth) outside of a person.[17] Everyone's particular humoral makeup determines their character and dictates the medical treatment they need, that is, how to rebalance their unbalanced humors. For the next 2,000 years, humoral theory and its evacuation

---

[13] Hippocrates, *Ancient Medicine*, ed. and trans. Paul Potter, Loeb Classical Library 147 (Cambridge, MA: Harvard University Press, 2022), 2, p. 11; 12, p. 31.

[14] Ibid., 8, p. 23.

[15] Hippocrates, *The Art*, ed. and trans. Paul Potter, Loeb Classical Library 148 (Cambridge, MA: Harvard University Press, 2022), 1, p. 191.

[16] On the close connections between Greek medical thought and philosophy, see Philip J. van der Eijk, *Medicine and Philosophy in Classical Antiquity: Doctors and Philosophers on Nature, Soul, Health and Disease* (Cambridge: Cambridge University Press, 2005) and Elizabeth M. Craik, "Teleology in Hippocratic Texts: Clues to the Future?," in *Teleology in the Ancient World: Philosophical and Medical Approaches*, ed. Julius Rocca (Cambridge: Cambridge University Press, 2017), pp. 203–16.

[17] Vivian Nutton argues that this particular constellation of humors was merely one variation among others. See "The Fatal Embrace: Galen and the History of Ancient Medicine," *Science in Context*, 18 (1) (2005), 111–21.

1 History: Medical Progress in Context

techniques – venesection, cupping, cathartics, emetics, sweating, and so on – provided an adaptable, personalized, and difficult-to-falsify framework for approaching disease. The medical art, then, was perceived as helping to restore a natural balance that had been disturbed, and in doing so imitating nature. Incremental improvements were framed in relation to the overarching powers of the natural world and the external limits to the progress of medicine, namely the health available to each sick person.

The notion of progress as occurring in relation to an external limitation influenced a shared sense of the aim and possibility of improvement in medicine. Aristotle, for example, in his ethics and politics develops the idea that each person has a unique state of health available to them.[18] For him, the medical doctor must act in a virtuous manner, namely react in a particular situation and context to bring the individual subject "to the highest perfection *of which it is capable*."[19] The final goal of health interventions therefore varies in different people according to their relative endowments, that is, gender, class – Aristotle considered women and slaves to have inferior constitutions – age, and so on, and the physician can never hope to achieve anything like "perfect health"; their objective, rather, must be the relative "golden mean" (*mesotês*) unique to each individual patient. Even if the art of medicine pursues health in an unlimited way, the end itself is a limit to medicine and other arts.[20] These views were closely aligned with Hippocratic thinking about progress, both in terms of the need for pragmatic action based on a specific sickness situation, the incremental nature of medical knowledge, and the inherent limits to medicine. For these reasons – and despite its depiction of medicine as having arrived at close to perfect accuracy – the Hippocratic idea of progress remained modest, and the limitations thereof are reflected in its canonical texts. Another passage on the art of medicine describes its inherent limits as follows:

---

[18] See Werner Jaeger, "Aristotle's Use of Medicine as Model of Method in His Ethics," *The Journal of Hellenic Studies*, 77 (1) (1957), 56.
[19] Theodore James Tracy, *Physiological Theory and the Doctrine of the Mean in Plato and Aristotle* (Berlin and Boston: De Gruyter, 2014 [1969]) pp. 317–18, citing *Nicomachean Ethics* 1333a29–30.
[20] See Aristotle, *Politics*, trans. H. Rackham, Loeb Classical Library (Cambridge, MA: Harvard University Press, 1932) book I, 1257b25–28, p. 45.

For in areas where we are able to gain the mastery by means of their nature or the tools of the art, it is possible for us to be craftsmen, but not in others. Thus when a patient suffers some evil more powerful than the means of the medical art, it cannot be expected that this should be in some way overcome.[21]

1.2 Health in Christianity and the Middle Ages

Ancient notions of progress were adapted by successive thinkers in a way that ensured both continuities and distinct legacies for medical progress. Much of the Hippocratic legacy was conveyed to Rome via Galen (AD 129–c. 216), who saw himself as both extending and popularizing the legacy of the Hippocratics. Galen was an experimenter and dissector, who was heavily invested in physical and anatomical explanations. At the same time, he conceived of all structures in a teleological perspective and of individual bodily humors and body parts as subject to life and celestial forces. But the transmission of the Hippocratic–Galenic tradition to the medieval world was fragmented; scientific theories and classical sources flowed through different channels, involving a complex process of cross-pollination between different local knowledges, religious views, and experience accumulated through practice. In the turmoil following the disintegration of the Roman Empire, Persian and Arab scholars preserved, systematized, and developed the medical knowledge of ancient Greek authors and Galen himself. In Europe, health-related knowledge remained mostly in the possession of families, lay healers, and religious orders.

The advent of Christianity altered previous patterns of care and medicine's theoretical framework. In early Christian anthropology, human nature and the body are defined by sin: After the Fall, humankind relinquished immortality and physical perfection and was marked by ill health, aging, and death. Similar to Greek thought, the human person and the world are organized in light of the moral ends of the highest order of being, the spirit or God. Yet a notable difference is the depiction in Judeo-Christian thought of history as linear and tending toward redemption and salvation, for example, as articulated by Augustine of Hippo (354–430).[22] Not only was this philosophy of history profoundly

---

[21] Hippocrates, *The Art*, 8, p. 203.
[22] On Augustine's influence, see Theodor E. Mommsen, "St Augustine and the Christian Idea of Progress: The Background of the City of God," *Journal of the History of Ideas*, 2 (3) (1951), 354–56. But on the dangers of

significant for conceptions of disease and their treatment, subsequent scholars have argued that much of the later history of the idea of progress amounts to a secularized version of Christian eschatology, reproduced as a general theme of historical development.[23]

From an etymological perspective, the modern concept of progress is indebted to several Latin terms and their connotations. The Latin *progressus*, the past participle of *progredi*, is derived from the preposition *pro*, which has the same Indo-European root as the ancient Greek, προ, and *gradi* – to step, walk – from the proto-Indo-European root *ghredh, to walk, go.[24] But the nonspecific use of *pro* in Latin, used to describe categories of motion including forward, from a position in the rear, out, as well as down before, meant that a word like *progrediente* could have a pejorative meaning. For example, Augustine's statement *genere humano progrediente atque crescente* (the human race advanced and grew) is a negative judgment because it refers to the ill-advised blending of the kingdoms of God and that on earth.[25] Another important term circulating in Latin for later theories of progress was *profectus*, a noun from the past participle stem of *proficere*, with the meanings of progress, success, and profit.[26] *Profectus*, as Augustine used the term in the sense of making progress and doing good, was able to resolve all of the world's contradictions. This *profectus*, however, was presented as outside of time and did not involve change per se, but rather a deepening of religious experience.[27] *Progressus*, therefore, was an ambivalent expression, and relative progress was rather described as *profectus* with a specifically religious meaning, as in a recurring description by influential Christian theologians and scholastics, *profectus hominis donum*

the oversimplification of a Judeo-Christian directed view of time, see Arnaldo Momigliano, "Time in Ancient Historiography," *History and Theory*, 6 (1966), 1–23.

[23] See Karl Löwith, *Meaning and History: The Theological Implications of the Philosophy of History* (Chicago: University of Chicago Press, 1957).

[24] "Progress, n.," *Oxford English Dictionary*, Oxford University Press, March 2024, https://doi.org/10.1093/OED/3034306464 and Douglas Harper, "Etymology of Progress," *Online Etymology Dictionary*, www.etymonline.com/word/progress.

[25] Augustine, *The City of God against the Pagans*, vol. 4, book 15, XXII, Loeb Classical Library 414, trans. Philip Levine (Cambridge, MA: Harvard University Press, 1966), p. 543.

[26] "Profit, n.," *Oxford English Dictionary*, Oxford University Press, March 2024, https://doi.org/10.1093/OED/6630322299.

[27] Koselleck, "Fortschritt," p. 364.

Dei est (man's progress is God's gift).[28] Medieval philosopher Peter Abelard (1079–1142), for example, discusses advancing by means of understanding (*intelligendo proficiens*), in the sense of improved ability to understand the scriptures.[29]

In medieval Europe dominated by the Church, individuals were encouraged to see earthly maladies as trivial compared to potential eternal rewards, and advances in the human arts and sciences played a secondary role. Prayer and humility were the most important means of addressing sickness, combined with local knowledge of healing plants and practices, including natural and magico-religious remedies of physicians and informal healers. The sequencing and weighting of these different approaches were crucial; a Christian could seek medical help while acknowledging their fundamental dependence on God, the ultimate healer.[30] This religious worldview informed the assumption that pain, as well as chronic and severe illness, was an opportunity for patiently accepting the will of God. In the case of physical torment, being able to deny one's own bodily needs and embrace suffering was what marked a person as able to identify with Christ, and therefore a higher order of being. Indeed, the markedly positive significance attributed to pain, for example, persisted until the early modern period; from the thirteenth to the fifteenth centuries, suffering was not to be dismissed or overcome, but rather felt with a deepening intensity.[31] To take one example, the death process of the archbishop of Canterbury, Hubert Walter, in 1205, was described as having been disrupted by a medical practitioner who favored physical remedies over spiritual ones.[32]

---

[28] See, for example, Isidorus (Isidore of Seville), *Sententiae*, 2, 5, *Monumenta*, http://monumenta.ch/latein/text.php?tabelle=Isidorus&rumpfid=Isidorus,%20Sententiae,%202,%20%20%20%205&level=4&domain=&lang=1&links=1&inframe=1&hide_apparatus=1.

[29] Tobias George, "From Reading to Understanding: Profectus in Abelard and Origen," in *Progress in Origen and the Origenian Tradition*, ed. Gaetano Lettieri, Maria Fallica, and Anders-Christian Jacobsen (Berlin: Peter Lang, 2020), p. 138.

[30] Gary B. Ferngren, *Medicine and Health Care in Early Christianity* (Baltimore: Johns Hopkins University Press, 2009), p. 61. A key biblical passage for such interpretations is Exodus 15:26, in which God says to Moses: "I am the Lord who heals you."

[31] Esther Cohen, *The Modulated Scream: Pain in Late Medieval Culture* (Chicago: University of Chicago Press, 2010), p. 4.

[32] Faye Getz, *Medicine in the English Middle Ages* (Princeton, NJ: Princeton University Press, 1999), p. 3 e passim.

1 History: Medical Progress in Context

In such cases, the point was not to focus on treating and curing the body, but rather on renouncing it and preparing the voluntary acceptance of death, as prescribed by the eschatology of salvation.

In this context, medicine was primarily seen as "assisting God in his works," in Hugh of Saint Victor's (c. 1096–1141) famous formulation.[33] Christ's healing miracles played a crucial role in the Christian faith; *salus* is the term for both health and salvation in Latin. While one's own physical torment was an opportunity for penitence, Christianity's ethical commitment to caring for the sick – associated with charity and the selfless love of fellow Christians – as well as remedying the anguish of others resulted in a sustained interest in practical medicine. In general, in addition to being the fruit of reason and individual experience, medicine was seen as a God-given way to address the earthly burden of having a body.

Translations of the medical texts of classical antiquity set the stage for more detailed and critical expositions, for example, by Persian philosopher and physician Ibn Sina (Avicenna). His *Canon of Medicine* (1025), a medical encyclopedia that proposed a systematic arrangement of the contemporary medical knowledge of the Islamic world, and integrated Graeco-Roman, Persian, and Ayurvedic traditions, went on to have an unparalleled influence. Various factors, including a more significant Western presence in former Byzantium, and the translation from Arabic into Latin of ancient Greek and Islamic medical texts, provided the foundation for a new reception of Galenism in Western Europe. The medicine of the late Middle Ages was marked by the rediscovery of authoritative texts, which enabled practitioners to deal with diseases in new ways and try to identify new pathologies, as well as changing ideas about novelty and progress.[34]

These shifts can be seen in, among other things, debates as to the relative importance of theory or practice in medicine.[35] *Medicina*

---

[33] See "Introduction," *The Didascalicon of Hugh St Victor: A Medieval Guide to the Arts*, trans. and intro. Jerome Taylor (New York and London: Columbia University Press, 1961), p. 31.

[34] See Chiara Crisciani, "History, Novelty and Progress in Scholastic Medicine," *Osiris*, 6 (1990), 118–39, and A. G. Molland, "Medieval Ideas of Scientific Progress," *Journal of the History of Ideas*, 39 (1978), 577.

[35] See John M. Riddle, "Theory and Practice in Medieval Medicine" (1974) in *Viator: Medieval and Renaissance Studies*, vol. 5 (Berkeley: University of California Press, 2020), pp. 158–85.

retained the connotation of a practical art gained through apprenticeship training and experience, while *Physica* is a natural philosophy associated with scholarly learning and reflections on the workings of the universe. The association between medicine and the term *physica* marked a change in priorities from the varieties and messiness of discovery and experience toward established learning. It also prompted a shift in the epistemological status of particular kinds of knowledge such as anatomy, physiology, and pathology because of their ability to be systematized. This association between medicine and particular kinds of science was a step with enormous consequences beyond the Middle Ages. It coincided with the solidification of the hierarchies between formally recognized (male) physicians who received academic training and other medical actors, including surgeons, barbers, dentists, and (female) midwives, who operated in local medical markets.

Christianity's transhistorical concept of progress, East–West translations and new knowledges, and the (re)valorization of theory – all these contributed to the sense that human beings can hope for a better life on earth and act so as to bring it about.[36] The idea of a progressive history gained particular impetus in northern France, where contemporary achievements in the arts and sciences were described as part of an overall forward movement; Bernard of Chartres (?-c. 1124), in a well-known formulation, referred to his contemporaries, "as dwarfs sitting on the shoulders of giants."[37] This implied that medicine could not improve merely by studying the teachings of the ancients but that it was necessary to supplement them. Henri de Mondeville (c. 1270–1325), a leading physician in his time, made this explicit when he wrote that: "It seems absurd and almost heretical to believe that sublime and glorious God would have given Galen a

---

[36] Stanley L. Jaki, "Medieval Christianity: Its Inventiveness in Technology and Science," in *Technology in the Western Political Tradition*, eds. Arthur M. Melzer, Jerry Weinberger, and M. Richard Zinman (Ithaca, NY and London: Cornell University Press, 1993), p. 46. See also Guy Beaujouan, "Histoire des sciences et philosophie au moyen âge: L'émergence médiévale de l'idée du progrès," *Bulletin de philosophie médiévale*, 30 (1988), 20–36, and Alistair C. Crombie, "Some Attitudes to Scientific Progress: Ancient, Medieval and Early Modern," *History of Science*, 13 (3) (1975), 213–30.

[37] See Robert K. Merton, *On the Shoulders of Giants: The Post-Italianate Edition* (Chicago: University of Chicago Press, 1993 [1965]).

1 History: Medical Progress in Context

great mind with the condition that nobody after him would be able to discover anything new."[38] But in speaking directly to Galen, de Mondeville created a history to accompany his particular narrative, skipping over, for example, ways in which Persian and Arabic contributions permitted the rediscovery of ancient medical treatises. In part, at least, progress inhered in this process.

De Mondeville's valorization of cumulative progress and enthusiasm for novelty existed alongside the imperative for order and symmetry and the need to integrate new cases and innovations into existing rational systems. The belief in the progressive cumulation of knowledge and confidence in ancient authorities, therefore, coexisted in the sense that accumulation occurred within a closed, predetermined framework. Around 1100, astrology – which purported to fuse mathematics, astronomy, and the patient's personal humoral situation – became an indispensable aspect of medical practice and remained so until well into the seventeenth century. Scientific approaches – such as Roger Bacon's (c. 1219–1292) emphasis on knowledge acquired through experience and experiment – were integrated into broader overarching visions of microcosmic human beings in a macrocosmic world order.[39] To be sure, there was a dynamic relationship between the framework and the "new," but it did not involve radical change. This conceptual apparatus for progress, in which persons were seen as a reflection of the celestial cosmos on a miniature scale, and illness explained in reference to its divine cause, was disturbed by the later findings of Copernicus and Newton. The old world in which matter held a spiritual meaning was slowly replaced by one in which material existence became increasingly important in and of itself. As a result, sustained attention to the mechanistic workings of the human body became increasingly central to notions of medical progress.

---

[38] Henry de Mondeville, cited in Plinio Prioreschi, "The Idea of Scientific Progress in Antiquity and in the Middle Ages," *Vesalius*, 8 (1) (2002), 38.

[39] See Lynn White Jr., "Science and the Sense of Self: The Medieval Background of a Modern Confrontation," *Daedalus*, 107 (2) (1978), 57. On Bacon and medicine, see Faye Marie Getz, "Roger Bacon and Medicine: The Paradox of the Forbidden Fruit and the Secrets of Long Life," in *Roger Bacon and the Sciences: Commemorative Essays*, ed. Jeremiah Hackett (Leiden and New York: Brill, 1997), pp. 337–64.

1.3 Progress and the Person in the Renaissance

In the accompanying conceptual revolution, medicine played an important metaphorical role. Historian Peter Gay describes how medicine was intimately linked to the scientific revolution from the beginning and how its proponents saw themselves as physicians, ministering to a sick civilization.[40] The sickness in question was the deference to antiquity associated with medieval thought and the belief – in the assessment of English philosopher Francis Bacon (1561–1626) – that an ambitious kind of progress was impossible.[41] Bacon's approach joined a utilitarian rationale that knowledge should be used for human good, with the joy inherent in discovering the truth. His attempt to undertake a total reconstruction of the foundations of all human knowledge was based on his disdain for his predecessors' attitudes to progress; the state of knowledge, he wrote, is "neither prosperous nor greatly advancing." Bacon did not break with a religious outlook so much as transform it; he depicts God as engaged in an "innocent and kindly" game of hide and seek with regard to knowledge and argues that if humans use their newly found knowledge "for the benefit and use of life," this will be sanctioned by God.[42] Bacon singled out medicine as a highly useful art that had much to gain by adopting the new empiricist scientific method and placed new emphasis on trying to understand how the body functioned.[43] In particular, because of its potential to affect human well-being, it was also crucial for human progress, understood as the advancement of God-sanctioned knowledge.[44]

---

[40] Peter Gay, *Enlightenment: An Interpretation*, vol. 2, *The Science of Freedom* (New York: Alfred A. Knopf, 1969), p. 13.

[41] Francis Bacon, *Novum Organum, or True Suggestions for the Interpretation of Nature*, ed. Joseph Devey (New York: P. F. Collier & Son, 1902), para 88, p. 67. On Bacon's commitment to progress more generally, see Robert K. Faulkner, *Francis Bacon and the Project of Progress* (Lanham: Rowman & Littlefield, 1993).

[42] Francis Bacon, "Preface to the Instauratio Magna," in *Prefaces and Prologues*, vol. 39, the Harvard Classics (New York: P. F. Collier & Son, 1909–14), available at www.bartleby.com/39/20.html.

[43] See Bacon's *The Advancement of Learning*, ed., William Aldis Wright (Oxford: Clarendon Press, 1869 [1605]), and his island utopia, *New Atlantis* (1626), in which he emphasized the importance of good health and the ways in which medical advances could improve human well-being.

[44] Marta Fattori, "*Prolongatio Vitae* and *Euthanasia* in Francis Bacon," in *Francis Bacon on Motion and Power*, eds. Guido Giglioni et al. (Switzerland: Springer, 2016), p. 124.

1 History: Medical Progress in Context

René Descartes (1596–1650) shared Bacon's desire to recast the conceptual foundations of progress, and his methodological skepticism, which separated an immaterial mind and a body that has a different order of existence, further challenged the integrated worldview of the Middle Ages.[45] Descartes himself was not a crude materialist, but in describing the body as made up of component parts – bones, nerves, muscles, veins, blood, and the like – independent of the mind, his work inspired reductionist currents of thought that sought to locate health squarely in the physical body.[46] Cartesian dualism, historian Klaus Bergdolt argues, meant in fact the secularization of the body and was reclaimed by those who sought to put physical and mechanical interventions at the center of theories of medical advance.[47] Descartes himself saw medicine as a prime field that could benefit from his method. He referred to health as "the first good [le premier bien] and the foundation of all other goods in this life" and argued that "if it were possible to find some means of rendering men wiser and more capable than hitherto, I believe we must seek it in medicine."[48] Concomitantly, his expectations of the progress of medical science were vigorously optimistic:

What we know is almost nothing compared to what remains to be known; we could be freed from innumerable maladies, of body and mind alike, and perhaps even from the infirmities of old age, if we had sufficient knowledge of their causes and of all the remedies which nature has given us.[49]

Based on such statements, Descartes has been interpreted posthumously as aspiring to nothing less than to use medicine to provide a solution to the human condition.

Bacon's and Descartes's ideas were widely discussed, but there was no single way in which the attitudes to progress they articulated

---

[45] Among the extensive literature on Descartes and medicine, see Gerrit Arie Lindeboom, *Descartes and Medicine* (Amsterdam: Rodopi, 1979), *Descartes and Medicine: Problems, Responses and Survival of a Cartesian Discipline*, ed. Fabrizio Baldassarri (Turnhout, Belgium: Brepols, 2023), and *Embodiment: A History*, ed. Justin E. H. Smith (Oxford: Oxford University Press, 2017).
[46] See William Barrett, *Death of the Soul. Philosophical Thought from Descartes to the Computer* (Oxford: Oxford University Press, 1987).
[47] Klaus Bergdolt, *Well-being: A Cultural History of Healthy Living* (Cambridge: Polity Press, 2009), p. 202.
[48] Descartes, *Discours de la méthode pour bien conduire sa raison et chercher la vérité dans les sciences* (Paris: Librairie Hachette, 1876 [1637]), p. 65.
[49] Ibid.

were integrated into medicine. The iatrochemical ideas of the Swiss physician Paracelsus (1493–1541), the insights of anatomist Andreas Vesalius (1514–1564), the description of blood circulation by William Harvey (1578–1657), and the mechanical worldview of the iatrophysicists of the seventeenth century – to name but a few – blended with Cartesian/Baconian theories, the humoral framework, and religious beliefs in complex ways. The medical knowledge of the ancients, and Hippocrates in particular, continued to be valorized, and medical progress was portrayed as the rediscovery of the past.[50] This tendency to view Hippocrates as the origin and ultimate goal of highly divergent concepts of medical progress was strengthened by both cyclical understandings of history and theories of degeneration. Hippocrates could be portrayed as the "dawn" of medical art, and the medical Renaissance a new dawn, or, in a theory of permanent degeneration, as the only dawn in the history of medicine. In England, for example, renowned physician Thomas Sydenham (1624–1689), a follower of Francis Bacon known as the "English Hippocrates," stressed the importance of on-the-ground experience and that his role lay in assisting nature. Yet while Sydenham operated in a humoral framework, and saw himself as contributing to and maintaining Hippocratism, he also laid the foundation for going beyond Hippocrates by suggesting that medicine should study not so much patients and their illnesses, but rather diseases as phenomena with an existence separate from the persons who suffered from them.

In general, from the seventeenth century onward, suffering was demythologized, and no longer considered a sign of communion with Christ.[51] The rise of Protestantism, which repudiated magical healing and religious practices allowed by the medieval Church, such as visits to sacred shrines and the use of holy relics, contributed to the decline of magical practices in medicine.[52] Yet spiritual worldviews, and the fact that salvation was anchored in Christ, continued to inform the meanings ascribed to suffering and to place them in a time frame that extended beyond punctual episodes of illness. For example,

---

[50] See Thomas Rütten, "Hippocrates and the Construction of 'Progress' in Sixteenth- and Seventeenth-Century Medicine," in *Reinventing Hippocrates* (London and New York: Routledge, 2001), pp. 37–58.

[51] Bergdolt, *Wellbeing*, p. 204.

[52] See Keith Thomas, *Religion and the Decline of Magic: Studies in Popular Beliefs in Sixteenth and Seventeenth Century England* (New York: Penguin Books, 1982).

1 History: Medical Progress in Context

historian Mary Fissell chronicled how in early modern England men and women attributed acute afflictions to incidents or sins committed years earlier.[53] For these patients, understanding the meanings of illness and health – which were linked to a divine plan and their personal religious beliefs – was more important than the cure or the curer and emphatically more relevant than the new experimental science.

New scientific insights, therefore, coexisted with traditional Hippocratic remedies, and the overall view of the body as a "divine machine," as Leibniz (1646–1716) had put it in his *Monadology* (1714).[54] Slowly, the religious meanings of *profectus* edged closer to a form of world-historical progress, without taking on all of the connotations that it would later on.[55] The dynamic process whereby ideas of progress influenced and reinforced medical practices was particularly visible in the so-called Quarrel of Ancients and Moderns in the latter part of the seventeenth century. This debate opposed those who believed that nothing in modern times reached the heights of antiquity and those who argued that modernity could be superior to classical times. For moderns, it became highly desirable to direct their efforts toward a goal located in the future, and they also enabled the articulation of what Nisbet calls the first secular statement of the idea of progress in modern Europe.[56] And this new idea of progress gave medicine a particular status.

1.4 Medical Progress, Self, and Enlightenment

It was during the Enlightenment that a mindset that no longer associated improvement with the recovery of the past, but rather with a

---

[53] Mary E. Fissell, *Patients, Power, and the Poor in Eighteenth-Century Bristol* (Cambridge: Cambridge University Press, 1991), pp. 34–35. See also Olivia Weisser, *Ill Composed: Sickness, Gender and Belief in Early Modern England* (New Haven, CT: Yale University Press, 2015).
[54] Leibniz, *Monadology* (1714), para 64, in Lloyd Strickland, *Leibniz's Monadology: A New Translation and Guide* (Edinburgh: Edinburgh University Press, 2014), p. 27.
[55] Koselleck, "Fortschritt," p. 368.
[56] Robert Nisbet, "Idea of Progress: A Bibliographical Essay," p. 17. See also Hans Robert Jauss, "Ursprung und Bedeutung der Fortschrittsidee in der 'Querelle des Anciens et des Modernes,'" *Die Philosophie und die Frage nach dem Fortschritt*, eds. Helmut Kuhn and Franz Wiedmann (Munich: Anton Pustet, 1964), pp. 51–72.

future goal orienting earthly life, really took hold. The most ardent proponents of the notion of progress during that era – such as Abbé de Saint-Pierre (1658–1743) and Turgot (1727–1781) – sought to popularize a view whereby human societies pass through stages, from hunting, pastoral life, and agriculture, becoming ever more perfect, as evinced by the cultural and material accomplishments of contemporary European society.[57] Marquis de Condorcet (1743–1794), whose work is generally referred to as the zenith of the idea of progress, adopted Turgot's idea of the law of progress enabled by reason and claimed that the progress of the sciences and the perfection (*perfectibilité*) of human faculties could proceed without limits.[58] Not only did key Enlightenment figures portray progress as expanding potentially infinitely but also as a harmonious whole, whereby progress in different spheres of life, including science, politics, economics, and morality, is mutually reinforcing.[59] The comprehensiveness of this view of history as proceeding upward in a same direction, and the interdependence between different spheres, meant that individual instances of progress were no longer viewed as ambivalent, but rather as part of a broad historical movement in a forward direction. It was also around this time that an important semantic shift took place and the spiritual *profectus* was replaced or superseded by the secular *progressus* and its derivatives.[60] From then on, progress was largely reduced to the notion of betterment; historian Christian Meier writes that "no progression toward something bad could be progress."[61]

From these premises, the potential of medicine – a field that was starting to be considered foundational for other forms of knowledge

---

[57] See Turgot, *Discours sur les progrès successifs de l'esprit humain*, (1750), *Institut Coppet*, www.institutcoppet.org/turgot-discours-sur-les-progres-successifs-de-lesprit-humain-1750/. On Turgot, see Jean-Pierre Poirier, *Turgot: Laissez-faire et progrès social* (Paris: Perrin, 1999) and Robert Nisbet, "Turgot and the Contexts of Progress," *Proceedings of the American Philosophical Society*, 119 (3) (1975), 214–22.

[58] See Condorcet's *Esquisse d'un tableau historique des progrès de l'esprit humain* (Paris: Masson et Fils, 1822 [1795]).

[59] See Nannerl O. Keohane, "The Enlightenment Idea of Progress Revisited," in *Progress and Its Discontents*, eds. Gabriel A. Almond, Marvin Chodorow, and Roy Harvey Pearce (Berkeley: University of California Press, 1982), pp. 21–40.

[60] Koselleck, "Fortschritt," p. 371.

[61] Christian Meier, *The Greek Discovery of Politics*, trans. David McLintock (Cambridge, MA: Harvard University Press, 1990), p. 191.

about persons and societies – was framed as transformative. Diderot (1712–1784), for example, wrote that it "is very hard to think cogently about metaphysics or ethics without being an anatomist, a naturalist, a physiologist, and a physician."[62] Medicine occupied a crucial place in the nascent discipline of the philosophy of history, and the optimism of the philosophes was reflected in histories of medicine that presented present-day practices as the embodiment of progress; Daniel Le Clerc's *Histoire de la médecine, où l'on voit l'origine et les progrès de cet art, de siècle en siècle* (*History of Medicine, Where We See the Origin and Progress of This Art, from Century to Century* [1696]) was a case in point.[63] For the philosophes, medicine continued to play an important symbolic role; its capacity to wage a campaign against disease was closely associated with the Enlightenment questioning of superstition and religion. Historian Peter Gay notes that Christianity was portrayed as an "infection," a "germ," and a dangerous source of contagion. In Enlightenment rhetoric, both the attempt to control nature and question revealed religion were framed as a struggle for health.[64]

Condorcet, in particular, had an exuberant faith in medicine as a means of human betterment and ascribed it a prominent place in his vision of how nature and earthly life are proceeding together toward truth, happiness, and virtue. He described reason as driving the potentially limitless nature of medical progress and concluded that it would be able to eliminate disease, and perhaps even death. He argues that:

> the progress of protective medicine (*médecine préservatrice*), which will become more efficacious with the progress of reason and of the social order, will mean the end of infectious and hereditary diseases and illnesses brought on by climate, food, or working conditions. It is reasonable to hope that all other disease may likewise disappear as their distant causes are discovered. Would it be absurd, then, to suppose that this perfection of the human species should be seen as indefinite progress; that the day will come when death

---

[62] Cited in Peter Gay, *The Enlightenment*, vol. 2, p. 15.
[63] (The Hague: Isaac van der Kloot, 1729 [1696]). Similar works include John Friend, *The History of Physic from the Time of Galen to the Beginning of the Sixteenth Century* (London: J. Walthoe, 1725) and Robert James, *A Medicinal Dictionary Including Physic, Surgery, Anatomy, Chemistry and Botany in All Their Branches Relative to Medicine* (London: T. Osborne, 1743), which includes a Preface "tracing the Progress of Physic."
[64] Peter Gay, *The Enlightenment: An Interpretation*, vol. 2, p. 16.

will be only due to rare accidents or to the ever-slower decay of vital forces, and that ultimately the average span between birth and decay will have no assignable value?[65]

This passage, written in 1793 as he was hiding from the Jacobins and two years before his untimely death in prison, exemplifies the divergence between the expectations placed on historical progress and the realities of flesh-and-blood life on earth.

In contrast to naïvely confident views of progress, or theories that human life is directionless, Immanuel Kant developed a particularly influential theory of progress grounded in a teleological conception of the universe.[66] Kant depicts nature as purposive and goal-directed and thought of this as a condition for the actions of moral agents to have meaning. For Kant, progress is conceived as an answer to the question "What can I hope for?." In developing the notion that we have a moral duty to hope for progress, he rejected sanguine hopes about the history of humanity proceeding in the direction of progress. In fact, he wants to show that the problem of progress cannot be resolved directly through experience and that knowledge of the development of history based on past facts is impossible.[67] The irrelevance of historical evidence for progress is justified by the fact that the hope for improvement, which every person feels, is enough to ensure progress.[68] Per Kant, we have an inborn duty to assume that progress is possible, even if history might suggest otherwise.

Beyond his account of hope, the significance of Kant's philosophy for the idea of progress further lies in his association between the human

---

[65] *Esquisse d'un tableau historique des progrès de l'esprit humain*, pp. 304–5.
[66] On Kant's different explanations for why we have the right to understand human history as a purpose-directed process of progress, see Axel Honneth, "The Irreducibility of Progress: Kant's Account of the Relationship between Morality and History," *Critical Horizons*, 8 (1) (2007), 1–17.
[67] Immanuel Kant, "An Old Question Raised Again: Is the Human Race Constantly Progressing," in *Religion and Rational Theology*, trans. and ed. Allen W. Wood and George di Giovanni (Cambridge: Cambridge University Press, 2012), p. 300. See also Pauline Kleingeld, "Kant, History and the Idea of Moral Development," *History of Philosophy Quarterly*, 16 (1) 1999, 59.
[68] See Kant, "On the Common Saying: 'This May Be True in Theory, but It Does Not Apply in Practice," in *Kant, Political Writings*, ed. and intro. Hans Reiss, trans. H. B. Nisbet (Cambridge: Cambridge University Press, 1991 [1970]), 2nd enlarged ed., pp. 88–89. See Sofie Møller, "Kant on Non-Linear Progress," *Ethics & Politics*, 23 (2), 127–47.

1 History: Medical Progress in Context

capacities for reason, morality, and freedom. In Kant's view, the human capacity for reason is what enables us to become conscious of our moral duty and of absolute principles of morality. Human will, thus conceived, is autonomous because it is capable of self-determination according to this freely chosen moral law discoverable by reason. Moral autonomy, in Kant's view, implies the ability to abstract from one's own, biased point of view – including emotions and inclinations – and to subject oneself to universalizable moral principles. This includes the ability to rationally detach oneself from an ailing body and identify principles that transcend an individual perspective. Kant argued that, since purposiveness in nature requires us to develop our reason and free will, it therefore helps human beings realize their freedom. His view of flawed, mutually antagonistic moral agents, combined with the existence of autonomy as a normative ideal, meant that Kant understood the human condition as a process of "incessant laboring and becoming," through which we try to improve ourselves.[69]

The intellectual history of medicine was profoundly influenced by these philosophical developments. For example, the text by German physician Johann Karl Osterhausen (1765–1839) *On Medical Enlightenment* (*Über medizinische Aufklärung* [1789]) – a direct reference to Immanuel Kant's *What Is Enlightenment?* (*Was ist Aufklärung?* [1784]) – describes medical Enlightenment as man's emergence "from his ignorance [*Unwissenheit*] in all matters concerning his physical well-being." And he advocated a physician-led movement designed to eradicate "errors, miracle cures, occult remedies and other silly tricks [*Alfanzereien*]" that he associated with previous medical regimes.[70] The belief in the possibility of progress informed various practices of the time, including the establishment of hospitals and a new interest in the collection of vital statistics (fertility, death, height, weight, criminal record, etc.) of the population as part of the nascent discipline of social statistics and analysis of disease patterns.[71]

---

[69] Immanuel Kant, *Religion within the Boundaries of Mere Reason and Other Writings*, ed. and trans. A. W. Wood and G. di Giovanni, intro. R. M. Adams, (Cambridge: Cambridge University Press, 1998 [1793]), 6:48.

[70] *Über medizinische Aufklärung* (Zürich: Heinrich Gessner, 1798), cited in Klaus Bergdolt, *Das Gewissen der Medizin: Ärztliche Moral von der Antike bis Heute* (Munich: C. H. Beck, 2004), p. 198.

[71] William Bynum, *The History of Medicine: A Very Short Introduction* (Oxford: Oxford University Press, 2008), p. 42. See also Ludmilla Jordanova,

The link Condorcet articulated between political and medical optimism was particularly evident in the American colonies and the new republic where the attachment to the idea of progress was widely shared. The expansive spaces of the American continent were themselves seen as able to provide new and highly valuable sources of medical knowledge. Inventor and statesman Benjamin Franklin (1706–1790) marveled in 1780 at rapid scientific progress and speculated that it was impossible to know where the powers of man over nature would stop. All diseases, he wrote, "may by sure means be prevented or cured, not excepting even that of old age, and our lives lengthened at pleasure even beyond the antediluvian standard."[72] Breaking with previous limits – either natural or God-given – was sometimes justified with reference to the philosophy of Adam Smith and Smith's claim that bodily desires were not evidence of decadence or moral degeneration and to be resisted, but rather could be harnessed for progress.[73] In contrast to Christian philosophers, who placed moral and social value on limiting rather than multiplying needs and desires, the modern conception of progress valorized material comforts and the creative ingenuity required to produce them. These achievements are not only evidence of human beings' godlike powers but also what assure their salvation. According to Christopher Lasch, this is a key moment in the history of progress since the modern conception of progress depends on a positive assessment of the proliferation of wants.[74]

But it would be unwarranted to attribute a simplistic optimism about progress to the Enlightenment era in general. Romantic thinkers, for example, were concerned that Descartes' reduction of the body to its component parts irrevocably damaged the ability of medicine to treat and understand the whole person. They drew attention to what they perceived as a spiritual vacuum in medicine and tended to view the self in terms of the multitude of relations it entertains with others. Johann Gottfried von Herder (1744–1803), for one, mocked the philosophers

---

"Reflections on Medical Reform: Cabanis' Coup d'Oeuil," in *Medicine in the Enlightenment*, ed. Roy Porter (Amsterdam: Rodopi, 1995), pp. 166–80.

[72] (modernized spelling) "From Benjamin Franklin to Joseph Priestley, February 8, 1780," *Founders Online*, National Archives, https://founders.archives.gov/documents/Franklin/01-31-02-0325.

[73] Adam Smith, *An Inquiry into the Nature and Causes of the Wealth of Nations*, ed. S. M Soares (Amsterdam: MetaLibri, 2007 [1776]), p. 133.

[74] Lasch, *The True and Only Heaven*, p. 45.

who had unguarded, simplistic ideas of progress and favored instead a vision of social life as an organic whole. He stated "if only it were true that everything proceeded prettily in a straight line and that every succeeding human being and every succeeding race got perfected according to his [the philosopher's] ideal in a beautiful progress."[75] He drew attention to Swiss physician Albrecht von Haller's conception of irritability (*Irritabilität* or *Erregbarkeit*) and sensibility (*Sensibilität* or *Empfindlichkeit*) as important concepts for determining health.[76] Jean-Jacques Rousseau (1712–1778), who was associated with the emerging cult of feelings, was sharply critical of future-oriented views of progress, contrasting the present with a state of nature where there was no need for medicines, and even less for physicians.[77] Rousseau embodies the view that nature is what conserves health, while sickness arises because of the corrupting influence of society. Various lifestyle choices – including urban living and book learning – associated with the Enlightenment itself were seen as creating nervous, hysterical hypochondriacs. Meanwhile, Rousseau's own views on health have been an inspiration for modern "naturist" medicine, from hydrotherapy to dietetics, which tends to associate progress with the rediscovery of natural rhythms.[78]

As developed in the eighteenth century, the modern concept of progress understands history itself as the embodiment of progress. At the same time, this approach creates a disjunct between lived, historical experience and the potentially limitless horizon of expectations for progress. It should come as no surprise, therefore, that the theories of progress discussed in the Enlightenment era were articulated in the context

---

[75] Cited in Slaboch, *A Road to Nowhere*, p. 14.
[76] See Frank W. Stahnisch "The Tertium Comparationis of the Elementa Physiologiae: Johann Gottfried von Herder's Conception of 'Tears' as Mediators between the Sublime and the Actual Bodily Physiology," in *Blood, Sweat and Tears: The Changing Concepts of Physiology from Antiquity into Early Modern Europe*, eds. Manfred Horstmanshoff, Helen King, and Claus Zittel (Intersections – Interdisciplinary Studies in Early Modern Culture, vol. 25) (Leiden and Boston: Brill, 2012), pp. 609–10.
[77] J. J. Rousseau, "Discours sur l'origine et les fondements de l'inégalité parmi les hommes," in Rousseau, *Discours sur l'inégalité parmi les hommes; Contrat social; Discours sur l'économie politique; Projet de paix perpétuelle* (Amsterdam: Marc-Michel Rey, 1776), p. 15.
[78] See Serge Thériault, *Jean-Jacques Rousseau et la médecine naturelle* (Montreal: Les Editions Univers, 1979) and Philippe Casassus, "Les idées de Jean-Jacques Rousseau sur la médecine," *Médecine*, 13 (7) (2017), 330–34.

of very high rates of sickness and mortality. Only smallpox was being treated somewhat successfully by inoculation, and various diseases such as rickets and tuberculosis contributed to high levels of sickness overall. It is reasonable to speculate that a sick person who consulted a physician in the eighteenth century had a worse chance of surviving than one who did not; in Enlightenment society, it was justified to be more concerned about the dangers of medical practice for patients than its benefits. Voltaire (1694–1722), for example, wrote that regimen is better than medicine, and that for a very long time, ninety-eight out of a hundred doctors were charlatans.[79] The disconnect, therefore, between visions of open-ended progress and the realities of medical practice was huge. But at the same time, these attitudes to progress provided momentum for the idea of large-scale historical transformation.

1.5 Nineteenth Century: Medical Progress and Civilization

The commitment to elaborating philosophical frameworks for progress continued unabated during the nineteenth century and witnessed the development of numerous social philosophies that aimed to become the "science" of progress.[80] Auguste Comte (1798–1857), for one, developed a schema of historical progress according to which society moved through theological, metaphysical, and positive stages of world history; in the positive phase, it is possible to discern the scientific laws of historical and societal development. Comte used various biological and medical analogies to describe the task of enlightened thought in the positive age; he considered society an organism and thought that if its equilibrium was disrupted, it became sick. Positive philosophers, therefore, were physicians able to restore society's health.[81]

---

[79] He did however refer to surgery as the "most useful of arts," "having undergone such swift and renown progress this century." Voltaire, "Histoire du Siècle de Louis XIV," ed. Gustave Masson and G. W. Prothero (Cambridge: Cambridge University Press, 1882), p. 124. Cited in J. D. Rolleston, "Voltaire and Medicine," *Proceedings of the Royal Society of Medicine*, 19 (1926), 25.

[80] See Piotr Sztompka, "Agency and Progress: The Idea of Progress and Changing Theories of Change," in *Rethinking Progress: Movements, Forces, and Ideas at the End of the Twentieth Century*, eds. Jeffrey C. Alexander and Piotr Sztompka (London: Routledge, 1990), p. 247.

[81] See Mary Pickering, *Auguste Comte: An Intellectual Biography*, vol. 3 (Cambridge: Cambridge University Press, 2009), p. 542.

By emphasizing the connection between scientific progress and social life, Comte laid the grounds for other theories that sought to link medical progress and the life of social collectivities.

Darwin's *On the Origin of Species*, published in 1859, further developed the possibility that personal growth is linked to progressive developments in nature. Darwin left open the possibility for interpreting his theory as progress, writing that "as natural selection works solely by and for the good of each being, all corporeal and mental environments will tend to progress toward perfection."[82] In his *Descent of Man* (1871), he made the link with medicine more explicit and, using the racialized discourses of the nineteenth century, articulated the widespread concern over the perceived degeneration of the human stock, and the ways in which improved medical interventions aggravate this. He wrote:

[w]ith savages, the weak in body or mind are soon eliminated; and those that survive commonly exhibit a vigorous state of health. We civilized men, on the other hand, do our utmost to check the process of elimination; we build asylums for the imbecile, the maimed, and the sick; and our medical men exert their utmost skill to save the life of everyone to the last moment. There is reason to believe that vaccination has preserved thousands, who from a weak constitution would formerly have succumbed to small-pox. Thus the weak members of civilized societies propagate their kind. [...] It is surprising how soon a want of care, or care wrongly directed, leads to the degeneration of a domestic race [...].[83]

Darwin demurred from unpacking the implications of these ideas in medicine; he argued that intentionally neglecting the weak and helpless would be profoundly evil and that sympathy for the suffering of the weak is the noblest part of human nature. But various subsequent iterations of Darwinism invoked the well-being of the social organism to justify why potentially successful medical techniques should not be applied to individual members of society with existing conditions that made them "deficient."

The term "survival of the fittest" was associated with political and social philosopher Herbert Spencer (1820–1903) who, drawing on

---

[82] Charles Darwin, *On the Origin of Species* (Minneapolis: Lerner, 2008 [1859]), p. 455.
[83] Charles Darwin, *The Descent of Man*, vol. 1 (New York: American Home Library, 1902 [1871]), pp. 180–81.

Comte, argued that organic progress is effectively the law of social progress.[84] While in the past, natural selection had performed the task of weeding out the weaker, "unfit" members of the population, modern medicine and welfare were now doing the opposite. In time, "Social Darwinism," an umbrella term referring to the application of natural selection to other areas of human life, became closely related to negative eugenics, a term referring to medical measures aimed at reducing or hindering the reproduction of all those deemed unworthy – including the "feeble minded," "racially inferior," criminals, mentally and chronically ill, or simply impoverished. Negative eugenics, as Peter Gluckman and others have shown, were seen as a modern, technological, and scientifically justified solution to a social problem. If science provided the tools to improve animal or plant breeds through selection, reproduction was seen as a natural extension of such "progress."[85]

In this way, racism, colonialism, and the exclusion of entire categories of people were bound up with the commitment to the idea and practice of medical progress.[86] Improved medical techniques were explicitly associated with issues of power and control, especially of marginalized groups. The first uses of various medical devices, such as the speculum, for example, were justified in reference to and tested on the most powerless members of society. The insistence on the physical insensitivity of slaves and their purported high tolerance for pain underpinned various instances whereby intrusive forms of examination were used in the name of medical advance.[87] The experience of prostitutes in France, Germany, and Britain, where the speculum was used as an instrument of surveillance by the medical police, further highlights how an intrusion into the body in the name of more accurate examination techniques and medical advances was a profoundly

---

[84] Herbert Spencer, "Progress: Its Law and Cause" in *Essays: Scientific, Political and Speculative* (London: Williams and Norgate, 1891), vol. 1, p. 10.
[85] See Peter Gluckman et al., *Principles of Evolutionary Medicine* (Oxford: Oxford University Press, 2016), pp. 332-35.
[86] See Robert A. Williams, *Savage Anxieties: The Invention of Western Civilization* (New York: Palgrave, 2012).
[87] Joanna Bourke, "Pain Sensitivity: An Unnatural History from 1800 to 1965," *Journal of Medical Humanities*, 35 (3) (2014), 301-19 and Deirdre Cooper Owens, *Medical Bondage: Race, Gender, and the Origins of American Gynecology* (Atlanta: University of Georgia Press, 2017).

political act.[88] Knowledge gained in controlling infectious disease could be used to control and even eliminate populations who lacked that knowledge. In such cases, those with access to medical advances purposefully withheld and/or selectively wielded medical knowledge in the name of civilizational "progress."[89]

At the time, most theoreticians of progress were utilitarian in that they were convinced that the health of the community took precedence over the health of individuals. But a broad commitment to Comte's laws of historical progress resulted in no single vision of medical progress. In Germany, for example, Comte's ideas influenced German pathologist and statesman Rudolf Virchow (1821–1902), a founder of scientific biomedicine. Virchow was both ambitious and optimistic about the powers of science, believing that his century embodied progress toward the scientific age.[90] Yet he also drew attention to the connection between the origins of disease and social conditions that could be addressed and remedied. In contrast to the eugenicist ideas associated with Social Darwinism, he called for moral and sociopolitical progress, which he associated with the principle of equal entitlement and public healthcare.[91] In the context of social legislation and the rise of welfare associations, physicians were portrayed as bearing considerable responsibility for addressing social questions.

These ideas about progress interacted with contemporary scientific developments, such as the disease theory of medicine, which developed in France in the first decades of the nineteenth century, and formalized what Sydenham had intimated, namely that each sick patient is affected by a unique disease phenomenon, and the task of the clinician is to recognize and treat the disease. Knud Faber, in an early

---

[88] See Ornella Moscucci, *The Science of Woman: Gynaecology and Gender in England, 1800–1929* (Cambridge: Cambridge University Press, 1990).
[89] See Gary Geddes, *Medicine Unbundled: A Journey through the Minefields of Indigenous Health Care* (Victoria: Heritage House, 2017), James Daschuk, *Clearing the Plains: Disease, Politics of Starvation, and the Loss of Indigenous Life* (Regina: University of Regina Press, 2014), and Samir Shaheen-Hussein, *Fighting for a Hand to Hold: Confronting Medical Colonialism against Indigenous Children in Canada* (Montreal: McGill-Queen's University Press, 2020).
[90] Virchow, "Lernen und Forschen: Rede beim Antritt des Rectorats an der Friedrich-Wilhelms-Universität zu Berlin," October 15, 1892 (Berlin: Angust Hirschwald, 1892).
[91] See his *Collected Essays on Public Health and Epidemiology* (Cambridge: Science History Publications, 1985 [1848]), p. 14 e passim.

study of nosography, disease classification, describes its significance in terms of how clinical medicine is, therefore, at work like the other natural sciences "at the great task of attempting to understand natural phenomena in an attempt to control them."[92] As a rule, the introduction of new techniques and theories was not perceived at the time as a simple triumph of progress over reaction, but rather as mixed blessings with drawbacks. Anesthesia, for example, was introduced in the 1840s, and with anesthesia, "the patient-as-a-person" was no longer present during an operation.[93] Robert Koch's (1843–1910) insights into how particular germs could cause disease, Joseph Lister's (1827–1912) use of antisepsis, and Louis Pasteur's (1822–1895) research on micro-organisms have been interpreted as harbingers of progress. In reality, all these had varying degrees of acceptance and effectiveness and existed in complicated relationships between the laboratory and medical practice.[94] The recognition of the mental dimensions of health and sickness and the valorization of prior experience of illness for healthy living continued to be widespread. Friedrich Nietzsche (1844–1955), for example, emphasized the limits of scientific knowledge and the ability to cope with suffering and illness as a key part of human life.[95] The nineteenth century also witnessed significant medical nihilism and denials of the effectiveness of medical treatments.[96] But it was also during these decades that traditional therapies associated with treating unbalanced humors started being questioned more actively. In 1833, a satirical lithograph by Honoré Daumier showed a doctor seated at his desk under a bust of Hippocrates and asking himself: "Why the devil do all my patients go off like this [in coffins] … I do my best by bleeding them, purging them, drugging them … I just don't

---

[92] Knud Faber, *Nosography*, 2nd ed., rev. (New York: Haber, 1930), 210ff, cited in Eric Cassell, *The Nature of Suffering and the Goals of Medicine* (Oxford: Oxford University Press, 2004), p. 6.
[93] See Martin A. Pernick, *A Calculus of Suffering: Pain, Professionalism and Anesthesia in Nineteenth-Century America* (New York: Columbia University Press, 1985).
[94] See, among others, *Medical Innovations in Historical Perspective*, ed. John V. Pickstone (New York: St Martin's Press, 1992) and Michael Worboys, *Spreading Germs: Disease Theories and Medical Practice* (Cambridge: Cambridge University Press, 2000).
[95] See his *The Birth of Tragedy*, trans. and intro. Douglas Smith (Oxford: Oxford University Press, 2008 [1872]).
[96] Jacob Stegenga, *Medical Nihilism* (Oxford: Oxford University Press, 2018), pp. 11–12.

1 *History: Medical Progress in Context* 61

understand it!"[97] Such depictions exemplify the change whereby doctors began fundamentally to challenge conventional Hippocratic remedies, thereby also contributing to new ideologies of medical progress.

1.6 Early Twentieth-Century Visions of Progress

In his comprehensive study, Robert Nisbet observes that there is no want of declarations by historians and intellectuals that the idea of progress "died with Herbert Spencer," "ended with the nineteenth century," and "was banished forever by World War I."[98] Yet writings from the time show that an enthusiastic belief in progress remained viable, paradoxically in light of World War I. In a period marked by military tensions and confrontations, the ethos of progress became bound up with engineering advances necessary to defend national priorities, as well as related corporate interests. During the Great Depression, this type of commitment to a business–military–engineering model of progress is evident. The world fair entitled "A Century of Progress" held in Chicago in 1933, and celebrating what has been called the "western, masculine perspective of technology" is just one event that contributed to defining a particular historical narrative of progress.[99]

In medicine too, the idea of progress became increasingly associated with medical science and technology. The influential Flexner Report *Medical Education in the United States and Canada* (1910) signaled a realignment of medical knowledge and practice with scientific disciplines including anatomy, physiology, pathology, and microbiology. In Flexner's view, the physician should act like a scientist: observe, make a hypothesis, and act to test their theory accordingly.[100] This enthusiasm for the physician-scientist prompted a return to the optimistic hope that scientific medicine could potentially overcome and eliminate disease. Writing in 1914, a physician observed that the student of scientific medicine "has possession of methods which ultimately will lead

---

[97] Cited in David Wootton, *Bad Medicine*, p. 142.
[98] Nisbet, *Idea of Progress*, p. 297.
[99] See Cheryl R. Ganz on the "western, masculine perspective of technology" in relation to the idea of progress, *The 1933 Chicago World's Fair: A Century of Progress* (Urbana, Chicago and Springfield: University of Illinois Press, 2008), p. 2.
[100] Abraham Flexner, *Medical Education in the United States and Canada*, intro. Henry S. Pritchett (New York: Carnegie Foundation for the Advancement of Teaching, 1910), p. 55.

to the solution of most if not all of our problems."[101] While we have seen that this utopian belief in the unlimited potential of medical progress existed regardless of medicine's practical capabilities, it was bolstered by the fact that early twentieth-century patients were starting to benefit from new methods of diagnosis – including X-rays, blood, and laboratory tests – and, eventually, the so-called "drugs revolution" associated with the discovery of penicillin in 1928. These technologies and interventions provided physicians with the confidence that – as one wrote in 1934 – "when I told my patient what was wrong, I *knew* that was what was wrong."[102] This belief was one further iteration of a limitless model of medical progress, seeking not only the improvement of human health but its ultimate mastery, and bound up with the faith that science could discover the causes of and cures for disease.

Alongside calls to understand medical progress in terms of scientific progress, another strand of thinking highlighted the evident social aspects of illness, including the high disease levels of immigrants, workers, and those with lower incomes generally. From its inception, socialist thought emphasized the adverse health effects of capitalism and incorporated them into a theory of progress; Engels's *The Condition of the Working Class in England* (1845) cited numerous medical reports and physicians cataloging terrible social circumstances and asked rhetorically "[h]ow is it possible, under such conditions, for the lower class to be healthy and long lived?"[103] Numerous socialist thinkers saw illness and premature mortality primarily as the product of a sick – that is, capitalist – society. Henry Sigerist, director of the Johns Hopkins Institute for the History of Medicine, admired "socialized medicine" and called for simultaneous scientific-technical and social progress to make medicine available to a maximum number of people.[104] Socially oriented liberalism also sought to reconstruct progress with reference

---

[101] H. S. Pritchett, "The Medical School and the State," *Journal of the American Medical Association*, 63 (8) (1914), 648.

[102] A 1934 medical graduate cited in Eric Cassell, *The Nature of Suffering and the Goals of Medicine* (New York and Oxford: Oxford University Press, 2004), p. 7.

[103] Frederick Engels, *The Condition of the Working Class in England in 1844*, trans. Florence Kelley Wischnewetzky (London: Swan Sonnenschein & Co., 1892 [1845]), p. 98.

[104] Henry Sigerist, "The Development of Medicine and Its Trends in the United States, 1636–1936," *The New England Journal of Medicine*, 218 (8) (1938), 328.

to the well-being and happiness of society, including its least fortunate members. Adopting and reappropriating Comte's metaphors of society as an organism, new liberals, including D. G. Ritchie (1853–1903), L. T. Hobhouse (1864–1929), and J. A. Hobson (1858–1940), argued that moral questions could be resolved with reference to the health of the social organism and elaborated a vision in which biological, social, and industrial progress all reinforce one another. As Michael Freeden has shown, the new liberal commitment to the better health and medical treatment of worker-citizens also amounted to an investment in social progress in a capitalist model.[105]

Different visions of social – and therefore medical – progress were supported by different understandings as to what constituted health. In America, Hermann M. Biggs, Commissioner of Health of New York State, declared in 1911 that the reduction in the death rate is the principal index of human and social progress.[106] But others questioned whether a longevity measure was fully able to capture the multiple facets of health. In a speech delivered in 1918, sociologist Max Weber differentiated between technical progress and moral life and highlighted medicine's particular role in bridging the two. He concluded that to the extent medicine is a technical art, it can make progress, but it cannot address ethical questions about how to live.[107] In essence, Weber argued that since health is bound up with the human condition, we are dealing with scientifically insoluble questions of value, and conventional conceptions of progress do not apply. Such critiques echoed within the medical establishment; in 1926, MD Francis Peabody at Harvard Medical School called for a return to considering patients as "whole persons" and observed that while young medical graduates have been taught a great deal about the mechanisms of disease, they do not know how to bring patients back to health: "They are too 'scientific' and do not know how to take care of patients."[108]

Alongside uncertainties as to whether health is an objective value that can be fully captured by science, social thinkers questioned visions

---

[105] See Michael Freeden, *The New Liberalism: An Ideology of Social Reform* (Oxford: Clarendon Press, 1986 [1978]), pp. 241–42.
[106] Hermann Biggs, "Public Health Is Purchasable," *Monthly Bulletin of the Department of Health of the City of New York*, 1 (10) (1911), 226.
[107] Max Weber, "Wissenschaft als Beruf," *Gesammelte Aufsätze zur Wissenschaftslehre* (Tübingen: 1922), pp. 524–55.
[108] Peabody, "The Care of the Patient," p. 877.

of progress based on ineluctable laws. Science, for example, was generally acknowledged as having progressed; its history was described by historian of science Georges Sarton in 1936 as the only history able to illustrate the progress of humankind.[109] Yet its aspirations to objectivity and progress were increasingly scrutinized. Georges Sorel, in his *Les illusions du progrès* (*The Illusions of Progress* [1908]), emphasized the utopian qualities of various progress doctrines and the mistaken expectations of science; science, he wrote, is not a "mill (*moulin*) into which you can drop any problem that faces you" or a "recipe" that produces outcomes that are automatically true.[110] Ludwik Fleck (1896–1961), in his study *On the Genesis and Development of a Scientific Fact* (1935), questioned the notion of a fact as an objective truth and considered progress of knowledge – including medical knowledge – as linked to shifting presuppositions or thought styles. Fleck's insights were crucial for ideas of progress since he argued that there is no vantage point from which one thought style can be deemed superior to another.[111] In doing so, he anticipated subsequent challenges to the notion of cumulative scientific progress, which profoundly affected ideas of progress in medicine.

1.7 Conclusion

By the 1940s, the experience of war, fascism, and a wider awareness of the domination of the less powerful in the name of progress meant that the concept had acquired a heavier connotation than it had in previous decades. Perhaps most famously, the oppressive nature of progress was summed up in Walter Benjamin's *Theses on the Philosophy of History* (*Über den Begriff der Geschichte*, 1940), which emphasizes that progress cannot be conceived independently of the sufferings and losses of those who are subjected to it. His analysis of Paul Klee's

---

[109] Georges Sarton, *The Study of the History of Science* (Cambridge, MA: Harvard University Press, 1936), p. 5.
[110] Georges Sorel, *Réflexions sur la Violence* (Paris: Marcel Rivière et Cie, 1908), p. 94.
[111] "Introduction," in *Cognition and Fact: Materials on Ludwik Fleck*, eds. Robert S. Cohen and Thomas Schnelle, Boston Studies in the Philosophy of Science, 87 (Dordrecht: Springer, 1986), p. xxiii. See also Fleck's "Some Specific Features of the Medical Way of Thinking (1927)," in Ibid., pp. 39–46.

1 History: Medical Progress in Context 65

painting "Angelus Novus" sought to capture the dialectical nature of the concept of progress from the viewpoint of its victims and concludes that the storm we call "progress" is actually a "single catastrophe that keeps piling wreckage upon wreckage."[112] The dualities of progress came to the fore in science, the field that just recently had been portrayed as exemplifying progress. Nuclear weapons marked a turning point in the assessment of whether inordinate increases in knowledge were always desirable and symbolized a new awareness of the darker consequences of scientific progress. Philosopher and psychiatrist Karl Jaspers (1883–1969) voiced his generation's concern that progress in different spheres was not harmonious and that the failure to recognize that progress in knowledge and technology did not lead to progress in the sum total of humanity could have horrific consequences.[113] Philosopher Theodor Adorno (1903–1969) linked progress in knowledge to the drive for "technification" and increased ability to control nature but a concomitant loss of capacity to understand the humanistic aspects of life.[114] Contributions from Jaspers, Adorno, and others all flagged the ambivalences of an optimistic, all-encompassing notion of progress that went on to have a profound relevance for medicine.

With the post-war period, we arrive at the beginning of this book's journey through the second half of the twentieth and twenty-first centuries. In essence, the history of the idea of progress in medicine reveals it to be as much an intellectual history as it is a history of different personalities and techniques. Ideas of progress themselves have influenced and shaped the practice of medicine, and they have done so by emphasizing not a single facet of personhood or health, but rather different facets at different times. If contemporary medicine is sometimes characterized as a field in which progress is assured, the history of the idea of progress shows the multiplicity of possible meanings medical progress can take on.

---

[112] Walter Benjamin, "Theses on the Philosophy of History," in *Illuminations*, ed. and intro. Hannah Arendt, trans. Harry Zohn (New York: Schocken Books, 1969), pp. 257–58.

[113] Jaspers, *The Origin and Goal of History* (London and New York: Routledge, 2021 [1949]), p. 136.

[114] *Minima Moralia: Reflections from Damaged Life*, trans. E. F. N. Jephcott (Frankfurt: Suhrkamp, 1951), p. 129.

2 | Medical Progress as Biomedical Knowledge Gains

As depicted in Chapter 1, a key component of Enlightenment visions of progress was the notion of progressive knowledge. What has been called "strong progress," which is the belief in sustained, linear advances in the human condition, was inextricably bound up with a particular kind of epistemic progress, namely progress in the knowledge of the natural world dating back to the Scientific Revolution.[1] In the course of the twentieth century, persistent trends questioning the progressive and cumulative nature of knowledge – including scientific and medical knowledge – were themselves linked with undermining the status of the idea of progress. In the paper "*Was ist Wissensgeschichte?* (What Is the History of Knowledge?)," historian Philipp Sarasin outlines the rise of approaches that conceive of knowledge as always circulating back and forth between different social spheres, institutions, and media, as well as between scientists and the so-called public.[2] Knowledge, in this view, is not fixed and cumulative but rather unstable, connected to power, contingent on highly variable conceptual presuppositions, and always has the potential to dissolve again.

In this chapter, I monitor the status of the medical example for proponents of new approaches to scientific knowledge and progress, as well as for the strong reactions it entailed.[3] Throughout, my aim is to show the implications for medical progress of larger debates about the progress of knowledge. Postmodernism, for example, forcefully questioned positivistic attachments to progress and presented the idea

---

[1] See Wagner, *Progress: A Reconstruction*, pp. 7, 23.
[2] Philipp Sarasin, "Was ist Wissensgeschichte?," *Internationales Archiv für Sozialgeschichte der deutschen Literatur*, 36 (1) (2011), p. 159. See also Lorraine Daston, "The History of Science and the History of Knowledge," *Know: A Journal on the Formation of Knowledge*, 1 (1) (2017), 131–54.
[3] In this chapter, I use the terms "biomedical" and "scientific" interchangeably with regard to knowledge. I do not mean to say that other approaches to health than the biomedical one are not scientific or cannot be analyzed scientifically.

of progress as a way of formulating a fundamental human need but one without a foundation in reality.[4] Medicine, for this collection of theories, was a powerful example demonstrating that there is no such thing as knowledge that continually approaches the truth, that even the body is historical, and that knowledge is always a tool of the powerful. Medical historians too wrote about problems associated with the belief in the improvement of medical knowledge and therapies.[5] From the medical side, some respondents were adamant that scientific knowledge about the body is rigorous and objective and that medicine could remain uniquely immune to the uncertainties inherent in relativistic accounts of knowledge. In what follows, I show how prominent representatives of the view that medical knowledge can improve are not immune from the epistemological critiques of the progress of knowledge developed in the past half-century, as well as highlight how an excessive focus on biomedical knowledge gains neglects other, important dimensions of medical progress. Taken together, these attenuate strong claims for progress in medicine based on progress in science.

2.1 The Importance of (Biomedical) Scientific Knowledge after War

I mentioned earlier the role of nuclear weapons in bringing the dilemmas of progress into sharp relief. But coexisting with the fear of their potentially devastating consequences was the awareness that World War II had been won precisely thanks to the scientific research program behind their creation. In the last months of the war, American President Franklin D. Roosevelt wrote to his advisor and Director of the Office of Scientific Research and Development, Vannevar Bush, asking how the same vision and boldness employed during the war could be during peacetime and, in particular, what could be done with particular reference to "the war of science against disease."[6]

---

[4] Patricia Waugh, ed., *Postmodernism: A Reader* (London: Hodder Arnold, 1992), p. 9.
[5] See Paul B. Beeson, "Changes in Medical Therapy during the Past Half Century," *Medicine*, 59 (2) (1980), 79–99 and S. J. Peitzman, "When Did Medicine Become Beneficial? The Perspective from Internal Medicine," *Caduceus*, 12 (3) (1996), 39–44.
[6] "President Roosevelt's Letter to Vannevar Bush," *U.S. National Science Foundation*, 1945, www.nsf.gov/about/history/nsf50/vbush1945_roosevelt_letter.jsp.

The response was Bush's report *Science, The Endless Frontier* (July 1945), which began with the statement that "progress in the war against disease depends upon a flow of new scientific knowledge." Bush called for increased government funding to science, identified medical progress with scientific progress, and positioned it as a foremost political concern, linked to national military security and public interest.[7]

This particular idea of progress in medicine resonated widely in North America at the time and was bound up with the sense of victory and new hegemony of the post-war period. In the political context of the Cold War, the continued advancement of science was perceived as both practically and ideologically necessary for maintaining the international status of Western powers and repackaged as essential for Western self-understanding and values. In the article "Science on the March" (1952), MIT President Karl Taylor Compton linked the exigencies of war, the joy of discovery, and the pioneer mentality to explain the scientific and technological breakthroughs of the past decades.[8] The United States' new identity as a nuclear power resurfaced in attempts to link the nation's progress not to westward migration but rather to a potentially limitless technological "frontier."[9] And if the darker sides of scientific knowledge had become more tangible, scientific progress continued to be associated with the desire to explore the unknown, rather than a heightened responsibility for the ethical implications of scientific discoveries. Testifying to a Congress committee on space exploration in 1958, rocket engineer Wernher von Braun observed that: "[p]eople are just curious [...] What follows in the wake of their discoveries is something for the next generation to worry about."[10]

---

[7] "*Science, The Endless Frontier,*" A Report to the President by Vannevar Bush, Director of the Office of Scientific Research and Development, 1945, *U.S. National Science Foundation*, www.nsf.gov/about/history/nsf50/vbush1945.jsp.

[8] Karl Taylor Compton, "Science on the March," *Popular Mechanics*, 97 (1) (1952), 120–25.

[9] Michael L. Smith, "Recourse of Empire: Landscapes of Progress in Technological America," in *Does Technology Drive History? The Dilemma of Technological Determinism*, eds. Merritt Roe Smith and Leo Marx (Cambridge, MA: MIT Press, 1994), p. 43.

[10] Cited in Ibid., p. 50. See also Roger Pielke Jr., "A 'Sedative' for Science Policy," *Issues in Science and Technology*, 36 (1) (2020), https://issues.org/endless-frontier-sedative-for-science-policy-pielke/.

2 Medical Progress as Biomedical Knowledge Gains 69

Post-war medicine had a special status in these discussions of scientific advance. Historian of medicine Roger Cooter describes a commonplace whereby medicine (along with the weapons industry) was considered the ultimate endorsement of Trotsky's saying that war is the locomotive of history, the locomotive of progress.[11] If surgeons, in particular, received intensive training during the war, medical practices and technologies with their roots in the West spread to a number of countries, enhancing Western medicine's sense of its global potential. In general, the period was characterized by widespread enthusiasm about the extent to which breakthroughs in scientific knowledge could successfully resolve health problems. New possibilities for medicine brought about thanks to the biological sciences included the synthetic production of penicillin, the development of chemotherapy, the first open heart surgery in 1952, better vaccines, and the chemical DDT and its insecticidal properties, for example for controlling malaria.[12] I do not want to list all the major medical events in the post-war period, but I do want to underline that they could be seen as embodying the promise of scientific medicine to guarantee human well-being. In reference to the era, physician Leon Eisenberg describes it as a time when "medicine as a source of human progress was an article of common faith."[13] Crucially, medical progress could both serve an ambitious political agenda and perform a stabilizing function. It offered an important means of projecting international power but without the direct threat of leading to war between major powers. The pursuit of progress in medicine also promised that life was getting better without requiring any substantial internal societal reorganization – as per the Communist model – or globally. Sociologist Paul Starr writes that the valorization of medical science "epitomized the postwar vision of progress without conflict. All could agree about the value of medical progress, and [theoretically, at least] all could benefit from it."[14]

---

[11] Roger Cooter, "Medicine and the Goodness of War," *Canadian Bulletin of Medical History*, 7 (1990), 149.
[12] On the controversial history of DDT see Elena Conis, "Beyond Silent Spring: An Alternate History of DDT," *Distillations* (Science History Institute, 2017), www.sciencehistory.org/distillations/beyond-silent-spring-an-alternate-history-of-ddt.
[13] Leon Eisenberg, "Medicine and the Idea of Progress," p. 46.
[14] Paul, *The Social Transformation of American Medicine* (New York: Basic Books, 1982), p. 336.

In this sociopolitical landscape, new knowledge of nuclear technologies sparked public imagination in terms of its potential for ambitious visions of better health and medicine. Future progress in medicine was a foundational part of how the "new world of tomorrow" was presented at the time.[15] Medicine was touted as the most promising field in the "atoms for peace" program that US President Dwight Eisenhower announced to the United Nations in 1953. The allure of harnessing the knowledge of the atomic world was associated with the resurgence of the idea of essentially limitless medical progress, as well as a potentially disease-free life. In an article that appeared in *American Magazine* in 1947, University of Chicago Chancellor Robert M. Hutchins suggested that the future atomic city "will have a central diagnostic laboratory, but only a small hospital, if any at all, for most human ailments will be cured as rapidly as they are diagnosed."[16] The National Education Association produced publications for students describing atomic energy as that which ensures the unlikelihood "that you or any of your classmates will die prematurely of cancer or heart disease, or from any contagious diseases, or from any other human ills that afflict us now."[17] Translated into medicine, the sense of breakthrough associated with the atomic era provides a powerful illustration of how an idea of progress emerges from the interaction between the scientific knowledge of a given time and concomitant political and societal interests.

Eventually, this early enthusiasm for atomic medicine faded. But the sense that it was specifically scientific knowledge that had the potential to improve human health to the point of defeating death and disease remained. A WHO pamphlet entitled *Ten Years of Health Progress* (1958) underlined the role of great scientific advances in the accelerated progress of the past years.[18] In the same year, WHO Director-General Marcolino G. Candau observed that:

---

[15] F. Barrows Colton, "Your New World of Tomorrow," *National Geographic Magazine*, 88 (4) (1945), 385–410.

[16] Cited in Paul Boyer, *By the Bomb's Early Light: American Thought and Culture at the Dawn of the Atomic Age* (Chapel Hill & London: University of North Carolina Press, 1985), p. 119.

[17] Cited in Ibid., pp. 119–20.

[18] "World Health: Ten Years of Progress," *The UNESCO Courier: A Window Open on the World*, 11 (5) (1099) (1958), 3.

2 Medical Progress as Biomedical Knowledge Gains

if the great advances gained in science and technology are put at the service of all the people of the world, our children and their children will live in an age from which most of the diseases our grandparents and parents took for granted will be banished.[19]

And he spoke of a new chapter in the history of medicine, replete with practices and experiences that until now belonged to the realms of fantasy and fiction.

Inevitably, overly optimistic claims about scientific knowledge as able to overcome disease and prolong life indefinitely were sharply criticized by contemporaries, and some of these critiques are similar to the ones canvassed in Chapter 1, including insufficient attention to all dimensions of health and overly simplistic ideas of progress. But the critique of medical progress as the scientific knowledge of body mechanisms occurred in the broader context of debates as to how and whether there could be progress in scientific knowledge at all. In the post-war decades, voices from within the medical establishment and the social sciences profoundly questioned whether scientific truth-seeking could translate into progress in medicine. Slightly later, these debates became incorporated into more general reflections as to what is meant by progress in knowledge. Relativistic positions took this challenge to its logical extreme, arguing that medical knowledge could not make progress because there is no such thing as progress in knowledge at all.

2.2 Challenges to Scientific Knowledge Progress from Medicine and the Social Sciences

Within the medical sciences, one prominent challenge to optimistic ideas of unlimited medical progress was related to insights into ecosystemic, holistic health. René Dubos (1901–1982), a microbiologist active in medical research, questioned the notion that medical progress could be reduced to the progress of laboratory sciences, a view that had heavily influenced ideas about progress in medicine since germ theory. Based on the insight that virulent pathogens are highly present in healthy individuals and yet rarely cause disease, he argued that the

---

[19] Cited in *The United States and the World Health Organization: Teamwork for Mankind's Well-Being. Report of Senator Hubert H. Humphrey* (Washington, DC: Government Printing Office, 1959), p. 35.

context is as important as any single microorganism – for example, a bacteria – in determining disease.[20] In doing so, he developed a non-linear, multifaceted notion of disease that called for understanding the whole person in their physical, social, and psychological contexts.

A concern with the patient as a whole person, an interest in the possibility of multiple causes of disease, and a cautious approach to accepted doctrines of medical science: Dubos shared these traits with many other researchers, but he underscored the ramifications of his concerns for narratives of medical progress. He welcomed the dramatic decreases in mortality rates of the past century but thought that they were largely misattributed to the knowledge of specific disease causes. Using a number of examples including leprosy, the plague, and typhus, he sought to revisit conventional ideas about progress by arguing that the most devastating infectious and nutritional diseases had all but disappeared in Europe before the advent of germ theory.[21] Not only had laboratory medicine been given undue credit for controlling infectious disease and reducing infant mortality – a phenomenon that Dubos associated with better nutrition and sanitation – but he also noted that little practical progress had been made toward addressing varied, ill-defined ailments including those of old age, which constitute such a large percentage of medical practice.[22] While Dubos readily conceded that new knowledge – for example of microbial diseases – had led to some spectacular successes, he emphasized that the accompanying rhetoric of progress obscured medicine's ultimate inability to eliminate the disease burden on society.[23] Progress against specific diseases, he argued, runs up against fundamental biological and knowledge limits.

---

[20] See Carol Moberg, "René Dubos: A Harbinger of Microbial Resistance to Antibiotics," *Microbial Drug Resistance*, 2 (3) (1996), 287–97 and Lauren N. Ross, "The Doctrine of Specific Etiology," *Biology & Philosophy*, 33 (37) (2018), https://doi.org/10.1007/s10539-018-9647-x.

[21] See, in particular, his *Mirage of Health: Utopias, Progress and Biological Change* (New York: Harper, 1959). Dubos echoed themes developed in Henry Sigerist's influential publications in the history and sociology of medicine on the need for progress in both technical and social spheres and anticipated Thomas Mckeown's later emphasis on the socioeconomic dimensions of health (see Chapter 4).

[22] *Mirage of Health*, pp. 23–24.

[23] See René Dubos, "The Evolution of Infectious Diseases in the Course of History," *The Canadian Medical Association Journal*, 79 (6) (1958), 448.

2 Medical Progress as Biomedical Knowledge Gains

Central to his argument is that medical knowledge transcends laboratory knowledge because it deals with the health of human beings who are fundamentally ecological, living in an environment that changes over time. Referencing contemporary books *Our Synthetic Environment* by Murray Bookchin (1962) and Rachel Carson's *The Silent Spring* (1962), he noted that technological advances bring with them harms to health that are revealed only after a certain amount of time, and even then often too late.[24] Health, Dubos believed, should be conceived as fitness to respond to various factors and that fitness is achieved through innumerable adaptations to those factors. Essentially, he challenged the view that diseases have remained more or less constant throughout human history, and what has changed is only our knowledge of them. He, therefore, was also skeptical of "utopian" views of progress that sought to acquire cumulative knowledge about a fixed disease entity. Since the body was engaged in constant adaptation, and disease could always arise when maladjustments occurred, the burden of disease, he wrote, "is not likely to decrease in the future, whatever the progress of medical research and whatever the skill of social organizations in applying new discoveries."[25] Dubos developed these arguments in his book, *The Mirage of Health: Utopias, Progress and Biological Change* (1959), in which he tells the reader: "Complete freedom from disease and from struggle is almost incompatible with the process of living," and that a related belief in progress is a coping strategy that "has provided mankind with solace in times of despair and with élan during the expansive periods of history."[26]

While he was concerned to point out the fundamentally misguided nature of a certain kind of scientific knowledge-seeking, Dubos was also interested in articulating what he saw as a viable, yet fundamentally limited view of progress. He muses that since it is impossible to know in advance the nature of the ecosystem that will be relevant for future diseases, what is left is the challenge of how medical knowledge can help individuals and societies become better able to face unpredictable problems. And he noted that this is an "ill-defined task," which

---

[24] See René Dubos, "The Conflict between Progress and Safety," *Archives of Environmental Health: An International Journal*, 6 (4) (1963), 449–52.
[25] René Dubos, "Medical Utopias," *Daedalus*, 88 (3) (1959), 411.
[26] *Mirage of Health*, pp. 1–2.

requires a much more nuanced assessment of both the possibilities of future progress and the achievements of the past.[27] Nevertheless, Dubos believed that this necessarily modest task was also a form of ideological protection against utopia. He drew attention to how the "restless" pursuit of specialized medical knowledge without "any clear statement of direction" would not lead to any viable conception of progress and could be harmful.[28] In a notable break with the view that progress in biomedical knowledge is inherently peaceful and beneficial, he warned that unless medical scientists take a long-range view of the consequences of their activities, they may very well come to know the anguish that atomic physicists experienced as they witnessed the tragic effects of their scientific triumphs.[29]

As Dubos was referring to bioscientific medical progress as a "mirage," a number of contributions from the social sciences documented how the knowledge categories and technologies of Western medicine did not have the universal appeal that had been optimistically assumed. Various inputs chronicled at length how local medical services were consistently preferred to Western biomedicine and concluded that this was largely due to the ways in which they were better adapted to local social structures. In the example of campaigns to boil drinking water, both the local populations who chose to do so and those who did not did so for differing motives, for example, because they were offended by the socially degrading implication that their hygiene was inadequate. Such cases heightened the interest of social scientists in the social and cultural contexts of medical knowledge and beliefs, as well as prompted them to question whether rational, progressive knowledge was the exclusive prerogative of Western scientific medicine.[30] Accordingly, a number of academics from the social sciences developed distinct theoretical approaches to investigate medical knowledge by integrating social factors into epidemiological and other medical research. And in doing so, they turned a critical eye on Western medicine's sense of itself as able to achieve progress by uncovering the truth about disease.

---

[27] "Medical Utopias," p. 420. [28] *Mirage of Health*, pp. 276–77.
[29] "Medical Utopias," p. 424.
[30] Benjamin D. Paul, "Introduction: Understanding the Community," in Benjamin D. Paul, ed., *Health, Culture, Community* (New York: Russell Sage, 1955), p. 5. See also Claude Lévi-Strauss, *Les Tristes Tropiques* (Paris: Plon, 1955).

2 Medical Progress as Biomedical Knowledge Gains 75

A major figure in this regard was sociologist Talcott Parsons (1902–79), who articulated, this time from a social science perspective, a theory of health as graspable only within a broad, systems perspective. Medicine itself, he points out, should be understood as a complex multilayered system made up of multiple actors, institutions, norms, and beliefs. Among the elements constituting this system, Parsons zoomed in on the prevalence of the belief in medical progress, which he saw as particularly developed in Western cultures. Parsons emphasizes that the belief in the accumulation of truths as able to overcome medical uncertainties was in large part cultural. And he criticizes the widely held view that the progress of scientific knowledge consists essentially in piling up discoveries and facts, describing how the "exact relation of the known to the unknown elements cannot be determined; the unknown may operate any time to invalidate expectations built up on analysis of the known."[31]

In doing so, Parsons reframes uncertainty not as something that knowledge-seeking can surmount but as something that coexists alongside and is even driven by progressive knowledge. Uncertainty, in this view, takes on a paramount importance in relation to knowledge generally. He argues that even as what is known increases, the physician is faced with inherent limitations of control, given that many medical conditions are essentially uncontrollable. The advances in medical knowledge, while remarkable, are far from eliminating such aspects of medical practice and are unlikely to do so in the future. On the contrary, increases in knowledge may resolve some uncertainties, but they also create new forms of uncertainty that did not previously exist, thereby shedding light on the extent of human ignorance. Years later, his former student Renée Fox – who went on to work extensively on medical uncertainty – summarized one of Parsons' key contributions as follows:

while medical scientific progress can reduce extant areas of uncertainty and limitation, it also identifies previously held misconceptions, uncovers fresh areas of ignorance, raises new questions, and brings in its wake side effects and iatrogenic harms that did not exist before.[32]

---

[31] Talcott Parsons, *The Structure of Social Action: A Study in Social Theory with Special Reference to a Group of Recent European Writers* (Glencoe, IL: The Free Press, 1949), p. 449.
[32] Renée Fox, cited in Evan Willis, "Talcott Parsons: His Legacy and the Sociology of Health and Illness," in *The Palgrave Handbook of Social Theory in Health, Illness and Medicine*, ed. Fran Collyer (London: Palgrave Macmillan, 2015), p. 217.

Parsons saw the desire to overcome uncertainty and enthusiastic claims about medical-scientific progress as bound up together and attributed this to the fact that health problems affect the most intimate aspects of patients' bodies and lives and are linked with physicians' own emotional involvement and responsibility. Drawing on the work of anthropologist Bronisław Malinowski (1884–1942), he notes that magical beliefs and practices cluster around situations involving a significant uncertainty factor and in which there are strong emotional interests in a successful resolution, for which health problems present a classic example.[33] Since scientific medicine precludes magic, rhetorical strategies and beliefs in the need for action rather than inaction tend to fulfill that function. He singled out his own country, the United States, as one in which the pressure on physicians and families to do everything possible is particularly strong. The notion of progressive knowledge as underpinning progress in medicine, therefore, cannot be dissociated from the specific coping strategies and expectations of both physicians and patients. These confirm optimistic bias in favor of intervention and reinforce beliefs about the possibility of truly controlling organic processes.

2.3 Challenges to Scientific Knowledge Progress from the Philosophy of Science

If these developments in the social and medical sciences posed a significant challenge to traditional ideas about the importance of progressive scientific knowledge for medicine, a further, distinct challenge came from the philosophy of science. Ludwik Fleck had argued in 1946 that contemporary science "is not closer to any objective picture of the world than the science of 100 years ago";[34] work by Thomas Kuhn, Paul Feyerabend, and Larry Laudan, among others, further contributed to questioning the view that science develops simply by adding new truths to established foundations in a linear progress format.[35]

---

[33] *Structure of Social Action*, pp. 468–69.
[34] Ludwik Fleck, "Problems of the Science of Science" (1946), in *Cognition and Fact*, eds. Cohen and Schnelle, pp. 113–27.
[35] See Paul Feyerabend, *Against Method: Outline of an Anarchistic Theory of Knowledge* (London: New Left Books, 1975), Larry Laudan, *Progress and Its Problems: Towards a Theory of Scientific Growth* (Oakland: University of California Press, 1977), and Karl Popper, *The Logic of Scientific Discovery* (London: Hutchison, 1959).

2 Medical Progress as Biomedical Knowledge Gains 77

In *The Structure of Scientific Revolutions* (1962), Kuhn develops a view of progress as problem-solving rather than achieving a potentially universalizable end and argued that knowledge should not be equated with an objective truth but rather seen as an intervention, able to illuminate specific aspects of the object of inquiry. He distinguishes between normal science – that is, scientific endeavors conducted within an accepted paradigm – and revolutionary science, in which different accepted truths compete and eventually generate a new paradigm. Progress that is cumulative and continuous could occur within the parameters of the research program of normal science, but this progress is always theory dependent; while Newton claims that an apple falls to the ground because of gravity, Aristotle says that it falls because it is seeking its telos. Kuhn writes that unless one simply defines approaching the truth as the result of scientific endeavor, "we cannot recognize progress toward that goal."[36] If the new paradigm produced following a revolution cannot be said to have made clear epistemological progress compared to the prerevolutionary paradigm, then progress across paradigms is difficult.

Kuhn drew attention to how hard it is for scientific knowledge to represent nature objectively by observing that scientists make decisions according to plural criteria, criteria that cannot be ranked in any impartial way.[37] Four years earlier, in 1958, historian of ideas Isaiah Berlin had argued that:

[i]f, as I believe the ends of men are many, and not all of them are in principle compatible with each other, then the possibility of conflict – and tragedy – can never wholly be eliminated from human life, either personal or social. The necessity of choosing between absolute claims is then an inescapable characteristic of the human condition.[38]

Building on Berlin's account of persistent ethical tensions, something that resonates in the normative framework for medical progress developed here, Kuhn's theory showed that there is no one way to resolve epistemic tensions and that choosing between values is an inescapable

---

[36] Thomas Kuhn, *The Essential Tension: Selected Studies in Scientific Tradition and Change* (Chicago & London: University of Chicago Press, 1977), p. 289.
[37] Thomas Kuhn, *The Structure of Scientific Revolutions*, 2nd ed. (Chicago: University of Chicago Press, 1970 [1962]), p. 185.
[38] Isaiah Berlin, "Two Concepts of Liberty," in *Liberty*, 2nd ed., ed. Henry Hardy, p. 214.

part of doing science.[39] Even if several values – accuracy, simplicity, and explanatory power, say – are relevant to a decision, we might still weigh these values in different ways and therefore arrive at different results. There may be no common measure for abstract values such as accuracy and simplicity; values may also be incommensurable, in that they cannot be compared. Thus conceived, the free exercise of human reason does not lead to one truth but rather to numerous competing truths since there is no correct way in which plural values should be ordered.

Not only do well-informed scientists arrive at different judgments about what is true, Kuhn also argued that extrascientific factors, such as politics, institutions, thought leaders, and the like, often dictate how scientific change takes place. In short, the paradigm in which progress occurs is itself dependent on values and determined by outside factors. Kuhn did not deny the possibility of progress per se, and in a postscript written in 1969, he clarified his position by remarking that later scientific theories "are better than earlier ones for solving puzzles in the often quite different environments to which they are applied. That is not a relativist's position, and it displays the sense in which I am a convinced believer in scientific progress."[40] Nevertheless, the consequences for overarching claims of scientific progress were profound across different fields. Kuhn's work has consistently been read as disputing the notion of orderly progress, for example, identifying instead "a secretive and non-cumulative sequence of scientific revolutions: an opaque world that neither reflects nor validates liberal ideals."[41]

2.4 No Progress in Medicine: Questioning Cumulative, Progressive Knowledge

Kuhn's work did not so much break with the notion of progress per se but rather drew attention to the problems of progress in the physical sciences. But his depiction of scientific revolutions, and the complications they pose for progress, motivated relativism, skepticism,

---

[39] See Thomas S. Kuhn, "Objectivity, Value Judgment and Theory Choice," *The Essential Tension*, pp. 320–39.
[40] Thomas Kuhn, *The Structure of Scientific Revolutions*, 2nd ed. (Chicago: University of Chicago Press, 1970 [1962]), www.marxists.org/reference/subject/philosophy/works/us/kuhn.htm.
[41] John A. Harrington, "The Idea of Progress in Medicine and the Common Law," *Social & Legal Studies*, 11 (2) (2002), 212.

2 Medical Progress as Biomedical Knowledge Gains 79

and a host of other positions that developed fundamental critiques of a truth-seeking idea of progress. The importance of these debates for ideas of medical progress and knowledge is difficult to overstate; according to Steve Fuller, postmodernism made it "no longer fashionable to believe in the idea of progress."[42]

For skeptical arguments, medicine is a privileged field to show how a widely shared belief in justifiable, universalizable progress is not compelling. Jean-François Lyotard, whose book *La condition postmoderne: rapport sur le savoir* (*The Postmodern Condition: A Report on Knowledge*, 1979) intensified these debates, defined the postmodern attitude as incredulity toward metanarratives and the idea of progress as a prime example thereof, representing how knowledge supposedly accumulates toward a good ethicopolitical end.[43] The emphasis on discourse and the socially contingent character of knowledge was bound up with an important relativist proposition, namely that linear accounts of the history of medical progress must be abandoned. Instead, Lyotard advocated a return to the *petit récit* (small narrative) informed by lived experience, distinctiveness, and complexity. In doing so, he articulated a representative suspicion of the privileged epistemic status of scientific knowledge and the way it should be reconceived as one among other competing forms of knowledge, all of which have their own validity. Rather, by highlighting the contingency and perspectival nature of beliefs – including reason – grounded in the normative preferences of particular societies, narratives that draw on "rationality," "science," and "truth" are inexplicable without reference to the cultural context in which they are articulated and, in particular, without the Enlightenment commitment to progress and the imperialism that underpinned its idea of civilizational advance. Pushed to their logical extreme, such contributions have been described as denying "the existence of progress, even in science and especially in medicine."[44]

Critiques of the privileged status of scientific/biomedical knowledge were articulated in a fast-changing landscape in which there was a rising awareness of the complexities of lifestyle, stress-related, and

---

[42] Steve Fuller, *Knowledge: The Philosophical Quest in History* (London: Routledge, 2015), p. 1.
[43] Jean-François Lyotard, *La condition postmoderne: rapport sur le savoir* (Paris: Minuit, 1979), pp. xxiii–xxiv, 30.
[44] Prioreschi, "The Idea of Scientific Progress in Antiquity and in the Middle Ages," p. 41, fn 4.

chronic diseases. Medicine as a field able to capitalize on scientific advances was questioned both because successes in infectious disease control were not replicated for noncommunicable diseases and because the increasing costs and commodification of medicine seemed to have become decoupled from health benefits. As monitored in Chapter 3, the image of the expert, benevolent physician also lost status: a certain antipathy to professional authority developed in response to concerns about abuses of power in the medical context. If scientific progress was previously at the center of public attention, it slowly was displaced by medicine's various economic and moral problems.

Indeed, the confidence in medical, scientific progress was undermined to such an extent that medical nihilism flourished in the 1970s.[45] For instance, Ivan Illich (1926–2002), a theologian and social critic, articulated a particularly resonant critique of widespread confidence in medical progress. Illich emphasized that the pursuit of medical knowledge without taking into account the richness and inherent fragility of the human condition is detrimental to health. For him, the widely praised progress of medicine was greatly exaggerated; a vast amount of clinical care is incidental to curing disease, while the damage done by medicine to health is very significant.[46] The empirical work that Illich drew on to support his claims largely concerns the historical evolution of disease patterns, the questionable effectiveness of some medical treatments, and improvements in procedures and devices – including contraception, vaccination, and treatment of water, sewage, and the like – that have significant health benefits but are not medical in a narrow sense. Extrapolating from these observations, he argues that medicine's current priorities increase human suffering because the medical system actually harms the patients it treats, the medical profession holds power to the detriment of other social groups, and the commodification of health fundamentally damages individuals' innate ability to cope with illness. In his terms, the construction of hospitals amounts to "castles turned cathedrals, built to protect us against ignorance, discomfort, pain and death," and he characterized this development as profoundly disabling.[47]

---

[45] See Stegenga, *Medical Nihilism*.
[46] Ivan Illich, *Medical Nemesis: The Expropriation of Health* (New York: Pantheon Books, 1976 [1975]).
[47] Ivan Illich, *Disabling Professions* (London: Marion Boyars, 1977), p. 12.

Illich describes his writings as trying to question the ontological status of health as a certainty or an axiom, which also acts as a pillar of contemporary society.[48] But they are also an attempt to question widely held views about the reliance of medical progress on scientific progress. In his view, many technical medical interventions were based on an excessively narrow, scientific conception of medical knowledge, which held that solving a problem simply meant that there was one less problem to worry about. Knowing in medicine, he pointed out, transcends isolated interventions because it requires understanding how they fit together in the larger fabric of human life. Technologies, as he portrays them, do not contribute to individual independence and judgment abilities but rather harm them because by delegating knowledge tasks to technologies we lose in individual comprehension.[49] Illich points out that the logic of scientific progress underpins a medical system in which resources are increasingly diverted toward expensive, high-tech hospital treatments and one that has unrealistic expectations of medicine's curative potential. And he criticized the faith that open-ended improvements in health are possible, something he saw as "sentimental" and as rooted in a "deep-seated need for the engineering of miracles."[50]

Illich's arguments were inspirational for various attempts to rethink the "medicalization" of specific health issues such as depression and for redistributing funds away from, for example, intensive care toward education, preventative medicine, and social programs.[51] Discussing Illich's contributions, Michel Foucault (1926–1984) notes that a particularly important aspect of his critique was to show that the rational practice of medicine itself, and not medical errors or accidents, can cause harm. Effectively, medicine could be dangerous, not due to ignorance or falseness, but rather through its knowledge, and precisely because it was based on science.[52] In his own work, and drawing on Nietzsche's account of knowledge as a tool of power, Foucault used

---

[48] Cited in Joseph E. Davis, "Ivan Illich and Irving Kenneth Zola: Disabling Medicalisation," in *The Palgrave Handbook of Social Theory in Health, Illness and Medicine*, ed. Fran Collyer (London: Palgrave Macmillan, 2015), p. 308.
[49] See *Disabling Professions*. [50] *Medical Nemesis*, p. 35.
[51] See, for example, Ian Kennedy's Reith Lectures, published as *The Unmasking of Medicine* (London: George Allen and Unwin, 1981).
[52] Michel Foucault, "The Crisis of Medicine or the Crisis of Antimedicine," *Foucault Studies*, 1 (2004 [1974]), pp. 8–9.

historical examples to show how the imposition of medical knowledge is an act of authority and that claims to medical progress are exaggerated. He saw societies as having certain forms of discourse that they accept and consider true, practices that validate these assumptions and strengthen the status of those whose views count as the truth. These insights rest on his view of the self as fundamentally relational, whereby individuals' ability to reason is molded and shaped by the variety of relations they entertain. In Foucault's theory, the body itself is fundamentally political and subject to power relations: the self dissipates and conforms, confronted by a "power that is law, the subject who is constituted as subject – who is 'subjected' – is he who obeys."[53] There is, therefore, no stable, perfectible idea of the self or of society that grounds medical interventions and can act as a standard for measuring progress. With these premises, he was able to shed light on the ways in which the commitment to certain kinds of medical progress and powerful interests were bound up together. Both the history of sexuality and the history of psychiatry display evidence of the "medicalization" of issues that are not a disease and the authority of medicine to determine what is normal. In Foucault's account, changing historical categories of madness – from excessive to unreasonable and insane – did not represent epistemic progress toward understanding a single phenomenon but are rather manifestations of social norms and transgressions that always take place in a specific context.

2.5 Pluralism, Information, and Knowledge

In the course of the twentieth century, positivistic attachments to progress and the perception of medical knowledge as engaged in incremental progress toward uncovering all the mysteries of health were significantly undermined. Early portrayals of the violence done in the name of progress were expanded in a stream of writings – some of which are discussed in Chapters 3 and 4 – that detail the harms done to specific individuals and groups in the name of progress. Yet the lack of a clear relationship between scientific progress (however defended) and medical progress also opened up new ways of interpreting and reacting to human illness. For one, laying bare problems

---

[53] Foucault, *History of Sexuality*, vol. I, An Introduction (New York: Pantheon, 1978), p. 85.

in different accounts of scientific progress increased the value allotted to the knowledge of nonscientists and to that of patients. In an early contribution, Sandra Harding comments on the emancipatory potential of acknowledging that contrary to the assumption that there is "a" world out there, graspable and explainable through science, "there are as many kinds of interrelated and smoothly connected realities as there are kinds of oppositional consciousness. By giving up the goal of telling 'one true story,' we embrace instead [...] permanent partiality."[54] This valorization of epistemic pluralism set the scene for the expansion of scientific inquiry into a wider array of issues not normally associated with the material of scientific knowledge – such as the body, power, discipline, and gender. And this extension of the scope of inquiry fundamentally questioned narrower assumptions about what constitutes scientific knowledge.

One effect of this turn toward pluralism was to show how trends, fashions, and popularity of medical knowledge often take the place of progressivity.[55] For this reason, narratives of progress can be thought of as having been engulfed by a flood of data, associations, information, and cross-references associated with the internet.[56] On the web, knowledge functions as a good that acquires its worth from supply and demand, and the desire for progress makes it particularly liable to be co-opted by profit incentives. Rather than specific medical truths that ground narratives of progress, we have contingent knowledge masquerading as convincing truth claims. To illustrate this process, one internet user commented at length on an article in the *Economist* magazine chronicling a changing consensus among medical experts as to whether saturated fat or sugar was worse for health.

joski65, June 3, 2014, 12:25
    Run. Don't run. Walk. It's better. Don't walk in the mornings, there's too much smog in the air. Walking in the evenings isn't good for digestion and

---

[54] Sandra Harding, *The Science Question in Feminism* (Ithaca, NY: Cornell University Press, 1986), p. 194.
[55] Nihan Bozok, *From Modern to Postmodern Medicine: The Case of Organ Transplants*, unpublished PhD thesis, Middle East Technical University, Ankara, 2015, p. 85.
[56] N. Katherine Hayles & Todd Gannon, "Mood Swings: The Aesthetics of Ambient Emergence," in *The Mourning After: Attending the Wake of Postmodernism*, eds. Neil Brooks and Josh Toth (Amsterdam & New York: Rodopi, 2007), p. 118.

there must be at least a 3 hour gap between walking and bedtime. Play. But don't play impact sports. Those would cause permanent damage to your knees and joints. Swim. But remember the water in most pools are not clean and will lead to skin damage. In any case, exercise does not really matter. Your diet does. Breakfast, like a King, lunch like a prince and dinner like a pauper. That's bullshit. Eat 5 times a day in small equal quantities. No. Focus on proteins. Eat white meat, avoid red meat. Eat only fish. Eat only chicken. Eat only eggs. make that only the egg white. That's a recipe for high cholesterol! Eat only fruits, veggies. Eat only leafy veggies. don't eat leafy veggies because they have worm eggs in them. Avoid other veggies they have high carbs and lead to gas attacks. Eat that ugly looking Brazilian jungle vegetable, it cures cancer. No avoid it! it leads to impotence. Stick to fruits but avoid the skin. No eat only the skin, they're rich in proteins. But don't eat the fruits which have red seeds they are poisonous and green fruits should be avoided if they were purple flowers. Drink milk. But not buffalo milk, drink cows milk. But make it skimmed. No skimmed is processed, drink goat milk no camel milk. Don't drink milk! the body cannot digest milk after the age of three. Drink mother's milk? only till three. Drink? Water. But not from the tap. Mineral water. Which is tap water only dirtier. No only water from the Alps. Drinking is good. Small quantity of alcohol helps keep the arteries from clogging. But drink only wine. Red wine. but only with white meat. But now since no white meat there can't be no wine. Drink only coffee and tea. No they cause damage over the long run. Drink green tea. No it causes prostrate problems. Don't smoke! it causes cancer. Smoke cigars less tar. Beedis are better. But cause ulcer. Smoking up is best. Pot is bad. It is medicine. Yogis smoke up. Yogi's go nowhere. Breathing the air in any city is equivalent to smoking 20 cigarettes.

Welcome to the age of information. You are now better informed about every aspect of your health and can take informed decisions about leading a healthier, happier and emotionally stable life.[57]

In making the list of competing kinds of health advice as long and wide ranging as possible, Joski65 is very much at odds with proponents of medical knowledge as cumulative, stable, and progressive. But this caricaturized depiction resonates both in arguments that decry

[57] joski65, June 3, 2014, 12:25, comment to "The Case for Eating Steak and Cream: Why Everything You Heard about Fat Is Wrong," review of Nina Teicholz, *The Big Fat Surprise: Why Butter, Meat and Cheese Belong in a Healthy Diet*, May 31, 2014, the *Economist*, www.economist.com/news/books-and-arts/21602984-why-everything-you-heard-about-fat-wrong-case-eating-steak-and-cream?zid=318&ah=ac379c09c1c3fb67e0e8fd1964d5247f.

2 Medical Progress as Biomedical Knowledge Gains 85

privileging biomedical knowledge over other forms and in those that draw attention to the persistent gaps between progress in knowledge and related progress in its application to medical problems.

"Pluralistic," a "social product," "historically situated," and "perspectivist"; post-Kuhn progress in scientific knowledge appeared "messy," "imprecise," and subject to values and therefore muted.[58] What is significant about these developments for my purposes is that they reveal the difficulty, and perhaps impossibility, of providing a compelling account of scientific progress that is highly relevant to progress in medicine. For one, the line between science and nonscience was no longer as clear as it had been.[59] Science studies disciplines show how science is a social process, influenced by economic, professional, and cultural values and constraints. They also reveal the extent to which particular canons of knowledge are constructed by active elimination and forgetting and involved in a permanent struggle to claim some sources of knowledge as superior to others and give them a privileged status. Effectively, the narrowly scientific identity of Western medicine, and view of itself as a source of universalizable and incontrovertible knowledge, had to reckon with its status as a form of knowledge among others.

Secondly, the relationship between scientific advances and medical progress needs to be rethought. What is referred to as scientific progress in normal times is progress in acquiring knowledge about the world within a particular theoretical framework. At the same time, beyond discoveries and technological innovations, it is major problems or crises that can trigger the elaboration of a new framework. Such shifts occur when a novel theory develops in response to

---

[58] See Solomon, *Making Medical Knowledge* for a summary of relevant features of post-Kuhnian literature in the philosophy of medicine, pp. 18–19. Recent contributions to scientific progress offer different accounts of what it entails, for example truth requirements or its ability to problem-solve. See Ilkka Niiniluoto, "Scientific Progress as Increasing Verisimilitude," *Studies in the History and Philosophy of Science*, 46 (2014), 73–77, Finnur Dellsén, "Scientific Progress: Knowledge versus Understanding," *Studies in the History and Philosophy of Science*, 56 (2016), 72–83, Alexander Bird, *Knowing Science* (Oxford: Oxford University Press, 2022), and Darrell Rowbottom, *Scientific Progress* (Cambridge: Cambridge University Press, 2023).

[59] See Dien Ho, *A Philosopher Goes to the Doctor: A Critical Look at Philosophical Assumptions in Medicine* (New York: Routledge, 2019), Chapter 1.

a crisis that cannot be resolved by normal problem-solving activities. Transcending and, perhaps, abandoning a given framework may have a larger impact on individual or population health than improving specific practices within an accepted framework.

Finally, just as medical knowledge has multiple sources, there are multiple instances in which progress can occur, but they may not all add up. Scientific understandings of health provide valuable insights, but they do not capture health in its entirety. There may be progress in the understanding of health and disease or in the effectiveness of medical interventions, or the status of modern medicine in relation to other areas of human life might change.[60] Crucially, progress can be made on one level independently of the others and does not necessarily reinforce or contribute to progress in a different aspect. In this way, refining the relationship between scientific progress and medical progress shows the necessity of a multidimensional account of progress in medicine.

2.6 Defending Progress in Medicine

Despite the above views, the denunciation of scientific medicine (*Schulmedizin*) as unable to provide certainties does not predominate in Western countries. The belief in scientific advances as the main drivers of medical progress is still a popular notion among the general public as well as for medical professionals, scientists, and engineers. The technical successes of medicine aimed at healing the body continue to be referenced as prime examples of the potential of scientific knowledge to improve human life more generally. Cultural theorist Nico Stehr observes that scientific progress in medicine and other applied fields is regularly "paraded as incontrovertible evidence of the usefulness and power of knowledge."[61] Regardless of the abovementioned critical voices – and to some extent as a reaction to them – the idea that objective progress by applying scientific reason in medicine is both possible and desirable continues to flourish.

---

[60] William Goodwin, "Revolution and Progress in Medicine," *Theoretical Medicine and Bioethics*, 36 (2015), 25–39. See also Donald Gillies, "Hempelian and Kuhnian Approaches in the Philosophy of Medicine: The Semmelweis Case," *Studies in the History and Philosophy of Biological and Biomedical Sciences*, 36 (2015), 159–81.
[61] "On the Power of Scientific Knowledge. Interview with Nico Stehr," *Epistemology & Philosophy of Science*, 55 (1) (2018), 19–22.

2 Medical Progress as Biomedical Knowledge Gains

In such debates about the progress of knowledge, medicine is not simply one example among others. Regardless of the centrality of medical examples for questioning progress, medicine is also portrayed as uniquely impervious to esthetic or ironic insights that question progress. Physicians, one neurosurgeon writes, consider medicine to have a unique situation among other branches of knowledge in terms of its ability to remain unaffected by the widespread uncertainties that relativistic thinking has injected into almost every other field.[62] Describing the demise of Enlightenment thinking about progress, and the faith that we can obtain an objective understanding of reality, physician Paul Hodgkin muses that medicine alone remains curiously immune to these epidemic uncertainties.[63] And as other fields have adopted practices and modes of thought that distance themselves from the idea of progress, medicine retains what an MD calls an anomalous position in contemporary culture. They describe medicine as an "island of rationalistic modernity" floating in a sea of subjectivism, relativism, and cynicism and conclude that medicine "has not abandoned ideas of progress, neither has it abandoned the idea of purpose."[64]

The arguments that medicine is largely immune to skeptical accounts of progressive medical knowledge fall into several categories. The first is that the biomedical dimension of health is simply the predominant one and trumps all others. The serious, urgent nature of some medical complaints has been put forward to illustrate how this simply discounts the desirability of "alternative"/unorthodox treatments, and only the very deluded could fail to believe in treatments approved by the present state of specifically biomedical knowledge. Hodgkin sums up this attitude as follows: "[s]urely the rationalist, scientific project of biomedicine is immune to all this postmodern relativistic junk where one version of reality is as good as another. After all, a diabetic coma requires specific actions to be taken which cannot depend on whim but are the same for all times and all places."[65] Medical successes

---

[62] Asem Salma, "Neurosurgery in the Post-Postmodernism Era: On the Upcoming Discourse of Medicine," *World Neurosurgery*, 82 (1–2) (2014), e395–96.
[63] Paul Hodgkin, "Medicine, Postmodernism, and the End of Certainty," *BMJ*, 313 (1996), 1568.
[64] Bruce Charlton, "Medicine and Post-Modernity," *Journal of the Royal Society of Medicine*, 86 (1993), 497.
[65] Hodgkin, "Medicine, Postmodernism, and the end of Certainty," pp. 1568–69.

including more effective surgical techniques, powerful antibiotics with minimal side effects, and new treatments for some cancers have all been used as examples thereof. While discussing the variety of healing practices in the United States, one MD argues that while constructionist practices may provide some insight into psychosocial diseases, there exists a common core of diseases to which they simply do not apply:

> What of major biochemical and pathologic disorders, such as pneumococcal pneumonia, diabetic ketoacidosis, critical aortic stenosis, fracture of the hip, and a multitude of other serious diseases? These have responded to therapies that have grown out of the modern (pre-postmodern?) bio-physical model of disease. Would an American with a ruptured appendix really choose the shaman over a skilled physician?[66]

Such points are often made by framing the importance of biomedicine and health itself in terms of their relevance for life and death. The situation in medicine has been described as analogous to the situation in war, in which survival is a priority.[67]

Another reason that progress in scientific knowledge is portrayed as crucial is that it resonates with a view that health and disease are objective and real. If health is not a fluid, moving target but rather a fixed and given state, then it follows that the goals of medicine and progress can be refocused on curing disease. If the purpose of medicine is to alleviate illness and cure disease, there is also a clear goal, and progress toward it can be objectively measured. This assumption is what underpins the Chan Zuckerberg Foundation's aim to support scientific research to cure, prevent, and manage all diseases in the next century.[68] Essential to this claim is the assumption that there are universalizable truths about health valid in different times and places. Jeremy Simon summarizes the importance of an epistemic attitude that presumes an objective understanding of reality for such progress in medicine:

> There really are diseases out there that we can come to know about just as there really are electrons, and it is medicine's goal to learn about these real diseases. Thus, we make progress in medicine whenever we discover a new

---

[66] Donald A. Sandweiss, "Letter Response to Varieties of Healing 1 & 2," *Annals of Internal Medicine*, 137 (2002), 217–18.
[67] Charlton, "Medicine and Post-Modernity," p. 498.
[68] Mark Zuckerberg, "Can We Cure All Diseases in Our Children's Lifetime?," September 21, 2016, *The Chan Zuckerberg Initiative*, https://chanzuckerberg.com/newsroom/can-we-cure-all-diseases-in-our-childrens-lifetime/.

fact about the medical part of the natural world. Discovering a new disease that is "really" out there is progress, and so is learning something new about one of those diseases, such as how to eliminate it from the body of someone who is stricken by it.[69]

Conversely, some so-called diseases are not real and therefore should not be of concern either to medical researchers and practitioners or to patients. The corollary of this argument is that there is a clear consensus as to what health consists in, and while there has been a sustained interest in alternative medicine, different forms of well-being, and the mind–body connection, "reality" will have the last word. Speaking to this point, an anesthesiologist observes that, in the field of health, it is completely normal to still hold "the nineteenth-century idea of progress."[70] Given the continuous and dramatic progress against all forms of disease in the twentieth century, it is perfectly viable to expect this progress to continue. Meanwhile, forms of postmodern/alternative medicine will be exposed as fraudulent and return to the shadows, along with voodoo, phrenology, and bleeding, where they belong.

Furthermore, in light of the complexities of disease and treatment, the idea of progress is a valuable motivating factor for researchers, physicians, and patients alike. While physicians practice in conditions of pervasive uncertainty, it is well known that they struggle to communicate ambiguity and ambivalence to patients; nor are they expected to. The conviction that physicians must present a "solution" or a truth exists as a fundamental premise underpinning the clinical encounter, related to the very act of diagnosis, a concept that lends itself toward an attachment to one knowable truth. For this reason, some physicians argue that it should be replaced by the concept of hypothesis, which references the fluidity and slippery nature of knowledge.[71] Medical education remains based on a cumulative view of knowledge, driven by rational inquiry, overcoming ignorance, and leading to objectivity or the truth. And while individual physicians readily concede that

---

[69] Simon, "How to Make Real, Constructive, Progress in Medicine," p. 847.
[70] James Lee Brooks, "Postmodern Medicine; Review of *PC, MD: How Political Correctness Is Corrupting Medicine*, by Sally Satel," *The Atlas Society*, (2010 [2001]), www.atlassociety.org/post/postmodern-medicine.
[71] Arabella Simpkin and Richard Schwartzstein, "Tolerating Uncertainty – The Next Medical Revolution?," *New England Journal of Medicine*, 375 (18) (2016), 1713–15.

uncertainty is often unavoidable, medical training mainly teaches that uncertainty is something to be minimized, ignored, or repudiated. One MD cites her own experience as a medical student during which she reported a cardiac exam to her superiors and stated:

"In my exam this morning I didn't hear any murmurs or extra sounds, but someone else should probably listen to him, just to make sure." I was quickly and firmly chastised with the words, "No one wants to hear what you don't know." You should say "the cardiac exam showed no murmurs or extra sounds" and leave it at that.[72]

In her telling, the way in which physicians crave certainty, and believe that intervention in conditions of uncertainty is constructive for patients, is merely another manifestation of the desire for progress.

The broader culture in which physicians operate is internalized by patients too. As a rule, patients want to identify the source of their medical problem, to know why it occurred, and hope that medicine provides a solution to overcome it. Referring to the patient perspective, Charlton observes that "a sick person wants the certainties of modernity."[73] From the point of view of the patient, even a diagnosis, which implies corresponding knowledge about a condition and acceptance into a bureaucratic system, can be perceived as therapy. Not all diseases have the same biological legitimacy; many disorders that medicine does not fully understand are not considered legitimate, with all the repercussions this entails. For this reason, Joseph Dumit refers to them as "illnesses you have to fight to get."[74]

For patients, faith in medical progress is based on hope for a good outcome and the possibility of overcoming uncertainties. Hope, that

---

[72] Ellen Fox, "Rethinking DoctorThink: Reforming Medical Education by Nurturing Neglected Goals," in *The Goals of Medicine*, ed. Mark J. Hanson and Daniel Callahan (Washington, DC: Georgetown University Press, 1999), pp. 186–87.
[73] Charlton, "Medicine and Post-Modernity," p. 498.
[74] Joseph Dumit, "Illnesses You Have to Fight to Get: Facts as Forces in Uncertain, Emergent Illnesses," *Social Science & Medicine*, 62 (2006), 577–90. For example, the diagnosis of attention-deficit hyperactivity disorder (ADHD) in children was several times described as relief (*Entlastung*) by affected parents, conversations with the author, 2017, *Kinder fördern. Eine interdisziplinäre Studie zum Umgang mit ADHS* (University of Fribourg, ZHAW, Collegium Helveticum). See also Annemarie Jutel, *Putting a Name to It: Diagnosis in Contemporary Society* (Baltimore: Johns Hopkins University Press, 2011).

is, the belief in the possibility of progress, allows patients to anticipate a desired future, and makes illness conditions more bearable.[75] Surgeon-turned-patient Paul Kalanithi remarks on how "a drop of hope" pushes back uncertainties and the "fog surrounding [his] life" and allows him to cope with his illness.[76] But hope and progress are bound up together in complicated ways. Reflecting on her incredible desire to see her very premature son survive, and her knowledge as a trained obstetrician-gynecologist that this was unlikely, MD Jen Gunter refers to hope as an "analgesic" better than anything science has to offer.[77] Hope, in this case, is a refraction of her desire for progress without a strong grounding in reality. Persistent uncertainties in medical knowledge and difficulties associated with its implementation temper hopes for progress. Medical interventions come replete with multiple problems and side effects, and there may well be fewer effective ones than most people assume.[78] It is possible to argue that extant beliefs in medical progress are based more on patients' hopes for progress and new therapies that will improve their lives than on a well-founded confidence in medicine's capabilities.

Physicians' and patients' desires for progress in medical knowledge are shaped by broader cultural pressures that valorize the idea of scientific progress in medicine. Take cancer research, for example. Unprecedented amounts of funding were made available for cancer research in the 1970s, based on the desire to gain new knowledge and improve the treatment and prevention of the disease. The possibility of winning the "war on cancer" is associated with targeted therapies based on knowledge of mechanisms designed "to strike with devastating consequences for the disease."[79] Since that time, the US National Cancer Institute alone has spent more than 100 billion dollars on cancer research, under the mandate of "leading the nation's progress against cancer" in which the advance of scientific knowledge and expensive

---

[75] Huber, "Looking Back, Looking Forward," p. 126.
[76] Paul Kalanithi, *When Breath Becomes Air* (New York: Random House, 2016), p. 135.
[77] Jen Gunter, "Mother of 3, Parent of 2. Reflections on the Saddest Sorority," July 7, 2017, https://drjengunter.com/2017/07/07/mother-of-3-parent-of-2-reflections-on-the-saddest-sorority/
[78] Stegenga, *Medical Nihilism*, p. 183.
[79] See Douglas Hanahan, "Rethinking the War on Cancer," *Lancet*, 383 (9916) (2014), 558–63.

treatments play a key role.[80] Yet, the gap between epistemological progress gained and using new knowledge to explain and treat cancer in a cost-effective way remains.[81] Stopping smoking is one factor that has a pronounced impact on decreasing cancer rates, but cancer remains the second leading cause of death in the United States overall and the leading cause among people younger than eighty-five.[82] At the same time, the discourse of progress and cancer largely prevails. The medical profession, those who market it, and the public at large share a general sense that cancer is largely preventable and that, if not prevented, it can usually be treated and even beaten.[83] Beyond the questionable empirical basis for this belief is the fact that such narratives play a powerful role in and of themselves. Medical researcher Robert Weinberg reflects that while the "overenthusiasm" and "reductionist triumphalism" associated with certain phases of the war on cancer were certainly ill-founded, perhaps he and his colleagues would never have begun their work had they known how complicated things would turn out to be.[84] In other words, the belief in progress is a powerful motivating factor in its own right.

Much of this chapter has chronicled insights by philosophers, historians, and others about the contingent nature of science and truth, as well as a persistent tendency to associate medical knowledge with an ambitious, progress-oriented view. In what follows, I want to discuss in more detail two exemplary answers to the question of what is medical progress today. In addition to shedding light on the knowledge we seek, the kinds of knowledge we value, and the technologies we associate with that knowledge, these examples illustrate how science itself exists in perpetual motion, continually challenging the knowledge it has created, and revealing new unknowns.

---

[80] "Leading the Nation's Progress against Cancer into the Future," National Cancer Institute, Professional Judgment Budget, Fiscal Year 2019, www.cancer.gov/about-nci/budget/plan/2019-professional-judgment-budget.pdf.

[81] Marta Bertolaso and Bernhard Strauss, "The Search for Progress and a New Theory Framework in Cancer Research," in *Rethinking Cancer: A New Paradigm for the Postgenomics Era*, eds. Bernhard Strauss et al. (Cambridge, MA: The MIT Press, 2021), pp. 13–40.

[82] R. L. Siegel, A.N. Giaquinto, and A. Jemal, "Cancer statistics, 2024," *CA: A Cancer Journal for Clinicians*, 74 (1) (2024) 12–49.

[83] Gina Kolata, "Advances Elusive in the Drive to Cure Cancer," *The New York Times*, April 24, 2009, www.nytimes.com/2009/04/24/health/policy/24cancer.html.

[84] Robert A. Weinberg, "Coming Full Circle – From Endless Complexity to Simplicity and Back Again," *Cell*, 157 (1) (2014), 268.

2.6.1 Reclaiming Progress I: Evidence-Based Medicine

As depicted above, the rejection of relativism and skepticism, and the affirmation that real, tangible, and useful knowledge exists, reinvigorated the idea of progress in medicine. In turn, this belief is reflected in the knowledge theories and methods underpinning medicine. Evidence-based medicine (EBM), in particular, has been prominently associated with progress as scientific knowledge. If improved medical knowledge and its applications are linked to objective knowledge, EBM is regularly cited as the best example in this regard.[85] In a *BMJ* article, Paul Hodgkin argues that EBM "promises certainty" and that knowable certainties imply progress; "[a]fter all, if there are knowable medical truths 'out there' then we should get our act together and apply them."[86] Beyond its specific capabilities and fallibilities, one of the most striking successes of EBM has been to associate itself with the desirable future of medicine.[87]

The rise of "evidence-based medicine" – the term was first used in the 1990s and is often commuted to evidence-based healthcare – blends with wider debates on evidence, measurement, and causal inferences that were already well established beyond medicine. A devotion to empirical methods and the study of evidence informs the idea of evidence-based progress from policymaking and economics to legal studies and business. And visions of progress based on evidence-based scientific generalizations played a particular role in the debates around progress in medicine. In a seminal article in the 1990s that signposted itself as marking the emergence of a new paradigm for medical practice, Gordon Guyatt and his collaborators challenged the previous authority of expert-based medicine, writing that rather than intuition and unsystematic clinical expertise, EBM stresses the best available scientific evidence.[88] From an epistemological perspective, EBM's proponents hold that careful design, methodological rigor, and replication are fundamental for limiting personal bias and gaining

---

[85] Salma, "Neurosurgery in the Post-Postmodernism Era," p. 396.
[86] Hodgkin, "Medicine, Postmodernism, and the End of Certainty," p. 1568.
[87] Desmond J. Sheridan and Desmond G. Julian, "Achievements and Limitations of Evidence-Based Medicine," *Journal of the American College of Cardiology*, 68 (2) (2016), 205.
[88] Evidence-Based Medicine Working Group, "Evidence-Based Medicine: A New Approach to Teaching the Practice of Medicine," *Journal of the American Medical Association*, 268 (17) (1992), 2420.

knowledge, thanks to systematic inquiries. Rather than a hodgepodge of the idiosyncratic opinions of individual physicians, the aim of EBM, as further refined by David Sackett and colleagues in 1996, "is the conscientious, explicit and judicious use of current best evidence in making decisions about the care of individual patients."[89]

EBM's commitment to epidemiological and biostatistical ways of thinking means that randomized controlled trials (RCTs) and meta-analyses thereof are at the top of its evidence hierarchy. The preference for evidence produced by clinical trials is bound up with the conviction that we can arrive at an objective measurement and understanding of reality, independent of time and place, and generalize these results to other settings. EBM observers Devisch and Murray represent this belief with the equation "[evidence] = truth = reality."[90] Modernism has been characterized by the faith in the existence of objectivity, determinacy, and impartial observation, and EBM espouses many of these traits.[91] In an article devoted to assessing "progress in evidence-based medicine," two of its founders, Benjamin Djulbegovic and Gordon Guyatt, explain that the "higher the quality of evidence, the closer to the truth," and that the "pursuit of truth is best accomplished by evaluating the totality of the evidence."[92] "Does 'anything go,' as some post-modernists would have it," they asked in a different publication:

or is there such a thing as the objective scientific methodology that can be universally accepted by everyone? EBM espouses those philosophical views that endorse a central role of evidence to serve as a neutral, objective arbiter among competing views, thereby aiming to generate agreement among rational observers.[93]

---

[89] David L. Sackett et al., "Evidence Based Medicine: What It Is and What It Isn't," *BMJ*, 312 (1996), 71–72.

[90] Ignass Devisch and Stuart J. Murray, "'We Hold These Truths to Be Self-Evident': Deconstructing 'Evidence-Based' Medical Practice," *Journal of Evaluation in Clinical Practice*, 15 (2009), 950–54.

[91] Sietse Wieringa et al., "Has Evidence-Based Medicine Ever Been Modern? A Latour-Inspired Understanding of a Changing EBM," *Journal of Evaluation in Clinical Practice*, 23 (5) (2017), 964–70.

[92] See Benjamin Djulbegovic, Gordon H. Guyatt, "Progress in Evidence-Based Medicine: A Quarter Century On," *The Lancet*, 390 (2017), 416.

[93] Benjamin Djulbegovic, Gordon H. Guyatt, Richard E. Ashcroft, "Epistomologic Inquiries in Evidence-Based Medicine," *Cancer Control*, 16 (2) (2009), 165.

As a method of producing knowledge, the goal of EBM is to use RCTs to measure the reliability of medical interventions and the claim that the increased use of such trials – as an objective, universalizable, and neutral kind of methodology – constitutes progress.

Yet even as the proponents of EBM aspire to remove it from the realm of human values and opinions and connect it with truth-seeking scientific inquiry, epistemological and ethical questions arise in relation to every aspect of its knowledge production. Evidence is probabilistic knowledge, and such knowledge is obtained as the result of conscious, deliberate human activities.[94] EBM presents a kind of evidence that depends on eliminating the cultural context and subjectivities of the researchers creating that knowledge. Claims about the neutrality of scientific evidence obscure the ethical, emotional, and cultural complexities of clinical decisions.[95] Rather than a simple equation between evidence and truth-seeking, EBM implies a commitment to specific quantitative practices and statistical analyses. While EBM did propose new epistemic standards in the form of the RCT, it also brought to light the substantial limitations of this knowledge and the ideas of progress that rely on it.[96]

EBM is not presenting a fundamentally new theory of medical progress, or even a framework in which such a theory is encouraged to develop, but rather offering a coherent structure for optimizing medical practice based on diligent attention to a specific kind of medical evidence. In a study that emphasizes historical tensions between rationalism and empiricism in medicine, Warren Newton writes that "[f]or all its rhetoric of novelty, Evidence Based Medicine represents a counter-revolution of traditional empiricism, draped in modern clothes

---

[94] See Daniel Weinstock, "'What Is Evidence?' A Philosophical Perspective," presentation at 2007 National Collaborating Centres for Public Health Summer Institute, *Making Sense of It All*, 20–23 August 2007.

[95] See Michael P. Kelly et al., "The Importance of Values in Evidence-Based Medicine," *BMC Medical Ethics*, 16 (69) (2015), doi 10.1186/s12910-015-0063-3.

[96] Critiques of EBM can be found in John Worrall, "*What* Evidence in Evidence-Based Medicine?," *Philosophy of Science*, 69 (3) (2002), 316–30, and John Worrall, "Evidence in Medicine and Evidence-Based Medicine," *Philosophy Compass*, 2 (6) (2007), 981–1022, and recent contributions to the debate include Cristian Larroulet Philippi, "There Is Cause to Randomize," *Philosophy of Science*, 89 (2022), 152–70, and Jonathan Fuller, "Epidemiological Evidence: Use at Your 'Own Risk'?" *Philosophy of Science*, 87 (5) (2020), 1119–29.

of statistics and multi-variate analysis."[97] In light of controversies as to what scientific progress actually is, Leen de Vreese observes that EBM fits with one particular approach to scientific progress, namely "problem-solving" rather than "knowledge-gaining."[98] Since EBM's progressive results are small gains in piecemeal knowledge rather than significant gains in understanding, de Vreese concludes that the advantages offered by RCTs must be balanced out by those associated with different methodologies. John Wu, meanwhile, has pointed to the self-limiting ambition of this particular form of empiricist thinking for progress: "If everything has to be double-blinded, randomised, and evidence-based, where does that leave new ideas?"[99]

If there are important kinds of medical knowledge that are not captured by RCTs, EBM's self-allocated role in driving medical progress may not be justified. Systematic reviews and meta-analyses have epistemic limitations because they rest on researchers' decisions and choices about which studies to include in such reviews, how to determine their quality, and how to compare them statistically.[100] Multiple problems arise when conducting randomized clinical trials in social contexts, and they are at times ethically questionable, which limits the ability of RCTs to capture the social determinants of health. The expense of trials, the tenuousness of diagnostic categories constantly subject to revision and refinement, the existence of evidence that is narrative and subjective in nature, or derived from intuitions and physician expertise – all these have contributed to EBM acknowledging some of its limitations, as well as the importance of qualitative research and patient values.[101] In practice, however, it remains committed to methodological progress in the form of the RCT and its ability to produce reliable evidence about medical interventions. As a result, it has devoted much effort to improving this particular method of gaining

---

[97] Warren Newton, "Rationalism and Empiricism in Modern Medicine," *Law and Contemporary Problems*, 64 (4) (2001), 314.

[98] Leen de Vreese, "Evidence-Based Medicine and Progress in the Medical Sciences," *Journal of Evaluation in Clinical Practice*, 17 (2011), 852–56.

[99] John Wu, Letter: "Could Evidence-Based Medicine Be a Danger to Progress?," *The Lancet*, 366 (2005), 122.

[100] Jakob Stegenga, "Is Meta-Analysis the Platinum Standard of Evidence?," *Studies in the History and Philosophy of Biology and Biomedical Sciences*, 42 (4) 2011, 497–507.

[101] See S. Joshua Thomas, "Does Evidence-Based Health Care Have Room for the Self?," *Journal of Evaluation in Clinical Practice*, 22 (2016), 502–8.

2 Medical Progress as Biomedical Knowledge Gains

medical knowledge, but the measured effect sizes of interventions have gotten smaller and smaller. This has led one epidemiologist to lament that we seem to be using "more and more advanced technology to study more and more trivial issues, while the major population causes of disease are ignored."[102] Properly assessing progress means coming to grips with the strengths and weaknesses of various kinds of medical knowledge. It also implies acknowledging the difficulty of passing from clinical research to providing care in a real-world situation, with all of the epistemic challenges this entails.

2.6.2 Reclaiming Progress II: Big Data and Huge Progress

At this point, I want to step away from evidence-based ideas to wider debates on progress in recent decades. Just as warnings that progress could not be unconditionally associated with any one kind of evidence became more acute, the term and concept became caught up in a different field where dreams of progress were about to explode. The artificial intelligence (AI) boom following the breakthroughs in the feasibility of deep learning in the early 2010s was associated from the beginning with unprecedented knowledge gains in medicine. Tech commentator Peter Sweeney observes that the knowledge we expect of AI is "truly revolutionary" and links this aspiration to "theory-free science" that enables medicine to progress.[103] Others highlight the extent to which knowledge progress in the digital era represents a historical rupture and could result in a kind of progress that is markedly different from previous eras.[104] AI excels at producing knowledge through inductive reasoning, that is, learning from observation, and more generally, AI technologies are seen as elements in a progression that have enabled machines to both mimic and surpass human intelligence. Data is crucial: Computer programs reveal patterns and relationships that scientists or clinicians might not otherwise see because

---

[102] See Richard R. Nelson et al., "How Medical Know-How Progresses," *Research Policy*, 40 (2011), 1339–44.

[103] Peter Sweeney, "The Pendulum of Progress," *Experfy* (August 14, 2018), https://resources.experfy.com/ai-ml/the-pendulum-of-progress/.

[104] Anton Korinek and Joseph E. Stiglitz, "Artificial Intelligence and Its Implications for Income Distribution and Unemployment" in *The Economics of Artificial Intelligence: An Agenda*, eds. Ajay Agrawal, Joshua Gans, and Avi Goldfarb (Chicago: University of Chicago Press, 2019), pp. 349–50.

they are able to interpret results from trillions of data points relevant to a particular problem. As Sweeney puts it: "Data-driven has come to mean *progress*. If you subscribe to dataism, then it follows that access to data and talent are the only factors impeding progress."[105]

Part of the hype surrounding knowledge progress via information technologies is associated with the notion of rapid exponential growth, whereby each development becomes a building block for future developments. The implications for progress are profound: In this framework, it accumulates and accelerates. Pronouncements of individual researchers have contributed to these expectations; Mo Gawdat, formerly head business officer at Google X, argues that we will not experience 100 years of AI progress over the next century; rather, at current rates, we will experience 20,000 years, and that is without considering an unforeseen technological revolution.[106] As a rule, it is a recurring theme in the knowledge and progress discourse of the digital era to highlight that we are at a unique juncture in the history of medicine, whereby the capacity of information technologies to provide understanding makes comparisons with previous eras largely irrelevant.[107] Even as the problem of the excessively rapid growth of scientific knowledge was identified a century ago – Cynthia Whitehead argues that since then each era portrays the "exploding knowledge" problem as newly discovered[108] – AI is depicted as both the motor behind progress and the crucial answer to information explosion.

The famous knowledge is power paradigm, whereby knowledge is the antidote to fear and uncertainty, has been described as the initial motivation for AI research in medicine.[109] And yet, progress in AI research raises a host of difficult questions for this paradigm as well as for the idea of progress in medicine. Human beings are flawed knowledge creators, but it does not follow that the knowledge of highly complex algorithmic machines trumps all others. Ideas of medical

---

[105] Sweeney, "The Pendulum of Progress," (italics in the original).
[106] Mo Gawdat, *Scary Smart: The Future of Artificial Intelligence and How You Can Save Our World* (London: Pan Macmillan, 2021).
[107] *Topol Review*, (2019), p. 6.
[108] Cynthia Whitehead, *The Good Doctor in Medical Education 1910–2010: A Critical Discourse Analysis*, unpublished PhD Thesis, University of Toronto, 2011, p. 90.
[109] Werner Horn, "AI in Medicine on Its Way from Knowledge-Intensive to Data-Intensive Systems," *Artificial Intelligence in Medicine*, 23 (2001), 6.

knowledge progress as achievable via AI involve a redefinition of knowledge along the lines of what a computer can do; a recent statement by computer researchers that information processing tasks are "the foundation of all knowledge work" is exemplary in this regard.[110] Such statements tap into previous trends that valorize particular kinds of knowledge bound up with measurement, breaking down the whole into constituent parts, and researchers' disengagement. British scientist William Kelvin expressed this thought in 1883 when he said that when you can measure something and express it in numbers, you can know something about it, but if not your knowledge is meager and unsatisfactory.[111] A century later, the notion that we can arrive at an unbiased, neutral position expressed in numbers was identified as a tenacious assumption of Western medicine.[112] Giving priority to digitally generated data and associating it with the truth mask the way that the progress of that knowledge is always constructed and embedded in human value systems.

In a variety of ways, the readiness to cede epistemic authority to big data and AI is based on an image of persons – both patients and physicians – as resembling computers. Computer scientist Geoffrey Hinton differentiates between rule-based algorithms that aim to master the facts of a case (knowing that) and learning algorithms able to perceive patterns that are formed (knowing how). But there is a third realm of knowledge – knowing why – and he emphasizes that "*asking* why" is our conduit to every kind of explanation, and crucial for progress in medicine.[113] While AI has huge potential for both mastering facts and perceiving patterns, it has less for investigating causes. By delegating increasing aspects of clinical practice to opaque learning machines, physicians' daily experience of mixing implicit and explicit forms of knowledge, knowing how, knowing that, and knowing why, fades. At the same time, asking why relates both to patients' existence as finite

---

[110] Erik Brynjolfsson, Andrew McAfee, *The Second Machine Age: Work, Progress, and Prosperity in a Time of Brilliant Technologies* (New York City: W. W. Norton & Company, 2014), p. 16.
[111] William Kelvin, "Electrical Units of Measurement," May 3, 1883, *Popular Lectures and Addresses*, Vol. 1 (London: Macmillan and Co., 1889), p. 73.
[112] Gordon, "Tenacious Assumptions in Western Medicine."
[113] Hinton cited in Siddhartha Mukherjee, "A.I. Versus M.D.: What Happens When Diagnosis Is Automated?," *The New Yorker*, March 27, 2017, www.newyorker.com/magazine/2017/04/03/ai-versus-md.

beings with unique lives and values and to the broader social relationships in which they find themselves. This kind of *Zusammenhangwissen* (integrated knowledge) transcends task-focused algorithms because it requires physicians to step back and assess whether what they are doing is what they ought to be doing.[114] This kind of knowing, in all its dimensions, is an essential kind of knowledge in medicine.

A further problem with epistemic dependence on AI is linked to the fact that increases in knowledge occur alongside higher standards for justification, that is, standards that have to be met so that a given correlation between data and phenomena holds. Here, big data can make things worse, as more data throws up an inestimably large number of associative links that can make understanding which associations are causal and which are simply correlational more difficult. For example, while acknowledging the number of potential risk factors, and the importance of a systems approach, researchers identified 108 variables and 304 causal linkages that may influence obesity.[115] At the same time, such a high number of relevant traits does not result in a commensurate increase in genuine understanding of the medical problem at hand. In such cases, we are faced with the problem that more information is not an unconditional good, as well as the fact that increases in knowledge can entail increases in medicalization. Information about a connection that was previously unknown has consequences for those who choose to treat such a data point as an opportunity for intervention. Progress requires understanding the challenges involved in data provenance and collection and recognizing the limitations of deep learning.[116]

A further problem hindering medical knowledge progress driven by AI is related to health inequalities and how the factors associated with the rise of health AI – such as access to computers and electronic health information – may be widening existing disparities. This is linked to the well-known problem of bias in both the creation and

---

[114] Lutz Wingert, "Knowing the Whole. A Note on 'Integrated Knowledge' (*Zusammenhangwissen*)," unpublished article, April 2017.
[115] Philippe Vandenbroeck, Jo Goossens, Marshall Clemens, "Tackling Obesities: Future Choices – Building the Obesity System Map," *Foresight Programme*, UK Government Office for Science, 2007, p. 14, https://assets.publishing.service.gov.uk/government/uploads/system/uploads/attachment_data/file/295154/07-1179-obesity-building-system-map.pdf.
[116] Fei Wang, Lawrence Peter Casalino, and Dhruv Khullar, "Deep Learning in Medicine – Promise, Progress, and Challenges," *JAMA Internal Medicine*, 179 (3) (2019), 294.

use of algorithms. Algorithms learn from data that may be of bad quality, not representative, or affected by human opinions and prejudices. AI systems are often trained on readily available datasets from the internet, which are neither complete nor unbiased. For this reason, big data has been labeled a regime of knowledge, power, and control, and internet studies scholars argue that algorithmic power reinforces oppressive social relationships, for example by creating new indicators of racial profiling.[117] In healthcare, the consequences are alarming. Deep learning algorithms trained using the data from homogeneous populations – often adult males of Caucasian origin – do not have the same accuracy for diagnosing and treating minorities. For example, an algorithm widely used in American hospitals to refer people to healthcare programs was found to be systematically discriminating against specific population groups.[118] In the assessment of one arts and technology researcher, such uses of AI in medicine sound more like the escalation of various societal conflicts than like progress in healthcare.[119] Meanwhile, some have sought to redefine medical progress so that it includes due attention to fairness in AI, practices of non-discrimination, and the protection of patients' rights.[120]

2.7 Conclusion

Intellectual historian H. Stuart Hughes observes that the confidence it is possible to gain objective knowledge of the past is characteristic of the nineteenth century and contrasts this with a more typically

---

[117] See Safiya Umoja Noble, *Algorithms of Oppression: How Search Engines Reinforce Racism* (New York: New York University Press, 2018), Virginia Eubanks, *Automating Inequality: How High-Tech Tools Profile, Police, and Punish the Poor* (New York: St Martin's, 2018) and *Artificial Intelligence and Its Discontents: Critiques from the Social Sciences and Humanities*, ed. Ariane Hanemaayer (Cham, Switzerland: Palgrave Macmillan, 2022).

[118] Heidi Ledford, "Millions of Black People Affected by Racial Bias in Health-Care Algorithms," *Nature*, 574 (2019), 608–9, and Jenna Wiens, Melissa Creary, Michael W. Sjoding, "AI Models in Health Care Are Not Colour Blind and We Should Not Be Either," *The Lancet: Digital Health*, 4 (6) (2022), 399–400.

[119] Mihai Nadin, "Aiming AI at a Moving Target: Health (or Disease)," *AI & Society*, https://doi.org/10.1007/s00146-020-00943-x.

[120] Renate Baumgartner et al., "Fair and Equitable AI in Biomedical Research and Healthcare: Social Science Perspectives," *Artificial Intelligence in Medicine*, 144 (2023), 4, https://doi.org/10.1016/j.artmed.2023.102658.

twentieth-century perspective, which pays increased attention to built-in disparities between external reality and the subjective appreciation of that reality.[121] In recent debates on this topic, medicine played a central though Janus-like role. Within science studies, the humanities, and medicine itself, various voices chronicled the complex processes of knowledge production underpinning medical practices and paid particular attention to how power structures conditioned their implementation as well as shaped the expectations of patients and the public. Scientific medical knowledge came to be seen less as making incremental progress toward more refined and better knowledge but rather as a series of constantly renegotiated claims, contingent on unarticulated conceptual presuppositions. Biomedicine, it has been argued, is neither inevitable nor a given, but rather the product of specific political and ethical choices. Pushed to the extreme, relativistic sympathies are reflected in the belief that science is merely one among multiple options that foster health. Despite the above tendencies, the most optimistic incarnations of the idea of progress continued to hold sway in medicine. For some, medical knowledge is a "politically neutral," "real" form of knowledge that embodies scientific progress for the benefit of human beings. The conviction that science will find ways to eliminate all health problems has been strengthened by spectacular scientific achievements; many modernist assumptions about scientific medical knowledge and its links to medical progress continue to flourish.

While we look to medicine to produce orderly, progressive knowledge, it relies on uncertain and imperfect science and a body of knowledge that is constantly changing. This is one of the reasons that Richard Horton, editor of *the Lancet*, has written "[t]he idea of progress is wrong, as is the idea of catastrophe. These are the wrong coordinates by which to judge our lives. There is no endpoint we are working towards. All there is is transition."[122] Health is anything but static, and complete, definitive knowledge of health and disease is impossible. This is not least because a biomedical approach to health is only one among others. As we shall see in the next chapter, questioning a

---

[121] H. Stuart Hughes, *Consciousness and Society: The Reorientation of European Social Thought, 1890–1930*, intro. Stanley Hoffman (New York: Routledge, 2017 [1958]), p. 16.

[122] Richard Horton, "Offline: Rebelling against the Dictatorship of Reason," *The Lancet*, 381 (9869) (2013), 790.

narrow focus on traditional, scientific ideas of health and progress was associated with a rise of interest in alternative and complementary medicines and holistic healing practices. It begins with interrogating the claimed authority of physicians and researchers in favor of lay knowledge and patients' subjective experience. And a significant motivation for this shift was a widespread sense that scientific knowledge gains themselves are not enough to amount to progress, what is needed is knowledge that is able to empower patients.

3 | *Medical Progress as Becoming Free*

The notion that increased scientific knowledge is what drives progress persists in contemporary medicine. While working on this book, I received an email directed to the McGill University community in which the Principal and Vice-Chancellor wrote as follows:

As we continue to tackle [the SARS-CoV-2] pandemic, our best arm is knowledge: acquiring knowledge and sharing it [.] And [let's] find a ray of hope in the words of [Steven] Pinker: "There is no limit to the betterments we can attain if we continue to apply knowledge to enhance human flourishing."[1]

This confidence in our ability to translate knowledge into human flourishing notwithstanding, in the latter half of the twentieth century, the conceptual relationships between progress, knowledge, and well-being were increasingly probed. This chapter begins by returning to a key moment for conceptions of medical progress in the context of civil rights movements when a new awareness of the insufficiencies of medical progress as "merely" scientific knowledge gains led to a sustained interest in knowledge that was empowering for patients. Amid the growing numbers of people who challenged the focus on scientific progress, many turned to freedom as a new concept for grounding medical progress. At times, this went together with more holistic views of personhood and health and the desire to put self-determination at the heart of theories of progress. Other, related trends acknowledged the potential contradictions between freedom and progress head-on and argued that taking individual freedom seriously meant challenging traditional, scientific/technological forms of medical progress. The chapter concludes with a detailed examination of the most recent instances in which

---

[1] Suzanne Fortier, "Message to the McGill Community Regarding COVID-19," April 29, 2020.

3 Medical Progress as Becoming Free

technological progress is presented as being highly compatible with personal freedom. To that end, I discuss the ways in which digital medicine promises to empower and liberate patients. As we shall see, the recent emphasis on digital empowerment revives old debates about the multidimensionality of health and progress.

Before I proceed, a word about terminology is in order. Freedom is a term that relates to an array of notions about which there is a vast literature, including autonomy, self-determination, empowerment, and liberty. In what follows, I pay attention to the specific context in which such terms are used, while retaining a classic distinction between two kinds of liberty as a useful conceptual framework for navigating the terminology and concepts that come into play here.[2] These are negative liberty, in the sense of a realm in which individuals can act unobstructed, and positive liberty, associated with self-determination and the power to exercise control over one's life. Negative freedom has been associated with the absence of barriers and called an "opportunity concept" that refers back to available options, whether one can exercise them or not.[3] The notion of positive freedom is characterized by the claim that the lack of impediments to action is never a sufficient condition for freedom. Rather, it is an "exercise concept," associated with individuals' ability and power to act, whether or not they are in charge of their lives, and whether they are able to accomplish what they aspire to do.[4] Positive freedom might, therefore, be hindered by a lack of resources, or internal, psychological barriers, or outside interference. Autonomy, in a minimal sense, is precisely this kind of self-determination, which is choosing to do what one wants to do, while in more demanding conceptions of autonomy, such as Kant's version, the notion of reflective and responsible choosing is built into the idea of choice.

These distinctions are important as the terminology of freedom in Western medicine possesses a range of meanings. For example, respect for patient autonomy is taught to medical students as one of the four principles of medical ethics, along with justice, beneficence,

---

[2] Isaiah Berlin formulated this distinction in his essay "Two Concepts of Liberty" (1958).
[3] Charles Taylor, "What's Wrong with Negative Liberty," in *The Idea of Freedom: Essays in Honour of Isaiah Berlin*, ed. Alan Ryan (Oxford: Oxford University Press, 1979), p. 177.
[4] Ibid.

and non-maleficence.⁵ In medical ethics, this principle is thought primarily binding on healthcare providers and has given rise to a range of practices such as the facilitation of choice, the doctrine of informed consent, respect for privacy, and assessments of mental competency. According to Ruth Faden and Thomas Beauchamp, autonomy in a medical context is identified with several discrete ideas, including privacy, self-mastery, choosing freely, choosing one's own moral position, and accepting responsibility for one's choices.⁶ In order to make sense of this variety, I retain the above distinctions regarding positive and negative freedom and return to how different theories of progress express particular visions of personhood.

3.1 From Technical Knowledge Gains to "Moral Knowing"

In the Introduction and Chapter 1 of this book, I summarized how progress was often associated with a particular logic and a set of interconnected changes, for example that technological innovation leads to material welfare and the establishment of more rational forms of social and political organization. Individual freedom is at the heart of these linkages. The Enlightenment portrayal of the mutually reinforcing relationship between the progress of knowledge and negative freedom is one in which the ultimate objective of progress is to increase individual freedom. But individual freedom to think and create was also at the origin of knowledge gains. Being free from constraints was thus the precondition for as well as the objective of progress, and technology was central to this narrative. It is possible to argue that the very notion of technology is unintelligible without taking into account the broader context of the faith in progress and commitment to humanity's self-liberation through its progressive dominance of the natural world. As we saw in Chapter 1, historically speaking, the arts were not perceived as exalting human capabilities and freedoms, as much as imitating nature, which was itself divine. However, with the rise of the modern idea of progress, a particular notion of free, self-development through technology arose. The

---

⁵ Tom Beauchamp and James F. Childress, *Principles of Biomedical Ethics*, 7th ed. (Oxford: Oxford University Press, 2013), pp. 101–49.
⁶ Ruth Faden, Thomas Beauchamp, and Nancy King, *A History and Theory of Informed Consent* (New York: Oxford University Press, 1986), p. 7.

removal of external constraints on the possibilities for human control amounted to a conceptual revolution in which each particular technology is part of humanity's broader development toward freedom and self-mastery.[7] According to these assumptions, unfettered, rational inquiry into the world is what leads to truth, progress, health, and further freedoms.

In medicine, the relationship between ideas of freedom and progress has a distinct history, even as it has been affected by the broadly liberal premises outlined above. As we have seen, by the end of the nineteenth century, the typical physician–patient relationship was a paternalistic one, in which most patients willingly subjected themselves to the authority of the physician. It was also a fiduciary relationship, governed not by market principles but by the physician's duty to promote the patient's well-being. Various nineteenth-century developments such as the germ theory of disease led to a shift away from the patient's perspective by focusing on increasingly specialized processes within the body and physicians' interpretations of those processes. Nevertheless, the notion that the consent of the subject was important for medical intervention was already present at the turn of the century and gained immeasurably in international ethical reflection following World War II and the Nuremberg Code. The emphasis on individual choice within the nascent discipline of bioethics can itself be seen as a reaction against Nazi eugenic rhetoric and practices. In Chapter 2, I traced how the 1950s "reveled in the progress of medicine" and that the medical advances of the time were seen as "undiluted goods."[8] It was also at this time that the perceived link between doing science in a democracy – the "free" way of doing science, as opposed to science under fascism – and its success solidified. To be sure, portraying Western science and freedom as synonymous glossed over the fact that citizens of democracies were not equally free and did not benefit equally from scientific results and that the commitment to scientific freedom in the West could be in tension with the aim of

---

[7] Arthur M. Melzer, "The Problem with the 'Problem of Technology,'" in *Technology in the Western Political Tradition*, eds. Arthur M. Melzer, Jerry Weinberger, and M. Richard Zinman (Ithaca, NY: Cornell University Press, 1993), pp. 298–99.
[8] Albert R. Jonsen, *The Birth of Bioethics* (Oxford: Oxford University Press, 2003), p. 12.

achieving global equality.⁹ Nevertheless, the perception of "scientific freedom" as both apolitical and morally superior was a crucial part of the self-definition of Western science during the Cold War.

These mental preconditions notwithstanding, in the 1960s and 1970s, a new understanding of the relationship between medical progress and freedom developed. One reason was that patients were struggling on various fronts for freedom from what was increasingly perceived as the tyranny of technology. New procedures for heart surgery and insufficient or damaging treatments for mental illness were just two of the issues that were hotly debated in terms of their effects on patient well-being and medical progress more generally. The ethos of medical ethics of the time has been characterized as a general attempt to reclaim human values from ever-encroaching technology and a materialistic worldview.¹⁰ During this time, the harmony between increased scientific medical knowledge and the possibilities of patient self-realization was increasingly scrutinized. In essence, a slow accumulation of concerns about the ramifications and ambiguities of scientific progress merged with the emerging concerns of bioethics, and the redefinition of progress was central to that endeavor.

This mood was reflected in various conferences and publications of the period. In 1960, an event entitled "Great Issues of Conscience in Modern Medicine," held at Dartmouth College in New Hampshire, aspired to pry apart the tendency to equate scientific progress with ethical advances.¹¹ At stake in this reexamination of progress were not simply questions of life and death, but rather what kind of survival and what kind of future? Instead of being seen as fundamentally protected from the "dark side" of scientific knowledge associated with the advent of the atomic era, it became increasingly clear that unbridled advances in medical knowledge and possibilities of intervention had their own drawbacks and even potentially devastating consequences.

---

⁹ See Audra J. Wolfe, *Freedom's Laboratory: The Cold War Struggle for the Soul of Science* (Baltimore: Johns Hopkins University Press, 2018).

¹⁰ Alfred I. Tauber, "Historical and Philosophical Reflections on Patient Autonomy," *Health Care Analysis*, 9 (2001), 303.

¹¹ "Opening Assembly: Selections from the Addresses and Panel Discussions of the Convocation, The Dartmouth Convocation on Great Issues of Conscience in Modern Medicine, 8–10 September 1960," *Dartmouth Alumni Magazine* (1960), https://archive.dartmouthalumnimagazine.com/article/1960/11/1/opening-assembly.

Another conference on "Man and his Future," held in London in 1962, cautioned that the world had been thoroughly unprepared for the ethical and political ramifications of nuclear power; now, recent progress in biological research posed similar risks to nearly every valued aspect of human life.[12] The first human heart transplant in 1967 was followed by sustained reflections on the extent to which increased possibilities of intervention and scientific gains were accompanied by loss and ambiguities. Observers emphasized that all discussions of medical progress need to engage with the question of being human, namely what is it about human life that is or should remain constant and inviolable, and what is subject to change?[13]

By the end of the 1960s, the moral problems of medicine were competing with the public focus on the benefits of scientific progress. Rather than welcoming unequivocally new kinds of scientific knowledge, there was a perceived need for a thicker, more ethically articulated concept of progress. In a widely read book written in 1971, *Bioethics: Bridge to the Future*, Van Rensselaer Potter, a biochemist and bioethicist, described the idea of progress as moving through three roughly chronological stages – a religious, a materialistic, and a scientific-philosophic one – and argued that wisdom or the knowledge of how to balance scientific knowledge with other kinds of knowledge is "moral knowledge" and the "most important of all."[14] One result of these reflections was more emphasis on freedom's positive dimension and the importance of moral deliberation for understanding how to manage scientific advances. The philosopher who had done the most to explore the links between self-determination, reason, and morality, Immanuel Kant, was duly invoked to supplement existing accounts of freedom. In 1966, at a conference in Oregon entitled "The Sanctity of Life," philosopher Abraham Kaplan referred back to Kantian self-determination as crucial for moral decision-making and argued that "free science" must be guided by moral autonomy.[15]

---

[12] *Man and His Future: A Ciba Foundation Volume*, ed. Gordon Wolstenholme (London: J. & A. Churchill Ltd., 1963), p. v.
[13] Kenneth Vaux, ed., *Who Shall Live: Medicine, Technology, Ethics*, Houston Conference on Ethics in Medicine and Technology (1968) (Philadelphia: Fortress Press, 1970), p. 151.
[14] Van Rensselaer Potter, *Bioethics: Bridge to the Future* (Englewood Cliffs, NJ: Prentice-Hall, 1971), p. 49.
[15] Abraham Kaplan, "Social Ethics and the Sanctity of Life: A Summary," in *Life or Death: Ethics and Options*, eds. Edward Shils and Daniel H. Labby (Portland, OR: Reed College, 1968), p. 164.

By returning attention to the individual person as a moral agent, this Kantian-inspired emphasis on moral will gave discussions of progress a different emphasis. It also made clear that the availability of options, that is, negative freedom, did not always lead to patients feeling free. In Kant's theory, autonomy is linked to human dignity and the potential of human beings to realize themselves as reasonable beings. By referencing Kantian theory in this way, early bioethicists laid the groundwork for other theories that associated freedom with the practical impact of realizing one's potential. And it was the nascent bioethics movement that further articulated the connections between medical progress, personal freedom, and the ability to choose reflectively and responsibly.

3.2 The New Bioethics: Progress as Patient Autonomy

With the shift in the locus of progress from the knowledge of scientists to the knowledge of moral agents more generally, patients took on an increasingly important role in assessing whether or not progress was actually being made.[16] This shift was all the more marked since, as Eric Cassell observes, until the late 1960s a patient was not a person.[17] Prior to that era, patients were not considered agents, nor were they expected to make healthcare decisions, a task incumbent on physicians, who were perceived as more detached and rational. In discussions of the moral dimensions of progress, a recurring theme was the need to treat the patient, not as subsidiary to the disease, but as a "whole person." A seminal text, Paul Ramsey's *The Patient as Person* (1970) – one that bears a marked Kantian influence – emphasized that the physician–patient relationship is a covenant, in which healers lessen the effects of sickness, while recognizing the person's dignity and rights. For him, it was precisely the moral character of the physician–patient relationship that enabled "medical progress as a human enterprise."[18]

---

[16] Mark Sullivan, "The New Subjective Medicine: Taking the Patient's Point of View on Health Care and Health," *Social Science & Medicine*, 56 (2003), 1595–1604.

[17] Eric Cassell, *The Nature of Healing: The Modern Practice of Medicine* (Oxford: Oxford University Press, 2013).

[18] Paul Ramsey, *The Patient as Person: Explorations in Medical Ethics* (New Haven, CT: Yale University Press, 1970), p. 37.

3 Medical Progress as Becoming Free 111

At around the same time, the view that patients' bodies had separate existences from their mental lives, as largely presumed by the sciences, became increasingly controversial. Alongside the environmental movements of the 1960s, some argued that the body could no longer be reduced to biochemical processes and genetic characteristics but should rather be seen in a more holistic, integrated perspective. Sickness was increasingly acknowledged as affecting different facets of personhood far beyond the body and suffering linked to patients' psychological and social lives. The clinical insight that – with the exception of some acute infections – all illnesses differ in their outset, course, and treatment depending on the nature of the persons who have them bolstered the idea of individualized treatments and the vision of persons as highly complex entities.[19]

A new openness to patients' emotional reactions, as well as a heightened understanding of the relationship between health and happiness, went together with assigning importance to those aspects of medical care focused on controlling symptoms and ensuring a good quality of life. Reflecting back on these developments, bioethicist Diego Gracia writes that perhaps the most important goal of bioethics was its attempt to link the idea of health with moral well-being and freedom.[20] One way in which the relationship between health and happiness was portrayed at the time was grounded in the capacity of persons to communicate what was important to them. The history of reproductive medicine, for example – the birth control pill was approved by US federal authorities in the 1960s – can be recounted within a narrative of progress toward individual autonomy. Bioethics, therefore, coalesced around the insight that respect for autonomy was an essential part of respecting patients. In this view, patients are not just bodies that can be studied and healed – no matter how benevolently – but rather persons with the capacity to choose the kind of medical progress that makes sense for them.

The desirability of choice in the medical context cannot be considered independently from wider social developments. Indeed, the notion of the freedom of the patient to choose what happens to them in care

---

[19] Eric Cassell, "Pain, Suffering, and the Goals of Medicine," in *The Goals of Medicine*, p. 114, and Cassell, *The Nature of Healing*, p. 115.

[20] Diego Gracia, "A Historical Perspective on the Ends of Medicine," in *The Goals of Medicine*, p. 95.

gained importance alongside broader social movements that claimed rights and earned entitlements. More broadly, civil rights movements, including women's and disability rights, offered a hopeful vision of the future which, notwithstanding the skepticism I have mentioned about the progressive development of history, gave new energy to ideas of progress as freedom. The introduction of the principle of autonomy in medicine was, therefore, framed as a necessary corrective measure that "returned power" to patients but was also the specific result of a much broader emancipation movement that placed increasing emphasis on individual rights.[21]

Autonomy in the medical setting was both the embodiment of a social commitment to freedom and a reaction to a technological, impersonal medicine that seemed increasingly hostile to individuality. Both of these contributed to the association between patient autonomy and the need to preserve a "negative" sphere of freedom from the paternalistic physician, who traditionally attempted to claim expertise in matters that were actually best decided on by the patient. Writing in 1985, American bioethicist and physician Howard Brody suggested that the physician must, in effect, back away and stand aside, presenting different options for consideration by the patient, and thereby avoid influencing their freedom of choice.[22] Standing aside, disengagement, patients' choice: the general ethos of freedom built into these concepts meshed well with a shift in medicine's priorities toward individual responsibility for health. And it fits easily with an attitude toward medical progress that stressed the work required by individuals to attain health.

With the rise of the risk factor model in the mid-twentieth century – identifying factors in patient behavior and habits suspected of contributing to the development of a disease – the capacity for disease management shifted toward the individual. As a consequence, individual responsibility for maintaining one's health was foregrounded.[23]

---

[21] Claudia Wiesemann, "Das Recht auf Selbstbestimmung und das Arzt-Patient-Verhältnis aus sozialgeschichtlicher Perspektive," in *Geschichte und Ethik in der Medizin. Von den Schwierigkeiten einer Kooperation*, eds. R. Toellner and U. Wiesing (Stuttgart: Gustav Fischer, 1997), pp. 67–89.

[22] Howard Brody, "Autonomy Revisited: Progress in Medical Ethics: Discussion Paper," *Journal of the Royal Society of Medicine*, 78 (1985), 381.

[23] Martin Lengwiler and Jeannette Madarász, "Präventionsgeschichte als Kulturgeschichte der Gesundheitspolitik," in *Das präventive Selbst: Eine*

Optimizing a personal healthy lifestyle was intimately bound up with the philosophy of neoliberalism that frames health as a personal matter, linked to individual behavioral and lifestyle choices.[24] But it also linked to a Kantian subtext, whereby knowing one's potential means liberating oneself from previously imposed boundaries. The expectation that people would manage their own health dovetailed with the emphasis on the right – and the responsibility – to make choices about their health. In the words of sociologist Nikolas Rose, in the course of the twentieth century, "[t]he very idea of health was re-figured – the will to health would not merely seek the avoidance of sickness or premature death, but would encode an optimization of one's corporeality to embrace a kind of overall 'well-being'[.]"[25] This enlarged desire for health thus became bound up with more general norms of enterprise and self-actualization and was amplified by the emergence of a rapidly growing consumer market for health. And as Rose and others have pointed out, (potential) patients seek health not because of an obvious form of coercion but because they "freely" choose to be healthy, fit, and responsible; the desire for optimization can be linked to the practical desire to know one's potential.

While not all contributions of the time depicted free choice as the fundamental principle of medical progress, the conceptual framework of bioethics nevertheless associated it with respect for persons, respect for the principle of autonomy, and the ability to do what one wants to do.[26] Emphasizing the particularity of this way of approaching freedom generally went together with reiterating the novelty of this development. That patients were encouraged to have decision-making authority over their health, including their care, could easily be framed as a marked change from preceding decades and as a necessary step in the direction of progress. Writing in 1981, medical ethicist Robert Veatch asserted that never before in the history of

Kulturgeschichte moderner Gesundheitspolitik, eds. Martin Lengwiler and Jeannette Madarász (Bielefeld: Transcript, 2010), pp. 11–28.

[24] See R. Crawford, "You Are Dangerous to Your Health: The Ideology and Politics of Victim Blaming," *International Journal of Health*, 7 (4) (1977), 663–80.

[25] Nikolas Rose, "The Politics of Life Itself," *Theory, Culture & Society*, 18 (6) (2001), 17.

[26] See Renée C. Fox, "The Evolution of American Bioethics: A Sociological Perspective," in *Social Science Perspectives on Medical Ethics*, ed. George Weisz (Dordrecht: Kluwer Academic Publishers, 1990), p. 206.

medicine had there been any acknowledgment of the patient as a dignified agent free to participate in and exercise self-determination over medical decisions.[27]

Such readings, of course, glossed over the extent to which emphasis on the "patient as a person" could be read as a revival of ancient Greek assumptions or how the demand for more accountability from those engaged in medical/human experimentation had nineteenth-century precursors. And progress in what has been called the "era of autonomy"[28] or "autonomy-centered medicine"[29] had its own unresolved issues and tensions. One of its problems was that it privileged a formal, juridical understanding of equal individual rights as a measure of progress. Emphasis on patient choice and independence did not necessarily acknowledge the extent to which a free person depends on social arrangements. And the fact of privileging autonomy was subsequently criticized for being overzealous, in that it neglected other important principles such as justice, non-maleficence, and beneficence.[30] Those interested in tracking the high point of medicine's autonomy era generally place it in the 1970s; writing in 1985, MD Mark Siegler reflected that the "Age of Autonomy" that began in the 1960s was coming to an end.[31] But he still framed it as a "progression" whereby patients gained in freedom and would never return to the previous model of unquestioned physicians' authority.

3.3 Challenges to Negative Freedom

As the above discussion illustrates, in the 1970s, the ideal of autonomy was not overly problematized but rather taken as a given. Personal autonomy, that is, self-determination through choice, was a desirable

---

[27] Robert M. Veatch, "Autonomy's Temporary Triumph," *The Hastings Center Report*, (1984), 38.
[28] Pär Salander and Clare Moynihan, "Facilitating Patients' Hope Work Through Relationship: A Critique of the Discourse of Autonomy," in *Configuring Health Consumers: Health Work and the Imperative of Responsibility*, eds. Roma Harris, Nadine Wathen, and Sally Wyatt (London: Palgrave Macmillan, 2010), p. 117.
[29] Toni C. Saad, "The History of Autonomy in Medicine from Antiquity to Principlism," *Medicine Health Care and Philosophy*, 21 (2018), 133.
[30] Charles Foster, "Autonomy Should Chair Not Rule," *The Lancet*, 375 (2010), 369.
[31] Mark Siegler, "The Progression of Medicine: From Physician Paternalism to Patient Autonomy to Bureaucratic Parsimony," *Archives of Internal Medicine*, 145 (1985), 714.

3 Medical Progress as Becoming Free

trait for patients, that enabled them to make sense of a clinical encounter in which technology was increasingly present and to resist the unfair authority of physicians. However, in a next phase, the formal value of patients' rights was the subject of critical investigation from a number of directions at once. That patient choice trumped paternalism says nothing about the relationship of freedom to the agent's internal, psychological situation. Nor does it engage with the relational aspects of autonomy or fully explore the responsibilities that come with freedom. In the years and decades that followed, widely accepted views of patients as choice-making, independent persons integrated the notion that human beings are both socially and historically situated, as well as have emotional and psychological conditions that are important for realizing freedom. As a rule, this move toward more positive conceptions of freedom was also framed as progress.[32]

These changes also reflect modifications in the patient–physician relationship. From the 1990s, that relationship was reconceived as a "partnership"; as one observer put it, patients were now seen to have "grown up at last."[33] The importance of this shift, whereby healthcare progressively acknowledged the validity of patients' opinions about what happens to them in care, is so great that it has been described as a Copernican revolution in medical practice.[34] And while progress was central to this "revolution," it was bound up with various questions, such as: What are patients' preferred forms of medical progress? What weight should patients' values have and how should clinicians accompany them to honor these values? As we shall see, even as patient freedom became increasingly central to narratives of medical progress, there was no single way in which they were linked together.

3.3.1 Self-Reflexiveness of Patients

One way of reconceptualizing medical progress did so by emphasizing patients' experiences and their inner lives. Work in the 1980s by medical historians Roy Porter, Dorothy Porter, and others tried to recover how patients actually felt as their authority in the medical encounter

---

[32] Brody, "Progress in Medical Ethics," p. 386.
[33] A. Coulter, "Paternalism or Partnership: Patients Have Grown Up – and There's No Going Back," *British Medical Journal*, 319 (7212) (1999), 719–20.
[34] Renaldo N. Battista, "Practice Guidelines for Preventative Care: The Canadian Experience," *British Journal of General Practice*, 43 (1993), 303.

declined.[35] These studies implied that truly capturing the "patient's view" provided a needed challenge to stories of biomedical progress. Within traditional narratives of medicine's progress, patient experience, at least in any extended, self-reflective form, had rarely been given space; now, some privileged patients were increasingly being heard.[36]

In addition to the greater emphasis by historians of medicine on patient experience, various narrative contributions by patients highlight how much suffering occurs in the context of clinical successes.[37] In doing so, these testimonials reveal the gaps and cracks in modernist, linear stories of progress. Instead of freedom, progress, and resolution, much illness experience reveals chaos, vulnerability, and ineffectiveness. Rita Charon and other contributors to narrative ethics have, therefore, argued for the importance of paying attention to patients' stories as a way of making "meaningful" progress.[38] Focusing on narratives for approaching progress also implies distinguishing between disease as a medical condition understood from the viewpoint of the practitioner and illness as a condition experienced by a patient. While disease is contained and possible to resolve, illness is broad and pervasive and can affect all aspects of patients' and families' lives.

Amid this narrative turn, the limitation of the idea of "options" or of choice as tantamount to progress was remarked on by both physicians and patients. Institutionalized practices such as informed consent aimed at respecting patient autonomy were often portrayed by patients as stressful decision-making processes, rather than opportunities to experience agency.[39] HIV and AIDS narratives, as well as accounts of forced choices – involuntary commitment and the end-of-life option to

---

[35] See, for example, Porter, "The Patient's View," 175–98 and Roy Porter and Dorothy Porter, *In Sickness and in Health: The British Experience, 1650–1850* (New York: Basil Blackwell, 1988).

[36] John Wiltshire, "Pathography? Medical Progress and Medical Experience from the Viewpoint of the Patient," *Southerly*, 66 (1) (2006), 27–28.

[37] Anne Hunsaker Hawkins, *Reconstructing Illness: Studies in Pathography* (West Lafayette, IN: Purdue University, 1993), p. 5.

[38] See Rita Sharon's *Narrative Medicine: Honoring the Stories of Illness* (Oxford: Oxford University Press, 2006) and Arthur Kleinman, *The Illness Narratives: Suffering, Healing, and the Human Condition* (New York: Basic Books, 1988).

[39] See, for example, Walter M. Robinson, "The Narrative of Rescue in Pediatric Practice," in *Stories Matter: The Role of Narrative in Medical Ethics*, eds. Rita Charon and Martha Montello (New York, London: Routledge, 2002), p. 109.

3 Medical Progress as Becoming Free

live on a machine or to die – played a prominent role in highlighting the existence of medical failures and futility in the context of ongoing technological progress. Instead of feeling free, and able to shape the process of illness as they might wish, patient accounts significantly complicate ideas about what progress in medicine means.

If patient narratives generally posited freedom and the self as located in the mind as much as the body, their authors sought to capture the importance of positive freedom by emphasizing the psychological and clinical conditions that prevent patients from doing what they want. This view of freedom, which acknowledges how difficult it is to take distance from a situation and to evaluate it critically, adds an additional dimension to the importance of a sphere of private choice.[40] The ability to find self-knowledge, and to engage in moral self-scrutiny, implies that healing illness involves more than acting according to whatever one's values happen to be in a particular moment. Progress of medicine, in this understanding, is analogous to patients' ability to understand the meaning of illness and recovery for themselves. Contributions from narrative medicine demonstrate that as ill people give up their bodies to medicine, they remain very concerned to shape their own stories. Medical sociologist Arthur Frank has framed this desire to hold on to one's own story as resistance, and therefore freedom. He writes that holding on to narrative independence is an important part of patients' self-reflectivity, which, in turn, creates an ideal against which the "progress of the body-self can be measured."[41]

3.3.2 Relational Approaches to Autonomy and Progress in Medicine

Beyond the fact that autonomy intersects with the moral life and sense of self of patients, other visions of progress incorporate the fact that free human beings are fundamentally dependent and deeply embedded in a social context. Further challenges to a negative view of freedom and valorization of privacy were rooted in what has been called a communitarian turn in ethics. This is associated with the concept of relational autonomy, which recognizes relational experiences as

---

[40] Louise Campbell, "Kant, Autonomy and Bioethics," *Ethics, Medicine and Public Health*, 3 (3) (2017), 381–92.

[41] Arthur Frank, *The Wounded Storyteller: Body, Illness, and Ethics* (Chicago: University of Chicago Press, 1995), p. 52.

an integral component of individuality and freedom.[42] And if social relationships, dependencies, and self-trust are integral to freedom, these are particularly visible in the medical setting and have profound implications for health promotion.[43] Care-based and patient-centered approaches to medical ethics, for example, supplement older accounts of autonomy by emphasizing the importance of trust and interdependencies.[44] They also bring to the fore the tortuous path by which individuals struggle with their own moral impulses and the social contexts in which "autonomous" wishes and desires are formulated or oppressed. Autonomy, then, can be reconceived as a way to foster medical progress through non-oppressive caring relationships, and part of the task is understanding how background material, cultural, and social conditions affect health.

The implications for progress of leaving behind traditional individualistic assumptions about patient autonomy and thinking of patients in a fundamentally social and relational way are profound. Medical progress must be evaluated in relation to the extent to which medical interventions support patients' existence as an autonomous subject in meaningful ways, something that is influenced by all dimensions of their life – body, personal biography, relationships with others, social environment, and so on.[45] Given the complex conceptual links between freedom and social norms, simplistic accounts of technological medical progress are misguided. Thus, Susana Magalhães argues that the more scientific and technological progress in medicine, the more powerful and the more vulnerable we become.[46] In this reading, a reconfigured idea of progress needs to acknowledge the extent

---

[42] See Catriona Mackenzie and Natalie Stoljar, eds. *Relational Autonomy: Feminist Perspectives on Autonomy, Agency, and the Social Self* (New York: Oxford University Press, 2000).

[43] See Susan Sherwin, "A Relational Approach to Autonomy in Health Care," in *The Politics of Women's Health: Exploring Agency and Autonomy*, ed. Susan Sherwin (Philadelphia: Temple University Press, 1998), pp. 19–47.

[44] See M. A. Verkerk, "The Care Perspective and Autonomy," *Medicine, Health Care and Philosophy*, 4 (2001), 289–94 and C. Ells, M. R. Hunt, and J. Chambers-Evans, "Relational Autonomy as an Essential Component of Patient-Centered Care," *International Journal of Feminist Approaches to Bioethics*, 4 (2) (2011), 79–101.

[45] Françoise Baylis, Nuala P. Kenny, and Susan Sherwin, "A Relational Account of Public Health Ethics," *Public Health Ethics*, 1 (3) (2008), 196–209.

[46] Susana Magalhães, "Looking behind the Veil: Why Narrative Medicine Matters in Times of Uncertainties," in *Health Humanities for Quality of Care*

to which vulnerability is related to power. The power of new medical technologies can inhibit people's freedom because it can interfere with individuals' ability to choose and act in ways that correspond to their goals and values. Relational autonomy theorists have pointed to the ways in which the ambivalent nature of technological progress in medicine does not necessarily enhance autonomy and the good life, but rather creates new dependencies and pressures to use technologies in the medical context.[47] Once individuals recognize the importance of social, political, and material pressures on their own decisions, a reconstructed idea of progress becomes clearer.[48] This revised vision of progress requires attending to patients in a more holistic sense, as people who must rely on others to be free, but who must also take critical distance from their surroundings to articulate their own conceptions of what a good life involves.

By expanding autonomy in this way, relational approaches have obvious synergies with visions of progress discussed in the next chapters that aim to promote equality (Chapter 4) and rely on an ecological approach to health (Epilogue).[49] Environmental barriers to autonomy, unjust social conditions, and power relationships should all factor into accounts of medical progress. But relational autonomy also provides the theoretical insights for understanding why social and ecological approaches to health need not diminish patient autonomy, but rather enhance it, and how this is linked to better health outcomes. Progress, in this view, is never complete since self-definition is an open-ended process of reflection and revision. An autonomous self is never finalized, but rather constantly being redefined and developed alongside others. Just as we are vulnerable to illness and death throughout our lives, finding self-respect and self-trust in the healthcare context is an ongoing, never-ending process.[50]

---

    in Times of COVID-19, eds. Maria Giulia Marini and Jonathan McFarland (Cham: Springer, 2022), pp. 25–36.

[47] Birgit Beck, "Infantilisation through Technology," in *Technology, Anthropology, and Dimensions of Responsibility*, eds. Birgit Beck and Michael Kühler (Stuttgart: J. B. Metzler, 2020), pp. 33–44.

[48] Jennifer A. Chandler, "'Obligatory Technologies' and the Autonomy of Patients in Biomedical Ethics," *Griffith Law Review*, 20 (4) (2011), 905–30.

[49] See also Alistair Wardrope, "Relational Autonomy and the Ethics of Health Promotion," *Public Health Ethics*, 8 (1) (2015), 50–62.

[50] Janet Delgado, "Re-thinking Relational Autonomy: Challenging the Triumph of Autonomy through Vulnerability," *Bioethics Update*, 5 (2019), 60.

3.3.3 Responsibility, Vulnerability, and Freedom

These insights from relational autonomy for progress were articulated alongside other key contributions to the intellectual history of progress and freedom in the medical context. A recurring aspect of reflections on (medical) technological progress was how the possibilities offered by technologies do not always make us freer and happier, but rather create new dependencies and multiply the reasons to be unhappy. Hans Jonas, an early contributor to bioethics, singled out medicine as the field in which the impetus for progress is particularly marked and linked this directly to human aspirations for a particular kind of freedom.[51] Yet he points out that, envisioned as a quest for unlimited, infinite progress, without a clear final goal, contemporary medicine generates new problems as fast as it resolves others.[52]

Jonas argues that striving for the ideals of progress and liberation ultimately endangers humanity because these ideals disrupt the solidarity and symbiotic relationship between the human and nonhuman natural world. Freedom of choice, for him, therefore needs to be tempered by a bioethical perspective that takes into account human survival on a finite planet and exists in close proximity to responsibility and wisdom.[53] As an action-guiding principle, Jonas proposed a new categorical imperative, namely that all should act so that the effects of that action are compatible with the permanence of genuine human life. And he refers to it as an ethics of preservation and protection that draws attention to the limitations of negative freedom and argues for a more positive view emphasizing adherence to a moral duty.

Jonas and like-minded thinkers emphasized the idea of progress in the medical context because of the way in which it combines the ontological (creating) capacities of technology and the claim that neither history nor the person has yet been fully realized. The result can be a utopian commitment to the higher person who is yet to come and the technology that can bring this about. And in its most ambitious form,

---

[51] Hans Jonas, "Philosophical Reflections on Experimenting with Human Subjects," *Daedalus*, 98 (2) (1969), 231. See also Giacomo Cortesi, "Hans Jonas, il progresso medico e le verità della scienza," *Humana.Mente* 7 (2008), 107–20.

[52] Hans Jonas, "Reflections on Technology, Progress, and Utopia," *Social Research*, 48 (3) (1981), 411–55.

[53] Hans Jonas, *The Imperative of Responsibility: In Search of an Ethics for the Technological Age* (Chicago: University of Chicago, 1984).

the commitment to progress aims at bringing about a disease-free earthly paradise. In particular, if the idea of medical progress becomes the cult of technological possibility without limits, it diminishes the freedom of individuals to choose a life of their own. By reflecting on the potential tensions between technological progress and human autonomy, such arguments caution against taking an instrumental approach to human life, for example in the case of genetic enhancement or continually extending life.[54] If people are not the full moral agents of their actions – for example because they have benefited from genetic enhancement – they are not truly free.

This particular conceptualization of freedom derives from the desire to recognize human beings as responsible authors of their own lives, capable of entering into relationships with others. This approach to progress implies that authentic self-determination involves questioning the dominance of any one technique or technology no matter how useful. In attempting to think through the ramifications of the latest technology for medical progress, we must constantly ask to what extent a technology reveals the patient's holistic nature and relations between human beings. This vision of progress is affiliated with what Lucien Sève has described as progress toward an authentically human existence or progress in humanization.[55] Ultimately, it suggests that freedom and progress in the medical context are far greater than what biotechnology can provide.

3.4 Taking Autonomy Seriously: Freedom versus (Technological) Progress

While the previous pages focused on the importance of philosophically refining the concept of freedom in order to achieve progress, the following examine the practical implications of taking patients' freedom – in all its forms – seriously and the challenges this poses for conventional visions of progress. This section, therefore, highlights some of the concrete ways in which the tensions between freedom and medical progress have surfaced. In effect, the commitment to freedom, and therefore the unpredictable nature of individual and

---

[54] See Jürgen Habermas, *The Future of Human Nature* (Cambridge: Polity Press, 2001).
[55] Lucien Sève, *Pour une critique de la raison bioéthique* (Paris : Odile Jacob, 1994), p. 181.

collective actions, poses a problem for any simultaneous commitment to progress.[56] Taking patient freedom seriously may go against conventional senses of medical progress – for example, choosing to refuse prescribed interventions pushes back against a technology-oriented view of progress – as well as enables unexpected forms of progress to emerge.

3.4.1 Progress and Debates at the End of Life

Debates around the end of life provide perhaps the starkest example of the potential tensions between freedom and some forms of medical progress. The Promethean ambition often associated with progress, namely the defiance and transcendence of fate, is in tension with the notion of inevitable, biological demise.[57] As mentioned earlier, death rates traditionally provided an ostensibly value-free measure for monitoring progress in medicine. Mortality reduction rates are absolutely central to narratives of medical progress and biomedical research. Yet in an era where technological progress often requires that patients or their families choose when to die, the end of life puts the tensions between freedom and progress in sharp relief.

In the course of the twentieth and twenty-first centuries, alongside an increase in the number of deaths occurring in hospitals and intensive care units, there have been a rising number of complaints about how people die. Both palliative care and assisted dying movements – as different as their methods and emphasis are – have sought to reclaim the freedom of terminally ill patients to avoid being subjected to further medical interventions.[58] Faced with death, some patients demanded freedom over their lives, including in decisions about when and how to end them. In particular, the fear of losing autonomy has been widely reported as a strong motive influencing patients to resist life-prolonging treatments. This rejection of certain kinds of medical interventions can, therefore, be framed as an expression of freedom, an act of holding on to freedom before it is taken away.

[56] See Peter Wagner, "Progress and Modernity: The Problem with Autonomy," *Sociología Histórica*, 7 (2017), 87–88.
[57] See Michael Ignatieff, "Modern Dying: The Soul Returns to the Sick Bed," *The New Republic* (26 December 1988), 32
[58] See Nina Streeck, *Jedem seinen eigenen Tod: Authentizität als ethisches Ideal am Lebensende* (Frankfurt, New York: Campus, 2020).

3 Medical Progress as Becoming Free

These considerations occurred alongside a number of attempts to refocus progress on reducing the morbidity of aging populations rather than increasing life expectancy and emphasizing quality rather than quantity of life. In the 1960s, palliative care pioneer Cicely Saunders argued that patients should have the authority to refuse medical interventions because of quality-of-life considerations. In doing so, she sought to reorient progress away from the extension of life and toward each individual patient's journey in which they are able to adjust to and accept what is happening to them.[59] Once medicine is released from the imperative to cure, it engages in other practices that generate forms of progress that would otherwise be lost.[60] Often, progress in palliative care is identified with the prevention and relief of suffering, important goals of medicine distinct from the goal of restoring health; palliative care advocates have tried to refocus medical progress on meeting those goals.[61] Progress in this sense does not aim to find a perfect cure, but rather to meet the complex needs of ill patients, what can be thought of as helping each individual achieve the right balance for themselves in a life that will ultimately end.

If palliative care privileges a very personal understanding of progress, assisted dying – a term that comprises both physician- and patient-administered death – offers a different view of the relationship between freedom and progress. Because of its valorization of personal choice, assisted dying has been referred to as the ultimate case of prioritizing autonomy in healthcare decisions.[62] The philosophical merits of choosing to determine one's own death have ancient roots; for the stoic philosopher Seneca, suicide was the only truly free act possible and therefore ennobling. In contemporary culture suicidality is condemned, but, in some jurisdictions and for some categories of patients, assisted dying is associated with the expression of individual freedom and agency.[63] A prominent Canadian physician active in

---

[59] Cicely Saunders, *Living with Dying: The Management of Terminal Disease* (Oxford: Oxford University Press, 1967), pp. 54–55.
[60] See Daniel Callahan, "Modernizing Mortality: Medical Progress and the Good Society," *The Hastings Center Report*, 20 (1) (1990), 28–32.
[61] Charles F. von Gunten, "Prevent and Relieve Suffering: Professional Palliative Care," *Cancer Investigation*, 21 (6) (2003), 963–64.
[62] Joel Anderson, "Regimes of Autonomy," *Ethical Theory and Moral Practice*, 17 (3) (2014), 362.
[63] See Baril, *Undoing Suicidism* (2023).

medical assistance in dying, Stefanie Green, frames it not as ending someone's life, but rather as empowering patients.[64] Assisted dying laws tend to portray the right to die with assistance as either a liberty or a claim right.

Some terminally ill patients highlight that it is precisely at the end of life, liberated from traditional forms of progress and the valorization of health, that they are able to achieve a kind of freedom unlike anything previously experienced. Swiss author Peter Noll, in his *Diktate über Sterben und Tod* (*In the Face of Death*, 1989 [1984]), recounts the reality of terminal cancer as providing freedom. Since life is what he holds most valuable, and it is being taken anyway, we are left with what Noll refers to as "a feeling of freedom, like a breath of fresh air. The tyranny of imagined needs – the career, the status symbols, the social pressures – becomes increasingly irrelevant, and we feel free."[65] And he notes that death forces us to think, really to think, which in turn is a part of freedom (*ein Teil der Freiheit*). In a contribution from America in a similar era, *Intoxicated by My Illness: And Other Writings on Life and Death* (1992) by Anatole Broyard, Broyard discovers a "tremendous, unprecedented freedom in being ill, a freedom (perhaps for the first time in his life) to say exactly what he wants, and to be just as crazy as he wants."[66]

Given the ways in which technological advances have shaped dying in our time, a liberation-based ethics, together with the option of palliative care, is associated with a good death.[67] And this kind of freedom and death can only be achieved by abandoning a narrative of biomedical progress. But despite calls to see the end of a life as a privileged moment of freedom and to question narratives of medical progress that relentlessly pursue health, the rights of patients to refuse lifesaving treatment or to end their own lives are controversial. From a religious perspective, it is easy to imagine how technological progress

---

[64] Stefanie Green, *This Is Assisted Dying: A Doctor's Story of Empowering Patients at the End of Life* (New York: Scribner, 2022).

[65] Peter Noll, *In the Face of Death*, trans. Hans Noll (New York: Viking, 1989), p. 100.

[66] "Foreward," Oliver Sacks to Anatole Broyard, *Intoxicated by My Illness: And Other Writings on Life and Death* (New York: Random House, 1993), p. xiv.

[67] Meiriany Arruda Lima and Camilo Manchola-Castillo, "Bioethics, Palliative Care and Liberation: A Contribution to 'Dying Well,'" *Revista Bioética*, 29 (2) (2021), 275.

3 Medical Progress as Becoming Free

and a related hubristic instinct, whereby individuals treat death as an occasion to express individual preferences, rather than a shared, cultural experience, can be portrayed negatively. But even without seeing death through a religious lens, observers in Western healthcare systems have drawn attention to the ways in which the reality of death often takes the form of a "wrenching choice" rather than a "deliverance of fate."[68] Another critique of the association between freedom and progress at the end of life has come from disability organizations and mental health professionals, who have highlighted the problems of permissive assisted dying laws for populations in precarious social situations. What is the freedom of the privileged to choose to die can become the oppression of the disadvantaged, who lack positive forms of freedom, such as the resources and support necessary to live well.[69] In such cases, people risk choosing an assisted death because they cannot cope with their living conditions. Even if, for some people, emancipation is associated with the freedom to choose to die, this is not the case for all, and a more nuanced depiction of progress is needed.

3.4.2 Disability Rights and Anti-psychiatry Movements

Traditional stories of medical progress have further been disrupted by theories of freedom within disability rights and anti-psychiatry movements. In the 1970s, the disability rights movement consolidated around the notion that prejudicial attitudes and exclusionary societal practices are far greater barriers to societal participation than the physical or mental impairments of people with disabilities.[70] In doing so, it challenged the "medical model," which views disability in terms of individual difference, deficit, or lack, and focuses on biomedical and technological progress to remedy disability. The movement critically scrutinized contemporary technological developments to address disability – cochlear implants, for example, were developed in the 1960s – that were simultaneously hailed as examples of

---

[68] Callahan, "Modernizing Mortality," p. 29.
[69] See Jonas-Sébastien Beaudry, "Somatic Oppression and Relational Autonomy: Revisiting Medical Aid in Dying through a Feminist Lens," *UBC Law Review*, 2 (53) (2020), 241–98.
[70] Richard K. Scotch, "Politics and Policy in the History of the Disability Rights Movement," *The Milbank Quarterly*, 67 (2) (1989), 380–400.

medical progress.[71] In the societal model they privileged, disabilities are caused by societal norms about access and conceptions of "normal"; ideas about difference and capacity are all defined in social circumstances, and while science remains important, the most important kind of progress is the one that occurs in social institutions and ways of thinking.[72] By invoking the freedom not to have their conditions medicalized, disability activists articulated a sustained critique of traditional forms of medical progress.

Empowerment was a key concept for disability rights movements and related conceptions of progress. Justin Dart Jr., an activist who eventually became known as the Father of the Americans with Disabilities Act, outlined a "revolution of empowerment," which he describes as the elimination of obsolete thought systems and the systematic recognition that every person should live up to their potential.[73] In the decades that followed, the critique of the medical model and accompanying ideas of progress continued to be refined as the disability agenda grew internationally. Rather than portraying disability as a medical problem to be solved, disability studies highlight how we live in a world of norms and how disability cannot be grasped without understanding the norm-generating practices of a given society.[74] The agreement that reductionist tendencies of scientific-medical progress underplay the contextual complexity that creates disability was central to this movement.[75] Advocates have pointed out that health is not an objective state and that curing an organism from a

---

[71] See John B. Christiansen and Irene Leigh, *Cochlear Implants in Children: Ethics and Choices* (Washington, DC: Gallaudet University Press, 2002).

[72] Juliet C. Rothman, "The Challenge of Disability and Access: Reconceptualizing the Role of the Medical Model," *Journal of Social Work in Disability & Rehabilitation*, 9 (2010), 194–222.

[73] See Fred Pelka, *What We Have Done: An Oral History of the Disability Rights Movement* (Boston: University of Massachusetts Press, 2012), p. 167, and Jeanne Hayes and Elizabeth "Lisa" M. Hannold, "The Road to Empowerment: A Historical Perspective on the Medicalization of Disability," *Journal of Health and Human Services Administration*, 30 (3) (2007), 364–66.

[74] Lennard J. Davis, "Constructing Normalcy: The Bell Curve, the Novel, and the Invention of the Disabled Body in the Nineteenth Century," in *The Disabilities Studies Reader*, ed., Lennard J. Davis (New York: Routledge, 1997), p. 3.

[75] See Tom Shakespeare, "The Social Model of Disability," in *The Disability Studies Reader*, ed. Lennard J. Davis, 5th ed. (New York and London: Routledge, 2017), pp. 195–203.

3 Medical Progress as Becoming Free

disease is not the same as establishing its health, as health refers to a complex state of affairs that includes individual experience. The Deaf community, for one, has addressed this issue by observing that Deaf individuals do not need to be "fixed" by cochlear implants.[76] The fact that many individuals are able to transform their medical disability into a cultural identity, as in the case of Deafness, and consider themselves as having good lives, is powerful evidence that not all technological breakthroughs can be equated with medical progress, nor can it be considered an unalloyed good. At the same time, the concept of empowerment remained central to narratives of disability history. In the early 2000s, buses emblazoned with the slogan "The Road to Freedom" conducted national awareness, multimedia campaigns about disability history and community.[77]

Another highly varied movement that consistently linked progress to freedom from medicine was the anti-psychiatry movement, which saw the reduction of medicalization as highly desirable and argued that mentally ill people paid a disproportionate price for the desire for medical progress.[78] In parallel to the disability rights movement, coalitions of people with mental disabilities reconceptualized liberation and progress, while also illustrating some of the ways in which freedom is in direct tension with conventional stories of progress. In the early 1970s, psychiatric survivors began to come together and call for a kind of self-determination that could not be found within the medical establishment. Psychiatric patients organized around the connecting theme of patients' rights and drew on other minority groups' use of the term "liberation" to call for their freedom from oppressive medicalization and institutions.[79] Also known as the ex-patient liberation movement, they sought to expose a system that forced patients

---

[76] Amelia Cooper, "Hear Me Out: Hearing Each Other for the First Time: The Implications of Cochlear Implant Activation," *Missouri Medicine*, 116 (6) (2019), 469–71.

[77] Disability Rights Education & Defense Fund, "Road to Freedom," https://dredf.org/2006/11/15/road-to-freedom/ and Gary Arnold, "ADA Legacy Tour: Get on the Bus!," Abilities.com, The Resource for the Disability Community, www.abilities.com/community/ada-bus-tour.html.

[78] See Andrew Scull, *Desperate Remedies: Psychiatry's Turbulent Quest to Cure Mental Illness* (Cambridge, MA: Harvard University Press, 2022).

[79] See Doris Zames Fleischer and Frieda Zames, *The Disability Rights Movement: From Charity to Confrontation* (Philadelphia: Temple University Press, 2011), p. 119.

to accept treatment against their will, including involuntary institutionalization, forced drugging, electroconvulsive therapy, and – most dramatically – lobotomies.

Patient-centered histories drew attention to how oppressive so-called medical progress was for those who experienced its effects firsthand. In 1978, Judith Chamberlin published *On Our Own: Patient-Controlled Alternatives to the Mental Health System*, an account of her mental health journey that contrasted the authoritarian way mental health services were traditionally structured with alternatives that she argued were far more suited to addressing patients' needs. If mental illness is associated with biological sources, that means the responsibility for resolving the problem lies with the individual and typically requires a pharmacological intervention, as opposed to a broader range of caring and social actions.[80] Chamberlin, together with other activists, put patient self-determination at the heart of their philosophical and political framework and emphasized the problems of a restrictive medical model of mental health, as well as those inherent in the inhumane treatment of patients. The primary objective of the mental health system, patient and activist Rae Unzicker wrote, should be to "put itself out of business."[81] A major impact of calls to resist the medical establishment in the name of freedom occurred in Italy, where a law passed in 1978 directly closed all psychiatric hospitals, though the brusqueness of the measure ended up being very hard on patients. The multifaceted public resources required to further progress by accompanying patients and providing community integration and support remained conspicuous by their absence.

3.4.3 Freedom to Refuse: Anti-vaccination Movements and Medical Progress

Before concluding this section on the potential ways in which individual freedom disrupts narratives of medical progress, I want to discuss one more example, that of anti-vaccination movements. Vaccines have been referred to as one of the greatest achievements of modern

---

[80] See Joseph E. Davis, *Chemically Imbalanced: Everyday Suffering, Medication, and Our Troubled Quest for Self-Mastery* (Chicago: University of Chicago Press, 2020).

[81] See Rae Unzicker, "On My Own: A Personal Journey through Madness and Re-emergence," *Psychosocial Rehabilitation Journal*, 13 (1) (1989), 76.

medicine as well as crucial for saving lives during the COVID-19 pandemic.[82] The history of vaccines reveals significant advances in understanding disease vectors and immunology, as well as in the ability to make and distribute vaccines at scale. And yet, anti-vaccine sentiments are on the rise. Vaccine hesitancy, which is also the rejection of a particular kind of medical progress, is currently described as a major risk to global public health.[83] Indeed, it has been portrayed as precisely what is undermining general progress trends in medicine.[84]

The arguments of vaccine skeptics, to be sure, are marked by their plurality, and the shifting reasons for vaccine hesitancy were all already present since the development of vaccines. Recent studies confirm that the decision to vaccinate is a complex process, in which both cognitive and emotional factors play a role.[85] But despite this complexity, the strand of thinking that rejects vaccines in favor of individual rights and autonomy gained new prominence in recent years.

Arguments for individual liberty and against vaccines cut across political and geographical divides. Traditionally, the anti-vaccination movement has been associated with a libertarian distrust of the medical establishment. Anti-vaccination sentiments have a large overlap with support for alternative medicine broadly conceived and a certain skepticism toward conventional medicine (*Schulmedizin*) and big pharma. They are also associated with the view that science is just one way of perceiving reality, among other valid ones. Compulsory vaccination is perceived as encroaching on people's liberty and contrary to the right of parental control, ideological arguments that have remained remarkably similar over time.[86] Discussing a vaccine bill in Colorado, one parent refers to the bill as "a step toward the complete

---

[82] See this comment by former US Surgeon General Jerome Adams, @JeromeAdamsMD, https://twitter.com/JeromeAdamsMD/status/1711912940721299584 and his book, *Crisis and Chaos: Lessons from the Front Lines of the War against COVID-19* (Nashville, TN: Post Hill Press, 2023).

[83] The World Health Organization, "Ten Threats to Global Health in 2019," www.who.int/emergencies/ten-threats-to-global-health-in-2019.

[84] Azhar Hussain et al, "The Anti-Vaccination Movement: A Regression in Modern Medicine," *Cureus*, 10 (7) (2018), e2919.

[85] Noni E. MacDonald, SAGE Working Group on Vaccine Hesitancy, "Vaccine Hesitancy: Definition, Scope and Determinants," *Vaccine*, 33 (34) (2015), 4161–64.

[86] Rob Boddice, "Vaccination, Fear and Historical Relevance," *History Compass*, 14 (2) (2016), 71–78.

erosion of our medical freedom."⁸⁷ The freedom they are referring to is the freedom of parents to choose whether or not to vaccinate their child, rather than being obliged to do so by medical institutions. Attributing responsibility for health to individuals and their immediate families, rather than healthcare institutions, reoccurs among those opposed to vaccines both today and in the past. It is heard in the "my body my choice" anti-vaccination slogan (originally a feminist slogan referring to women's rights to reproductive choices), the Swiss *Freiheitstrychler* (Freedom ringers), and in posters with messages like "freedom not fear," "we do not consent," and so on.

In addition to a general skepticism of conventional narratives of medical progress, anti-vaccine sentiments are associated with a more general distrust of public institutions, which emphasizes individual experience and liberty while questioning the validity of "expertise."⁸⁸ The freedom not to vaccinate is a manifestation of the more general concern not to have the government impose one specific vision of progress. But the freedom invoked by anti-vaccine advocates tends to be much less concerned with the implications of that refusal for the freedoms of others, namely the health and well-being of society at large. In most cases, the arguments in favor of freedom do not take due account of the necessary tension between different freedoms in society and the need to find a compromise between them. Neither do they acknowledge the extent to which the free person depends on social arrangements, in particular the social solidarity offered by a well-functioning health system.

Even as anti-vaccine advocates are often portrayed as opposed to medical progress, their concerns for safety and capacity to provide civic oversight have had positive effects. For example, relatively high rates of vaccine hesitancy among certain communities have shed additional light on preexisting problems of healthcare, such as institutionalized racism.⁸⁹ The existing strategic interests of various stakeholders and the legacies of colonialism have been made newly visible

---

⁸⁷ Cited in Arthur Allen, "How the Anti-Vaccine Movement Crept into the GOP Mainstream," *Politico*, May 27, 2019, www.politico.com/story/2019/05/27/anti-vaccine-republican-mainstream-1344955.
⁸⁸ See Maya J. Goldenberg, *Vaccine Hesitancy: Public Trust, Expertise, and the War on Science* (Pittsburgh, PA: Pittsburgh University Press, 2021).
⁸⁹ See the Wellcome Trust-funded project, *Healthy Scepticism*, www.healthyscepticism.com.

in various large-scale vaccination campaigns.⁹⁰ The vaccine success story is, therefore, marred by imperialism and paternalism and in general reflects broader structural failures across global health. But in general, vaccination is a field in which the potential tensions between the constraints imposed on individual behavior and the well-being of all have played out. As examples of major public health issues, vaccination campaigns illustrate particularly well the tensions between different kinds of medical progress – between the freedom of individuals and the health needs of society at large, between the scientific power of the few, and the complexities that come with using that power to improve health outcomes for all.

3.5 Reclaiming Progress as Freedom

Despite the tensions and oppositions described above, and the fact that the emphasis on freedom points toward no single practice or action for medicine, the political association between freedom and progress has remained considerable. Patient autonomy remains the best-known principle of medical ethics and a widely accepted value for defining medical progress. Philosopher Somogy Varga holds that medicine's final aim is to enhance human autonomy; meanwhile, "[t]he more autonomy in medicine, the more progress" has been described as one of the main presuppositions of contemporary medicine.⁹¹ Indeed, as a rule patient freedom is portrayed as highly compatible with medical progress. And this compatibility is a key part of the so-called "liberation mythology" that associates digitalization with both progress and patients being empowered to take control of their health.⁹²

Since the early 2000s and the advent of Web 2.0, mobile devices like smartphones, tablets, and wearables have all had a significant

---

[90] Mosoka P. Fallah & S. Harris Ali, "When Maximizing Profit Endangers our Humanity: Vaccines and the Enduring Legacy of Colonialism during the COVID-19 Pandemic," *Studies in Political Economy*, 103 (1) (2022), 94–10.

[91] Ignass Devisch, "Progress in Medicine: Autonomy, Oughtonomy and Nudging," *Journal of Evaluation in Clinical Practice* 17 (2011), 857. See Somogy Varga, "The Aim of Medicine. Sanocentricity and the Autonomy Thesis," *Pacific Philosophical Quarterly*, 104 (4) (2023), 720–45 and Somogy Varga, *Science, Medicine, and the Aims of Inquiry* (Cambridge: Cambridge University Press, 2024).

[92] On liberation mythology, see Nicholas Carr, *Utopia Is Creepy and Other Provocations* (New York: W. W. Norton & Company, 2016).

impact on how individuals experience and perceive health. So too have social media platforms, citizen science initiatives, and platforms such as PatientsLikeMe, HealthBoards, or WebMD, which allow patient communities to gain and share information. The digital prosumer, a term coined to show how the distinction between producers and consumers of (online) content has been fundamentally blurred, has also emerged as one uniquely able to drive progress. The health data that is continuously generated from patients' devices contains a vast amount of potentially useful knowledge. Part of the hype is linked to the accessibility and democratization of knowledge: If rapid information acquisition and knowledge sharing without geographical constraints are possible for a larger number of people, these processes can be portrayed as increasingly democratic and egalitarian and reframed as human progress.[93] While the doctor has traditionally been the gatekeeper for medical knowledge and making medical decisions, in the artificial intelligence era, this hierarchy is portrayed as having been overcome; it is possible that medical knowledge that forms the basis of decision-making will be as accessible to the patient as to the doctor.[94]

In this worldview, progress is associated with encouraging people to voluntarily undertake practices to improve their health and fitness. As one enthusiast puts it, the old thinking "My health is the responsibility of my physician" is fundamentally outdated; the new thinking is that "My health is my responsibility, *and I have the tools to manage it*" (my emphasis).[95] These "digitally engaged"[96] patients are portrayed as at the forefront of this particular type of medical progress. As depicted in the influential *Topol Review*, a report for the British National Health System on its digital strategy, individuals will increasingly generate their own health data, and AI will transform this data into clinically useful information and empower patients to manage their own health

---

[93] Brynjolfsson and McAfee, *The Second Machine Age*, p. 86.
[94] Xiaoxuan Liu, Pearse A. Keane, and Alastair K. Denniston, "Time to Regenerate: The Doctor in the Age of Artificial Intelligence," *Journal of the Royal Society of Medicine*, 111 (4) (2018), 115.
[95] Melanie Swan, "Health 2050: The Realization of Personalized Medicine through Crowdsourcing, the Quantified Self, and the Participatory Biocitizen," *Journal of Personalized Medicine*, 2 (2012), 108.
[96] Deborah Lupton, "The Digitally Engaged Patient: Self-Monitoring and Self-Care in the Digital Health Era," *Social Theory and Health*, 11 (3) (2013), 256–70.

3 Medical Progress as Becoming Free 133

or seek appropriate support.[97] Digitalization and the deciphering of the genome are consistently portrayed as underpinning one of the most profound disruptions in medicine ever experienced. And related trends toward the decentralization of care and decision-making are consistently framed as game-changing forms of progress; the head of a major Montreal hospital, Dr. Lawrence Rosenberg, argued in a 2019 workshop that they are precisely what enable patients, for the first time ever, to take control of their health.[98]

3.5.1 Personalized, Participatory Medical Progress

Within the broader recasting of digital medicine and narratives of progress, personalized medicine plays a unique role. Personalized medicine aims to develop therapies based on individuals' unique molecular, clinical, and lifestyle information, using emerging, data-intensive means to do so. It is also the product of developments in biology that made it possible to carry out molecular analyses of and interventions in fundamental biological processes. Looking at organisms, their health and disease, through a genetic and biochemical lens, has been called a "molecular revolution" with multiple practical applications.[99] Capitalizing on this enthusiasm for a new way of framing disease, the editors of a recent book on its ethics observe that the term personalized medicine has become "the symbol of medical progress" and a label for better medical care in general.[100]

---

[97] *The Topol Review. Preparing the Healthcare Workforce to Deliver the Digital Future: An Independent Report on Behalf of the Secretary of State for Health and Social Care*, NHS Health Education England, February 2019, p. 47.

[98] Lawrence Rosenberg, "Disintermediation," Presentation Given at *Workshop: Medicine without Doctors? Disintermediation and Patient Agency*, 4th Workshop on the Impact of Technological Change on the Surgical Profession, May 8, 2019, Jewish General Hospital, Montréal.

[99] Michel Morange, *The Black Box of Biology: A History of the Molecular Revolution*, trans. M. Cobb (Cambridge, MA: Harvard University Press, 2020) and Robert Olby, "The Molecular Revolution in Biology," in *Companion to the History of Modern Science*, eds. G. N. Cantor et al. (London: Routledge, 1996), pp. 503–20.

[100] Jochen Vollmann, Verena Sandow, Sebastian Wäscher, and Jan Schildmann, eds., *The Ethics of Personalised Medicine: Critical Perspectives* (Farnham: Ashgate, 2015), p. 1. See also George Annas, "The Songs of Spring: Quest Myths, Metaphors, and Medical Progress," in *Ethics and the Arts*, ed. Paul Macneil (Dordrecht: Springer, 2014), p. 226.

These references to a conceptual revolution help explain why the hyperbolic language of progress so significant it will eliminate all diseases has resurfaced in reference to molecular biology and digitization. At an event marking the completion of the first draft of the human genome, US President Bill Clinton claimed that it is now conceivable that "our children's children will know the term 'cancer' only as a constellation of stars," while British Prime Minister Tony Blair characterized this "revolution in medical science" as having implications that "far surpass even the discovery of antibiotics."[101] Advocates of personalized, also called genomic, medicine maintain that it represents revolutionary progress not just in treatment possibilities but also in how patients are empowered to take control of their health. Francis Collins, a prominent figure in genomics research in the United States, describes the success of personalized medicine as developing alongside the need for each individual to take responsibility for their own health. And he uses the language of revolution and "paradigm shift" to underscore both the novelty and the possibilities of citizens living "life to the fullest" by harnessing this new research for health.[102]

Personalized medicine capitalizes on the language of empowerment, but it gives freedom a different meaning beyond individual rights in healthcare decisions. Advances in DNA sequencing, combined with the emergence of large biobanks in the 1990s, were linked with a shift from individual choice and control to concepts such as partnership and participation.[103] As a rule, the need for a participatory approach in medicine has been persistently characterized as the extension of what honoring patient autonomy really entails. In 2015, Barack Obama launched the Precision Medicine Initiative, which aimed to inaugurate a new era of medicine as well as to empower patient-participants.[104] Specifically, patient engagement has been portrayed as driving the progress of more personalized and efficacious medical

---

[101] "Remarks made by the President, Tony Blair, Francis Collins, and Craig Venter," The White House, Office of the Press Secretary, June 26, 2000, www.genome.gov/10001356.

[102] Francis Collins, *The Language of Life: DNA and the Revolution in Personalized Medicine* (New York: Harper Perennial, 2011), pp. xxiv, 275.

[103] See Alessandro Blasimme and Effy Vayena, "Becoming Partners, Retaining Autonomy: Ethical Considerations on the Development of Precision Medicine," BMC Medical Ethics, 67 (2016), 2.

[104] The Precision Medicine Initiative, The White House, President Barack Obama, https://obamawhitehouse.archives.gov/precision-medicine.

products. Medical progress is regularly framed as personalized, preventative medicine that relies on patient choice and participation.[105]

Participating in processes that affect one's life is a key element of positive freedom. But despite the rhetoric of participation and sharing, personalized health is associated not so much with open, representative spaces as with commodified ones. Among those who are empowered or likely to be given more opportunities by personalized medicine are those patients who are interested in their genomic data and can afford to access it. The line separating voluntary health promotion practices, individualized health states, and government and corporate strategies is increasingly blurred.[106] Powerful private actors, such as Google and genetic testing companies, also profit. The equation these companies propose between participation and empowerment serves their commercial interests, as they go on to benefit from access to valuable biomedical resources, profit from public funding, and yet are not accountable to the public.[107] Claims about empowering patients are associated with the notion of the consumer-patient, who is able to receive test results directly and make health decisions while bypassing doctors. It also creates demand, using the rhetoric of empowerment to give patients a stake in the movement itself. In doing so, the language of predictive, preventive, personalized, and participatory medicine intentionally avoids the word patient in favor of the client[108] and thereby disrupts the traditional fiduciary nature of the physician–patient relationship in which the patients' interests are paramount (in contrast to caveat emptor or buyer beware). It also shifts the responsibility for healthcare away from collective forms of freedom, as guaranteed by social and political structures, and onto individual patients.

---

[105] Margaret Anderson and K. Kimberly McCleary, "From Passengers to Co-pilots: Patient Roles Expand," *Science Translational Medicine*, 7 (291) (2015), 291fs25 and Matthias Orth et al., "Redefining the Role of the Physician in Laboratory Medicine in the Context of Emerging Technologies, Personalised Medicine and Patient Autonomy ('4P Medicine')," *Journal of Clinical Pathology*, 72 (3) (2019), 194.

[106] Tamar Sharon, "Self-Tracking for Health and the Quantified Self: Re-articulating Autonomy, Solidarity, and Authenticity in an Age of Personalized Healthcare," *Philosophy of Technology*, 30 (2017), 93–121.

[107] See Donna Dickenson, *Me Medicine vs. We Medicine: Reclaiming Biotechnology for the Common Good* (New York: Columbia University Press, 2013).

[108] Matthias Orth et al., "Redefining the Role of the Physician," p. 195.

To recall, what genomic science can provide is, first, probabilistic knowledge about a patient's possible chances of being affected by various ailments and, second, information about a patient's potential response to specific treatments. The prospective empowerment of patients, therefore, must be compared with other information relevant to understanding, preventing, or treating disease and other types of choices that may be more significant with regard to health.[109] Biostatistician Melody Goodman has spoken to this issue by highlighting the way in which personalized medicine does not fully capture the social determinants of health and noting that, in fact, zip codes are a better predictor of health than genetic codes.[110] A further problem from the perspective of patient autonomy is how incidental findings should be managed and whether the patient should be informed about them.[111] This is linked to the fact that patients tend to have very little control over what kinds of personal data are collected and how they go on to be used, for example by insurance companies.

Genomic technologies capitalize on the language of medical progress in several ways. The association between personalized medicine, the self-actualizing individual, and the "personalism" of a caring physician–patient relationship offers a rhetorically powerful view of progress. Personalized medicine in the sense of genomic medicine has profited from this vagueness, without offering a clear commitment to holistic, person-centered care.[112] Another way in which genomic technologies have been associated with an idea of progress is through their aim to provide both high-quality individualized care and increasingly accessible health services for all. In a special issue devoted to personalized medicine, the President of ETH Zürich Lino Guzzella claims that "medicine for all" is soon going to become a reality and links

---

[109] Eric Juengst, Michael A. Flatt, and Richard A. Settersten, Jr., "Personalized Genomic Medicine and the Rhetoric of Empowerment," *Hastings Center Report*, 42 (5) (2012), 35.

[110] Melody Goodman, cited in "Zip Code Better Predictor of Health than Genetic Code," News, Harvard T. H. Chan School of Public Health, 4 August 2014, www.hsph.harvard.edu/news/features/zip-code-better-predictor-of-health-than-genetic-code/.

[111] G. de Wert et al., "Opportunistic Genomic Screening. Recommendations of the European Society of Human Genetics," *European Journal of Human Genetics*, 29 (2021), 365–77.

[112] See Miriam Solomon, *Making Medical Knowledge* (Oxford: Oxford University Press, 2016).

3 Medical Progress as Becoming Free

personalized medicine with the impressive medical progress of the past decades.[113] The twin promise of better health outcomes and lower costs recurs in the current enthusiasm for digital technologies and for genomics in particular. Yet just how accessible these tools are remains to be seen; so far, the increased costs associated with personalized medicine are considerable.[114]

3.5.2 Human Enhancement as Progress and Liberation

One further domain that is portrayed as the final frontier of the liberation of human beings through progress in medicine is human enhancement. Enhancement refers to a range of technological (i.e., cosmetic/plastic surgery), psychopharmaceutical, or genomic interventions to improve human beings, allowing them to function beyond a normal range, and therefore can blur with personalized medicine.[115] Preventative and enhancing medicine have been described as inseparable, and both are associated with the rise of personalized medicine and the existence of active and informed healthcare consumers who want to exercise choice in the medical context. Both enhancement and personalized medicine emphasize the shift within the physician–patient relationship toward the patient-consumer, the ways in which digitalization facilitates this shift and associated freedoms.

At the simplest level, to enhance something is to improve it; the concept of enhancement thus contains in itself the notion of progress. Like many forms of medical progress, enhancement explicitly aspires to overcome limitations, in this case, those associated with human biology. It is possible to argue that enhancement is the logical extension of medical progress itself, which is constantly aggrandizing medicine's traditional therapeutic mandate.[116] As discussed previously, medical

---

[113] "Medizin Nach Mass: Mit Personalisierter Medizin zur Gesundheit von Morgen," *ETH Zürich Globe*, 1 (2018), 3.
[114] Elvio Baccarini, "Personalized Medicine, Justice and Equality," in N. Bodiroga-Vukobrat et al., eds., *Personalized Medicine in Health Care Systems* (Switzerland: Springer Nature, 2019), pp. 137–47.
[115] See Philip Brey, "Human Enhancement and Personal Identity," in *New Waves in Philosophy of Technology*, eds. Jan Kyrre Berg Olsen, Evan Selinger, and Søren Riis (New York: Palgrave Macmillan, 2008), pp. 169–85.
[116] Ulrich Körtner, "The Challenge of Genetic Engineering to Medical Anthropology and Ethics," *Human Reproduction and Genetic Ethics*, 7 (1) (2001), 22.

progress is responsible for determining what counts as normal human functioning; without the insights of bacteriology, "normal" human life span and health look different from what they are now. Some have associated precisely the blurring between therapy and enhancement with the implicit goals of biomedical progress, namely a definitive understanding of the causes of disease, as well as the indefinite extension of human life.[117]

The concept of freedom is inevitably front and center in the debate over human enhancement, which has been characterized as essentially a debate about human freedom.[118] This focus on freedom has been associated with a perceived harmony between choosing among different options and positive freedom in the sense of a self-ruled life. Bioethicist John Harris, for example, has argued that enhancement will allow humans to live more freely because they will not fear illness, pain, and premature death to the same extent; it will therefore allow them more control over their bodies and their destinies.[119] Being free can be equated with using technology to do what humans have done throughout history, namely to try and improve/enhance their lives using different means.

Proponents of enhancement have argued, furthermore, that the rationale for enhancement harmonizes the requirements of freedom and justice.[120] Harris, for one, argues that we are obligated to pursue human enhancement, as he sees biotechnological means as simply the most recent in a long series that human beings have used to improve themselves.[121] If arguments in favor of enhancement typically rely on an understanding of freedom as increasing human control, the close association they posit between freedom and control elides an easy

---

[117] However, for a distinction between enhancement and therapy, see Robert Sparrow, "Better than Men? Sex and the Therapy/Enhancement distinction," *Kennedy Institute of Ethics Journal*, 20 (2) (2010), 115–44.

[118] Ramez Nam, *More than Human: Embracing the Promise of Biological Enhancement* (New York: Broadway Books, 2005), p. 9 and Jan-Christoph Heilinger and Katja Crone, "Human Freedom and Enhancement," *Medicine Health Care and Philosophy*, 17 (1) (2014), 13–21

[119] John Harris, *Enhancing Evolution: The Ethical Case for Making Better People* (Princeton, NJ: Princeton University Press, 2011).

[120] Allen Buchanan, Dan W. Brock, Norman Daniels, and Daniel Winkler, *From Chance to Choice: Genetics and Justice* (Cambridge: Cambridge University Press, 2000).

[121] John Harris, *Enhancing Evolution*, p. 9.

distinction with justice. In general, advances in medicine have made addressing what was previously considered "natural" a requirement of justice. As Martha Nussbaum has clarified, many things that may previously have been considered a given now appear as things that people can change and may even have an obligation to change.[122]

At the same time, there are descriptive and normative reasons to challenge the notion that the enhancement of individuals will be empowering for all patients. For example, gene editing that enables parents to make important decisions regarding their children's health for enhancement purposes remains controversial. In this case, the perceived difference between therapy and enhancement is crucial in the minds of the public; 83 percent of citizens in a US public opinion survey found that genetic modification to make a baby smarter would be "taking medical advances too far."[123] Furthermore, implying that health exists in a stable way, and that attaining it is our shared goal, mistakenly assumes that one particular kind of medical progress can achieve it. In practice, however, if the specific technologies of enhancement are used to assess progress toward a purportedly stable goal, they can narrow our understanding of what means we have to achieve health. Bioethicist and disability studies professor Rosemarie Garland-Thomson, reflecting on the dangers of devalorizing variations between humans through enhancement techniques, calls, not for upgrading humans to fit better with the world, but rather for improving the world so that it can be more welcoming to all human experiences. This, she observes, could be done by using insights from disability culture, theories of justice, and inclusive technologies to make a shared world welcoming to the widest range of users.[124]

Other critics of enhancement point out that the freedom of some is not consistent with justice for all. When deployed in existing, unequal social contexts, enhancements are more likely to exacerbate rather than

---

[122] Martha Nussbaum, "Review of Allen Buchanan, Dan W. Brock, Norman Daniels, and Daniel Winkler, *From Chance to Choice* (2000)," in *Philosophical Interventions: Reviews 1986–2011* (Oxford: Oxford University Press, 2012), pp. 234–45.

[123] Antonio Regalado, "Engineering the Perfect Baby," *MIT Technology Review*, 118 (3) (2015), 26–33.

[124] Rosemarie Garland-Thomson, "Welcoming the Unexpected," in *Human Flourishing in an Age of Gene Editing*, ed. Erik Parens and Josephine Johnston (Oxford: Oxford University Press, 2019).

alleviate social injustices.[125] Those who can initially afford these technologies will see their privileges amplified by enhancements, whether physical, cognitive, or psychological, and existing social inequalities will increase. Neither is it a given that today's major health problems are being well served by proposed enhancement technologies. If human enhancement is a question of improving some aspects of health with expensive, scarce technologies, it has very little relevance to the health needs of the general population. Health goals that are achievable in the present may be undermined when funds are spent on a future health goal, the ramifications of which are unclear and potentially give rise to unwanted results. Ultimately, defining what counts as progress and liberation remains a question of power.

3.6 Conclusion

Since roughly the 1970s, ideas about freedom and medical progress are bound up together in new ways. The ambiguities inherent in increases in scientific medical knowledge led to the development of a new idea of progress that shifted in focus and content. Against the notion of a technologically deterministic idea of fate, and of paternalistic physicians deciding what was best for their patients, progress was henceforth connected to the idea of patients as persons, with their own values and choices. This development dovetailed with the broader emphasis on individual rights in the context of various emancipation movements.

However, freedom played a fluid and at times unruly role in discussions of progress. Part of this is due to the fact that there is no single understanding of the relationship between positive and negative forms of freedom, and arguments for freedom were used both for and against technological forms of medical progress. The initial move to (re)install the patient at the center of healthcare, and the birth of bioethics that paid due attention to patient beliefs, was marked by optimism. In subsequent years, a number of challenges to the predominance of individual rights in healthcare came from various sources. From the philosophical side, a new emphasis on the relationality of

---

[125] Tamara Garcia and Ronald Sandler, "Enhancing Justice?," *Ethics and Emerging Technologies*, ed. R. L. Sandler (London: Palgrave Macmillan, 2014).

3 Medical Progress as Becoming Free

autonomy questioned whether freedom could be honored with the provision of treatment options or whether it needed to be rethought much more collectively. Others questioned whether authentic freedom could even be obtained in a cultural mindset that privileged technological progress. Further, deep-seated challenges came from those who saw the affirmation of freedom as their right to oppose various forms of progress.

Yet the Enlightenment dream of an uncomplicated relationship between freedom and progress continues in many instances to thrive. Digital medicine is full of references to how particular technologies and applications will liberate patients and empower them through their own participation in medical treatment. Pushed to the extreme, these assumptions about freedom point in the direction of human enhancement and genetic engineering and a new view of selfhood for the digital age. The most sustained critiques of these particular views of progress emphasize the role of the state and society in ensuring the self-determination of their citizens. In the next Chapter, I want to turn to a particular form of this critique, one that emphasizes health in a community and argues that not freedom, but rather justice is the correct concept to anchor theories of progress in medicine.

4 "Health for All"
Medical Progress as Justice

In the first decades of the twenty-first century, the visions of medical progress I monitored in previous chapters remain intact. Medical progress as increased biomedical knowledge of the body, as taking charge of one's own health; these are important instantiations of the belief in progress in medicine. There is, however, another idea of progress, informed by research on different forms of oppression, including racism, sexism, and classism, that became increasingly prominent in discussions about how to improve human health. In the context of neoliberal policies of the 1990s, the idea that people are a product of intersecting circumstances beyond their control (re)emerged as a topic with implications for health, illness, and well-being. The related notion of progress was associated not so much with the "endless frontier" of knowledge, as Vannevar Bush described it,[1] nor with individual empowerment. Rather, it is connected with addressing powerlessness and social action to ensure that medical advances are more equitably shared.

As researchers from different fields used various tools and methods to shed additional light on long-standing health inequities, they (re)expanded the scope of the idea of progress in medicine beyond the narrow provision of care to a wide range of social and economic factors affecting health. The terminology also shifted from (narrow) medical progress to (wider) health progress, and this shift reflects a diminished role for specifically medical resources in ensuring better health. For this reason, while access to medical progress strictly speaking remains important, it is increasingly seen as only one of multiple factors determining health and illness. Some used the idea of health justice to create a new language of progress whereby any advance or forward movement should be judged according to roughly left-wing standards. The first World Health Organization (WHO) Commission

[1] See Chapter 2.

on Social Determinants of Health, established in 2008, published a report stating that social injustice is "killing people on a grand scale" and demanded progress toward "closing the gap."[2] For other actors, however, the idea of progress is too associated with irreversible meliorative change, which has little bearing on the persistently precarious health situations they want to bring into view. Finally, various critiques analyze the assumptions underpinning progress as health justice and argue that causality between equity and health is overstated or that action to address social inequalities involves inflating the notion of health to the extent that it loses meaning. Reappearing in these analyses are both the harmony-based and pluralistic visions of progress I have traced throughout this book.

This chapter tracks debates on progress and social justice as they evolve from the post-war period, but it focuses particularly on the late 1980s onward. While the social model of health had various influential early proponents, it was in the early 1990s that the notion of addressing health justice garnered enough momentum to challenge fundamentally previous ideas of medical progress in academia and beyond. The critique of a medical marketplace, the perceived need to dismantle an autonomy-based notion of progress, and a certain sociopolitical optimism all contributed to reimagining medical progress by placing social factors beyond healthcare front and center. As in previous chapters, I monitor transnational developments pertaining to the idea of progress, but with a special emphasis on medicine. Part of the story told in this chapter is the extent to which increased knowledge of the social determinants of health is portrayed as embodying progress. But the story is, of course, incomplete without reference to how this knowledge can be channeled into action to mitigate illness. Here, the question of action proves a particularly thorny one, as despite the strong evidence for the health impacts of social inequities, attempts to make cumulative progress on these issues have been fraught. I end the chapter with a case study of the COVID-19 pandemic. While I cannot analyze these events from a distant historical perspective, they nevertheless offer a powerful illustration of the way in which several ideas discussed here play out in real time. The extent to which COVID-19

---

[2] Commission on Social Determinants of Health, *Closing the Gap in a Generation: Health Equity through Action on the Social Determinants of Health*, Final Report (Geneva: World Health Organization, 2008), p. 26.

revealed existing social fractures and determinants of ill health in societies that think of themselves as at the vanguard of medical progress, the realities of the global vaccine rollout; these provide further material for a vision of health as occurring in a much larger ecosystem than previously thought and corresponding ideas of progress as social justice.

4.1 Progress as Medical Access: Origins

The previous chapter scrutinized some visions of social progress achieved through global markets and driven by new technologies; many are associated with the belief that capitalism is a powerful agent of collective progress. Indeed, many neoliberal philosophies of progress frame both the advancement of science and practices of self-improvement as inherently contributing to the public good.[3] The idea of progress I pursue in what follows takes a rather different perspective. In its modern iteration, it can be traced at least to dialectical socialism and the Marxist notion that capitalism has significant costs. Here, the idea of progress is not diminished and may even be paramount – socialism, to recall, is firmly committed to future progress – but it did take on a different form. It focused on protesting injustice and oppression; ill health was not merely a random absence of health, but rather something unjust that deserved to be rectified.

Of course, the insight that humans are equal beings who experience injustices because of power dynamics, and that rectifying these amounts to progress, is not new. As Simon Griffiths observes, the most common understanding of progressivism is that progress is concerned with some form of social justice.[4] And as depicted in Chapter 1, the development of medical care has long been linked to ideas about social progress. Nineteenth-century physician Rudolf Virchow, for instance, called physicians the natural advocates (*Anwälte*) of the disadvantaged and thought that the majority of diseases were attributable to defects in society.[5] Similarly, public health reformers of the early twentieth

---

[3] See Bobby M. Wilson, "Social Justice and Neoliberal Discourse," *Southeastern Geographer*, 47 (1) (2007), 97–100.
[4] Simon Griffiths, "What Was Progressive in "Progressive Conservatism"?," *Political Studies Review*, 12 (2014), 29.
[5] R. Virchow, "Was die 'medicinische Reform' will," *Medicinische Reform*, 1 (1848), reproduced in *Gesammelte Abhandlungen aus dem Gebiete der*

4 "Health for All": Medical Progress as Justice

century referred to the "social machinery" that would allow every individual a sufficient level of health as progress.[6]

Indeed, as the successes of bacteriology and laboratory medicine were shaping ideas of progress in medicine (Chapters 2 and 3), alternative visions bound up with the socioeconomic factors affecting health were present as well. They are visible, for example, in the establishment of the WHO in 1948 and its founders' interest in social medicine. These include Belgian professor René Sand (1877–1953) and Andrija Štampar (1888–1958) from Croatia, who shared the opinion that individualized medicine was in crisis and that the Organization must tackle the environmental and social roots of illness.[7] Henry Sigerist, a Swiss medical historian who advocated for both technological and social progress, was a close friend of Štampar and had an indirect influence on the WHO's initial priorities and definition of health.[8] Sand as well thought of medicine as an art that took into account the reciprocal relations between health and living conditions. In his book *Health and Human Progress* (1936), he approvingly quoted Descartes' claim for medicine's exceptional ability to further human progress, but gave medicine a decidedly social ethos:

We observe that nothing remains individual. Everyone borrows from the community. Production and sale, education and assistance, become collective functions calling for a rational organisation. Henceforth can medicine be anything but a social service?[9]

Sand was highly attentive to health inequalities, observing that death and disease increase down through social ranks and that narrowing the gap between the death rates of different social classes was a measure

---

öffentlichen Medicin und der Seuchenlehre, vol. 1 (Berlin: August Hirschwald, 1879), p. 4.

[6] See, for example, Charles-Edward A. Winslow, "The Untilled Fields of Public Health," *Science*, 51 (1306) (1920), 30.

[7] Though see Patrick Zylberman, "Fewer Parallels than Antitheses: René Sand and Andrija Stampar on Social Medicine, 1919–1955," *Social History of Medicine*, 17 (1) (2004), 77–92.

[8] S. Bok, "Rethinking the WHO Definition of Health," *International Encyclopedia of Public Health*, ed. H. K. Heggenhougen (Amsterdam: Elsevier, 2008), p. 594. See Henry E. Sigerist, *Civilization and Disease* (Chicago: University of Chicago Press, 1970 [1943]) and *Medicine and Human Welfare: The Terry Lectures* (New Haven, CT: Yale University Press, 1941).

[9] René Sand, *Health and Human Progress: An Essay in Sociological Medicine* (New York: Macmillan, 1936), pp. 3–4.

of progress.[10] These sensibilities were reflected in the WHO's famous 1948 constitution, which defined health as "a state of complete physical, mental, and social well-being," thereby articulating its own version of the view that health is a holistic concept with physical, mental, and social aspects.[11]

Sand's insights coincided with contemporary scientific investigations of health inequalities and their causes. In one early study, British researcher J. W. B. Douglas and his coauthors demonstrated that the incidence of disease occurs as a gradient within all socioeconomic levels. They used their results to contest the view that class differences in health result merely from inadequate medical care for the less well-off, as well as to suggest a new view of progress that privileged a more directly sociomedical approach.[12] A post-war US study further considered the link between physical illness and what it termed "social pathologies" and emphasized the connection between health problems and social situations.[13] Several years later, anthropologist Gordon MacGregor published a study entitled "Social Determinants of Health Practices," suggesting that clusters of health problems occur among family members, as do social problems that are linked.[14] But a number of factors, including major drug discoveries and the legacies of colonization, hampered the widespread implementation of the WHO's biopsychosocial health model; for political reasons, emphasis on a social model of health had ideological implications that were quite simply unwelcome in the context of Cold War politics.[15]

---

[10] Ibid., p. 260.

[11] "Constitution of the World Health Organization," in *Basic Documents*, 49th ed. (Geneva: World Health Organization, 2020), https://apps.who.int/gb/bd/PDF/bd47/EN/constitution-en.pdf?ua=1. On this definition, see Thomas Schramme, "Health as Complete Well-Being: The WHO Definition and Beyond," *Public Health Ethics*, 16 (3) (2023), 210–18.

[12] J. W. B. Douglas, "Social Class Differences in Health and Survival during the First Two Years of Life; the Results of a National Survey," *Population Studies*, 5 (1) (1951), 56.

[13] Zdenek Hrubec, "The Association of Health and Social Welfare Problems in Individuals and Their Families," *Milbank Memorial Fund Quarterly*, 37 (3) (1959), 251–76.

[14] Gordon McGregor, "Social Determinants of Health Practices," *American Journal of Public Health and the Nation's Health*, 51 (11) (1961), 1713.

[15] A. Irwin and E. Scali, "Action on the Social Determinants of Health: A Historical Perspective," *Global Public Health*, 2 (3) (2007), 237. Henry Sigerist, for example, was forced to leave the United States in the McCarthy era.

An attractive and operational alternative to a full-scale socialized notion of health was increased emphasis on the fact that every person should have equal access to healthcare services.[16] In the post-war period, expenditures on healthcare were themselves often described as social progress.[17] As a rule, the focus on healthcare system reform in accordance with the requirements of justice occurred in a period that was marked by optimism that economic growth "lifted all boats" and that civil rights and social welfare policies were effectively reducing various inequalities simultaneously. By the 1970s, the belief in public healthcare and insurance policies was translated into universal access to medical care in almost all Western countries.[18] In associating the expansion of the healthcare system with progress, advocates were well aware that health was one issue for which the richest would likely be willing to accept taxation for the sake of the less well-off. Meanwhile, making the health system more accessible also constituted a goal that did not require a drastic overhaul of current medical practices. On the contrary, it offered a sufficientarian view of justice premised, not on equality as an end in itself, but rather on a sufficient threshold of health and well-being available to a maximum number of individuals. This promised improved health for low-income members of society while allowing the affluent to retain their medical privileges, including access to fashionable and expensive physicians and treatments.

4.2 Progress on Health Equity I: Primary Care and "Health for All"

The tendency to privilege a view of progress that focuses on optimizing existing resources, and distributing them more equitably, was reflected

---

[16] Gene Outka, "Social Justice and Equal Access to Health Care," *The Journal of Religious Ethics*, 2 (1) (1974), 11–32.

[17] See, for example, Joseph F. Follman, *Medical Care and Health Insurance: A Study in Social Progress* (Homewood, IL: R. D. Irwin, 1963) and T. R. Marmor, M. L. Barer, and R. G. Evans, "The Determinants of a Population's Health: What Can Be Done to Improve a Democratic Nation's Health Status?," in *Why Are Some People Healthy and Others Not? The Determinants of the Health of Populations*, eds. Robert G. Evans, Morris L. Barer, and Theodore R. Marmor (London and New York: Routledge, 1994), p. 220.

[18] On the exceptional U.S. case, see Ronald L. Numbers, "The Third Party: Health Insurance in America," in *The Therapeutic Revolution: Essays in the Social History of American Medicine*, eds. Morris J. Vogel and Charles E. Rosenberg (Philadelphia: University of Pennsylvania Press, 2017), pp. 177–200.

in the variations of universal care for all citizens, implemented and consolidated in Western Europe, Canada, Australia, and New Zealand in the twentieth century. In a classic discussion, philosopher Bernard Williams made the case for equality in healthcare access, arguing that the provision of healthcare services should be based on health needs.[19] Trying to operationalize these and similar insights, proponents of national healthcare programs argued that healthcare is a social good that ought to be provided to all independently of income. Another philosophical influence on the idea of progress as health justice was John Rawls, whose theory of justice comprised a basic optimism about the ability of free and equal citizens to live together. Rawls did not theorize health justice; he did not think of health as something socially produced, but rather a product of random luck.[20] But while the effects of luck cannot be abolished entirely, and certain kinds of inequality are unavoidable, the negative impacts of bad luck can be softened. In an article devoted to "Medical Progress and National Health Care," philosopher Loren Lomasky observes that everyone should have access to medical technological progress and that the absence of health is rarely an indication of culpability; rather it is bad luck, and justice implies rectifying this.[21]

Given Rawls' importance to social justice theorizing, and his confident assumptions about the possibility of the lasting improvement of social institutions, several contributions subsequently refined his conception of justice to incorporate medical progress specifically.[22] Philosopher Norman Daniels, to take one prominent case, argues in his book *Just Health Care* that health and medicine have a special

---

[19] Bernard Williams, "The Idea of Equality," in *Problems of the Self: Philosophical Papers, 1956–1972* (Cambridge: Cambridge University Press, 1973), p. 240.

[20] John Rawls, *A Theory of Justice* (Cambridge, MA: Belknap Press, 1971); see also his *Justice as Fairness: A Restatement* (Cambridge, MA: Belknap Press, 2001) and *Political Liberalism*, expanded ed. (New York: Columbia University Press, 1996).

[21] Loren E. Lomasky, "Medical Progress and National Health Care," *Philosophy & Public Affairs*, 10 (1) (1981), 72. See also Charles Fried, "Equality and Rights in Medical Care," *Hastings Center Report*, 6 (1) (1976), 29–34.

[22] See, for example, John C. Moskop, "Rawlsian Justice and Human Right to Health Care," *Journal of Medicine and Philosophy*, 8 (1983), 329–38, as well as Lu Ann Aday and Ronald M. Andersen, "Equity of Access to Medical Care: A Conceptual and Empirical Overview," *Medical Care*, 12 (19) (1981), 4–27.

status because they affect the equality of opportunity in society. Daniels attributes objective characteristics to health, defining it as the absence of disease and diseases as deviations from normal functioning, and he defends both a right to healthcare and the social obligation to provide adequate healthcare to all. To that end, he argues that it is necessary to make a clear distinction between health preferences and fundamental needs, as well as to acknowledge problems of bias toward identified, recognized patients as opposed to more abstract, statistical ones. Daniels thus stipulates that progress consists in the provision of the basic medical services needed to maintain, restore, or compensate for the loss of species-typical functioning – that is, health – which determines fair equality of opportunity. By confining his argument in that way, Daniels says little about how to remedy the fact that larger social injustices are reflected in his definition of health or how factors beyond medical care affect health. But by offering an account of the societal obligation to provide equal access to health services, he articulates an influential theory of progress necessary to produce a more equitable healthcare system.[23]

Despite these theoretical contributions, as well as some real increases in the availability of care based on need, rather than the ability to pay, socioeconomic inequalities in health remained. Various examples from states with universal health systems demonstrated that access to health services is not sufficient for eliminating or even reducing health disparities; in fact, in some cases, these were widening. Scientific studies on such questions were conducted against the background of an increasing sense that improved healthcare access and distribution were not sufficient to address the health needs of people at risk. This interrogation of medical progress was associated with questioning sizable expenditures on sophisticated medical technologies whose overall implications for population health were unclear. While progress through scientific medicine was a tangible reality, in countries that financed medical services for all, its diminishing marginal returns were progressively chronicled. At the global scale, many preventable and treatable health problems related to drinking water, nutritious food, and hygiene practices remained. The aim of eliminating disease through biomedical research and therapies was criticized

---

[23] Norman Daniels, *Just Health Care* (Cambridge: Cambridge University Press, 1985), p. 229.

for its inability to improve health equity within countries and between countries themselves. British physician and public health officer N. R. E. Fendall captured this mood early on when he wrote in 1972:

> If I were asked to compose an epitaph on the twentieth century, it would read "Brilliant in its scientific discoveries, superb in its technical breakthroughs, but woefully inept in its application of knowledge to those most in need." [...] [T]he "implementation gap" must be closed.[24]

Progress, essentially, was being inequitably distributed. Part of the necessary reorientation involved acknowledging that medical knowledge did not need to be pursued without end. In fact, there was already enough specialist knowledge, as well as resources and qualified personnel, to improve people's health. Rather, what was required was a conception of medical progress that took into account not just formal equality, but rather a thicker, more substantive kind of equity, in order to make sure that communities facing barriers were able to benefit from medical progress. Only by including different background circumstances influencing health, and allocating resources accordingly, would it be possible to make real progress. A crucial corollary of this insight is that the entire scientific-medical community should recalibrate its priorities in a utilitarian fashion to ensure that medical progress is felt by the greatest possible number of people.[25]

In the late 1970s, the WHO became a vocal proponent of this way of thinking, and its concern with health equity underpinned a vision of progress based on the philosophy of primary healthcare. In 1978, the Alma-Ata conference sought to define the provision of primary healthcare for all, that is, basic healthcare with a spectrum of societal services, as the nearest thing approximating measurable medical progress.[26] The meeting concluded with the famous slogan, "Health for All

---

[24] N. R. Fendall, "Auxiliaries and Primary Medical Care," *Bulletin of the New York Academy of Medicine*, 48 (10) (1972), 1291–300.

[25] See M. Manciaux and T. M. Fliedner, "World Health: A Mobilizing Utopia?," in eds. S. W. A. Gunn et al., *Understanding the Global Dimensions of Health* (Boston: Springer, 2005), p. 79.

[26] "Declaration of Alma-Ata," International Conference on Primary Health Care, Alma-Ata, USSR, September 6–12, 1978 available at *World Health Organization*, www.who.int/teams/social-determinants-of-health/declaration-of-alma-ata. See Kenneth W. Newell, "Selective Primary Health Care: The Counter Revolution," *Social Science and Medicine*, 26 (9) (1988), 903–6 and

by the Year 2000"; even when commuted into "primary health care for all," it provided a singularly ambitious vision of medical progress centered on fighting health inequities by addressing social inequities more broadly. In 1981, Halfdan Mahler, a Danish physician and WHO Director-General from 1973 to 1988, reemphasized the links between progress and health justice when he wrote that a minimal level of health is essential and that health and social awareness must go hand in hand, progressively reinforcing one another. "Health for all," he noted, depends on continued progress both in medical care and in public health. But the kinds of medical services Mahler had in mind went beyond more conventional medical problems such as insufficient numbers of doctors, hospital beds, or drugs, to include the elimination of malnutrition, bad drinking water, and insalubrious housing. Health for all, Mahler wrote, is a holistic concept calling for efforts in agriculture, industry, education, housing, and communications, as much as in medicine. And he emphasized the shifting locus of health progress by observing that actions undertaken outside the health sector can affect health to a much greater extent than those within it.[27] By privileging comprehensive primary care accessible to all, over specialist care accessible to the few, the WHO ethos reimagined the stage for an idea of health progress that advocated community-based – rather than hospital-based – health and care.[28] It also channeled, once again, the idea of a disease-free future, based on harmonious progress in different spheres of life; the development of a country, the WHO Executive Board wrote, has to proceed harmoniously "any positive result in one field will be beneficial in others, just as any deficiency in one sphere will inevitably retard progress in the others."[29]

Susan B. Rifkin, "Alma Ata after 40 Years: Primary Health Care and Health for All – from Consensus to Complexity," *BMJ Global Health*, 2018, 3 (3), e001188.
[27] Halfdan Mahler, "The Meaning of 'Health for All by the Year 2000'," *World Health Forum*, 2 (1) (1981), excerpted in "Voices from the Past," *American Journal of Public Health*, 106 (1) (2016), 36–38.
[28] See Dave A. Chokshi, Louise Cohen, "Progress in Primary Care – From Alma-Ata to Astana," *Journal of the American Medical Association*, 320 (19) (2018), 1965–66.
[29] WHO Executive Board, *Organizational Study on "Methods of Promoting the Development of Basic Health Services,"* Report of the Working Group (Geneva: World Health Organization, 1973), p. 19.

4.3 Progress on Health Equity II: Upstream Determinants of Health

At roughly the same time that this WHO agenda was being developed, epidemiologist John B. McKinlay introduced the term "upstream determinants" in a contribution committed to reorienting the location of progress in health. McKinlay uses the analogy of a physician so busy helping struggling patients as they float downstream that they do not have the opportunity to look up and see what pushed them into the river in the first place. In a direct response to the "lifestyle approach" (see Chapter 3), McKinlay and like-minded colleagues attempted to reorient public opinion from downstream health problems to more pressing upstream ones. He observed that his approach:

> highlights the fact that a clear majority of our resources and activities in the health field are devoted to what I term "downstream endeavors" in the form of superficial, categorical tinkering – in response to almost perennial shifts from one health issue to the next, without really solving anything.[30]

McKinlay concluded that fighting the battle downstream was based on a misguided idea of progress that was not only futile but also led to exhaustion and disillusionment. Focusing attention upstream, on the contrary, would reveal the different actors – including interest groups and corporations – that push people into the river and then erect healthcare structures downstream to address the same health needs they have been complicit in creating. McKinlay, therefore, provides a critical reading of the dominant views of medical progress of his day, while also emphasizing the complexities and social nature of health.

McKinlay's research was largely sympathetic to the interventions of British physician and epidemiologist Thomas McKeown (1912–1988) who argues that twentieth-century trends toward financing high-tech curative medicine were a misguided diversion of resources away from prevention-oriented health programs.[31] Writing during decades in

---

[30] John B. McKinlay, "A Case for Refocusing Upstream: The Political Economy of Illness," *Interdisciplinary Association for Population Health Science Occasional Classics*, 1 (2019 [1975]), p. 1. The title echoes M. Mankoff, ed., *The Poverty of Progress: The Political Economy of American Social Problems* (New York: Holt, Reinhart and Winston, 1972), cited by McKinlay.

[31] On McKeown's impact see James Colgrave, "The McKeown Thesis: A Historical Controversy and Its Enduring Influence," *American Journal of Public Health*, 92 (5) (2002), 725–29.

4 "Health for All": Medical Progress as Justice

which formal access to healthcare – for example via Britain's National Health Service – was firmly established, McKeown's research further resonates with the idea that there are significant determinants of health beyond medical care narrowly understood. In particular, he challenged existing medical progress narratives that portray steady increases in life expectancy in the Global North as of the nineteenth century as attributable to technological interventions and biomedical research.[32] McKeown acknowledges the enormous improvements that occurred but links health progress to better standards of living, nutrition, and hygiene.[33] In his examples, McKeown conclusively shows that many of the most serious diseases had all but disappeared in England and Wales before relevant scientific medical knowledge and related innovations were available. While certain aspects of his thesis have been discredited – public health measures such as vaccination and access to clean water played a bigger role than he acknowledged – his challenge to previous understandings of medical progress still holds today. As public health historian Simon Szreter observes, McKeown effectively demonstrated that the advances we associate with clinical and hospital medicine played only a minor role in the historic decline in mortality levels.[34] The long-term outcome of McKeown's research, then, was to highlight the existence of an alternative progress narrative, whereby social conditions broadly construed had the power to effect meaningful and long-term improvements in health. Eventually, his analysis became foundational for the nascent field of population health, which focused on the social determinants of health, including early childhood care, education, employment, discrimination, poverty, housing, environmental hazards, and the like.

A final intervention of note for the model of progress as health justice that I want to mention here is the 1980 Black Report, published by the UK Department of Health and Social Security. The report was commissioned to investigate the effects of universal access to healthcare and found that increased access had not eliminated health disparities between classes. If individual care is what drives medical

---

[32] Thomas McKeown, *The Role of Medicine: Dream, Mirage, or Nemesis?* (Princeton, NJ: Princeton University Press, 1980), p. 156.
[33] Ibid., for example pp. 184–85.
[34] Simon Szreter, "The Importance of Social Intervention in Britain's Mortality Decline c. 1850–1914: A Re-interpretation of the Role of Public Health," *Society for the Social History of Medicine*, 1 (1988), p. 2.

progress, then a universal system with virtually free treatment for all should have made huge progress in improving the health of people vulnerable to poverty and raising it to a level comparable to the health of the affluent. It had not, and as various observers have gone on to elaborate, if the progress of biomedical knowledge combined with the availability of healthcare for individuals did not result in significant health improvements, then other powerful factors must be at play.[35] The Report itself concludes that while medical care plays an important role for health, numerous other factors related to everyday life are of greater importance. And it calls for a relative improvement in living standards for people at risk of bad health, together with measures to prevent new structures and technologies from undermining their existing living conditions.[36] By raising the importance of social life and diminishing the power of medicine, this assessment had potentially radical implications for ideas of medical progress. If medical interventions narrowly speaking only have a marginal influence on health progress more broadly, why should they occupy a central place in such theories?

4.4 Progress, the Social Determinants of Health, and Health Justice

As the idea of medical progress shifted beyond the technological prowess of healthcare – indeed, actively questioned it – and beyond the notions of accessibility and participation, it opened up to a much wider constellation of social factors that were newly acknowledged as crucial for improving health. But it was following the HIV/AIDS epidemic of the 1980s that debates about progress and health as a fundamentally social matter took on a new momentum. In the early years, AIDS symbolized how the causes of illness are not simply biological but rather social and highlighted the suffering of minority groups, whether gay men or women disadvantaged by poverty. Using life expectancy as a proxy, researchers and advocates further pointed

---

[35] See Sean A. Valles, *Philosophy of Population Health: Philosophy for a New Public Health Era* (London and New York: Routledge, 2018).

[36] *Inequalities in Health: The Black Report*, Chapter 9, para. 9.2, available at *Socialist Health Association*, www.sochealth.co.uk/national-health-service/public-health-and-wellbeing/poverty-and-inequality/the-black-report-1980/black-report-chapter-9-policies-to-reduce-health-inequalities2-a-wider-strategy/

4 "Health for All": Medical Progress as Justice

out that health occurs on a gradient in every society and that health and longevity correlate with socioeconomic status.[37]

As of the 1990s, the idea that social conditions produce disease and need to be addressed in any theory of medical progress gained much wider resonance. New insights into genetics refined the knowledge of how interactions between disease and various physical, environmental, and social factors occur. There was also an increased awareness of how technologies are used to further sexism, racism, homophobia, and oppression generally.[38] The medical knowledge of different publics, including knowledge that was previously left out, for example in relation to gender and race, began circulating more widely. In keeping with the notion that new knowledge requires a new mindset, epidemiologists remarked that the widespread existence of the social gradient in health changes both the most pressing scientific questions about health and the policies needed to address the problem.[39] The missing knowledge – related to understanding how an array of social factors influences health – was associated with a more complex and nuanced framework for judging medical progress.

In the early 1990s, epidemiologist Richard Wilkinson published a piece illustrating what he termed the strong relation between a society's income distribution and the average life expectancy of its population. In it, he develops the thesis that income redistribution would have little effect on the health of wealthy people, even as the end result would be to improve the average health of the population as a whole.[40] Wilkinson's research, coming as it did at a particularly

---

[37] See M. G. Marmot et al. "Health Inequalities among British Civil Servants: the Whitehall II Study," *The Lancet,* 337 (8754) (1991), 1387–93 and M. G. Marmot, G. Rose, M. Shipley and P. J. Hamilton, "Employment Grade and Coronary Heart Disease in British Civil Servants," *Journal of Epidemiology and Community Health,* 32 (4) (1978), 244–49.

[38] See Sandra Harding, *Whose Science? Whose Knowledge?: Thinking from Women's Lives* (Ithaca, NY: Cornell University Press, 1991).

[39] Michael Marmot, Richard Wilkinson, eds., *Social Determinants of Health* (Oxford: Oxford University Press, 2005), p. 2. See also Anne-Emmanuelle Birn, "Making It Politic(al): Closing the Gap in a Generation: Health Equity through Action on the Social Determinants of Health," *Social Medicine,* 4 (3) (2009), 166–82 and Barbara Starfield, "Are Social Determinants of Health the Same as Societal Determinants of Health?," *Health Promotion Journal of Australia,* 17 (3) (2006), 170–73.

[40] R. G. Wilkinson, "Income Distribution and Life Expectancy," *BMJ,* 34 (1992), p. 165.

propitious moment for that type of argument, was followed by a torrent of papers on the social, economic, and political determinants of health and disease. Around that time, health progress became widely associated with tackling health inequalities head-on.[41] As one *BMJ* editorial put it, if progress is to be made, it is necessary to address the fact that rising health inequalities are a consequence of an increasingly polarized society.[42] Medical progress was now associated explicitly with political and economic social choices.[43] It was around the same time that a vision of medical progress, namely that preventable death and disability ought to be minimized, gained momentum as what has been called a "dream of social justice."[44]

In the first decades of the twenty-first century, the notion that medical progress only makes sense in relation to an ecosystemic way of thinking about health gained in popularity, and the vocabulary of the social determinants of health became increasingly widespread. In 2008, a WHO Commission acknowledged that while societies have traditionally looked to the health sector to deal with health and disease, much of the illness burden responsible for unnecessary death is largely attributable to the conditions in which people are born, grow, live, work, and age, and they termed these conditions collectively the social determinants of health. In its report, *Closing the Gap in a Generation: Health Equity through Action on the Social Determinants of Health*, the Commission concluded that social injustice is killing people on a grand scale and named health equity as a marker of progress.[45] Research contributions reflecting on these findings point to evidence suggesting we can make massive progress toward closing the health gap by improving these conditions and also note that in order to do

---

[41] See Tony Delamothe, "Social Inequalities in Health," *BMJ*, 303 (1991), 1046–50.

[42] George Davey Smith and Jerry Morris, "Increasing Inequalities in the Health of the Nation," *BMJ*, 309 (1994), 1453.

[43] Marshall H. Becker, "A Medical Sociologist Looks at Health Promotion," *Journal of Health and Social Behaviour*, 34 (1993), 1–6.

[44] Dan E. Beauchamp, "Public Health as Social Justice," in *New Ethics for the Public's Health*, eds. Dan E. Beauchamp and Bonnie Steinbock (Oxford: Oxford University Press, 1999), p. 105.

[45] Commission on Social Determinants of Health, *Closing the Gap in a Generation*, pp. 1, 111. See also Michael Marmot et al., "Closing the Gap in a Generation: Health Equity through Action on the Social Determinants of Health," *The Lancet*, 372 (2008), 1661–69.

so, we must deal with inequities in power, money, and resources, as social injustice itself is a threat to health. In 2012, epidemiologist Michael Marmot summed up the mood as one that acknowledges the need to "address the wider determinants of health in order to make progress."[46]

The above remarks are representative of a larger debate, namely the revitalization of the notion of progress to address the collective experience of excluded, marginalized, and oppressed members of society and to resist and challenge dominant ideas of progress. The (re)discovery of progress as social justice was driven by a reinforced concern with uncovering and documenting the web of connections that binds us together in our collective existence. Social scientists have drawn attention to the uneven and fragile nature of progress, as well as the fact that we are all connected, and that inequalities both within and across countries threaten to fundamentally damage our social fabric. In doing so, they have reimagined the core values of progress to include equality of opportunity, mutual support and care, and sustainability.[47] Such perspectives emphasize the extent to which one's place in society determines our convictions about whether progress has the potential to benefit us. They, therefore, point to the inescapably political aspects of traditionally technology-focused visions of progress, portraying them as merely one way – and not a particularly fair way – of distributing limited resources within an unequal society. They also draw attention to the ways in which a shared commitment to the progress of science and technology can serve as a surrogate for social action.[48]

Among the various critics who hold that such progress is necessary today, many of them emphasize the insufficiencies of basing an idea of progress on an abstract notion of individual autonomy and personal responsibility. Critical theorist Axel Honneth observed in 2017 that,

---

[46] Michael Marmot, "Fair Society, Healthy Lives," *Public Health*, 126 (2012), p. 10. See also Michael G. Marmot, "Global Action on Social Determinants of Health," *Bulletin of the World Health Organisation*, 89 (2011), p. 702.

[47] See, for example, Nancy Folbre et al., "The Multiple Directions of Social Progress: Ways Forward," in *Rethinking Society for the 21st Century*, Report of the International Panel on Social Progress, vol. 2 (Cambridge: University of Cambridge Press, 2018), p. 818.

[48] See Daniel Sarewitz, *Frontiers of Illusion: Science, Technology, and the Politics of Progress* (Philadelphia: Temple University Press, 1996).

while up until recently the leitmotif of almost all progress was the idea of expanding individual autonomy, at present it must become collective autonomy.[49] Other contributions have linked the idea of progress to an emancipated social space and a notion of the self as driven by a concept of solidarity that involves responsibility for other people's welfare.[50] In such accounts, progress is linked to a concept of justice that takes into account the demands of equality between different social groups and generations. Not only societal progress but moral progress too has been associated with the expansion of the scope of justice and the aim of creating broadly inclusive communities. Accordingly, those who stand to gain have been vocal in promoting these conceptions of progress. Progress can, therefore, be seen as a kind of resistance, a demand on behalf of or from those who have been oppressed, or whose lives have been marked by injustice.[51]

One concrete manifestation of these philosophical sensibilities is the capabilities approach, developed by Amartya Sen and Martha Nussbaum and applied more specifically to health by Sridhar Venkatapuram, which emphasizes that being healthy has an intrinsic value, as well as increases our capacity to achieve our ends. Health, in this view, is no longer merely a primary good but rather an "actual freedom," and health justice promotes positive freedom, that is, our ability to pursue the projects that we choose. In an associated idea of progress, we can and should take measures that promote and sustain the capability to be healthy in a way that is commensurate with the equal dignity of human beings.[52] While enlarging shared perceptions of health in this way, critics also emphasized its importance among

---

[49] Axel Honneth, "How to Envision Social Progress Today," *Social Imaginaries*, 1 (2018), p. 165.
[50] R. C. Smith, *Society and Social Pathology: A Framework for Progress* (Cham, Switzerland: Palgrave Macmillan, 2017). See also Lea Ypi, *Global Justice and Avant-Garde Political Agency* (Oxford: Oxford University Press, 2011).
[51] See Rainer Forst, "Zum Begriff des Fortschritts," in *Vielfalt der Moderne – Ansichten der Moderne*, ed. Hans Joas (Frankfurt am Main: Fischer, 2012), p. 43. See also Rainer Forst, "The Justification of Progress and the Progress of Justification," in *Justification and Emancipation: The Critical Theory of Rainer Forst*, eds. Amy Allen and Eduardo Mendieta (State College, PA: Penn State University Press, 2019) and Marc Fleurbaey et al., *A Manifesto for Social Progress: Ideas for a Better Society* (Cambridge: Cambridge University Press, 2018).
[52] Sridhar Venkatapuram, *Health Justice: An Argument from the Capabilities Approach* (Cambridge: Polity Press, 2011), p. 8.

social goods. Sen argued in the 2002 Tanner Lectures "Why Health Equity?" that in any discussion of social equity, illness and health must figure as major concerns.[53] His words were not devoid of political significance; on the contrary, they point to the need for a fairer society with profound policy implications concerning how we think about, fund, and organize medicine. In 2005, former International Monetary Fund economist Ken Rogoff made the political stakes explicit when he asserted that health and life expectancy will be at the center of the next big battle between socialism and capitalism.[54] Progress as justice is not inevitable, but rather actively influenced by political and economic choices.

In academic circles, a vision of progress that sought to allocate medical resources more fairly in the pursuit of health has been widely taken up. Various policy frameworks and projects concerned with framing the mandate of physicians do so in terms of their social relevance and ability to meet "societal needs."[55] The shift to an expanded vision of health is evident in how Norman Daniels, rather than produce a second edition to his book *Just Health Care*, wrote an entirely new book called *Just Health: Meeting Health Needs Fairly*, implying that healthcare is the tip of the iceberg and that health progress requires looking beyond formal medical care to social justice issues.[56] There is a widespread agreement that the best predictor of good health in affluent countries is not access to biomedical technologies but social factors including education levels and material well-being. There is also a large assortment of evidence that children who grow up in a nurturing environment and receive a good education have better health, as do adults who have fulfilling employment and support structures.

---

[53] Amartya Sen, "Why Health Equity?," *Health Economics*, 11 (2002), 659–66.
[54] Cited in Richard Horton, "Marx and Medicine," *The Lancet*, 390 (2017), p. 2026.
[55] See Cynthia R. Whitehead, Zubin Austin, Brian D. Hodge, "Flower Power: The Armoured Expert in the CanMEDS Competency Framework?," *Advances in Health Sciences Education*, 16 (2011), p. 686.
[56] (Cambridge: Cambridge University Press, 2007). See also Norman Daniels, "Justice, health, and health care," in *Medicine and Social Justice: Essays on the Distribution of Health Care*, eds. R. Rhodes, M. P. Battin, and A. Silvers (New York: Oxford University Press, 2002), pp. 6–23 and Norman Daniels, Bruce P. Kennedy, and Ichiro Kawachi, "Why Justice Is Good for Our Health: The Social Determinants of Health Inequalities," *Daedalus*, 128 (4) (1999), 215–51.

Researchers have also shown that there is something about income inequality itself, as a different phenomenon from poverty, that lowers the health of both individuals and populations.[57]

These considerations have led some to contend that taking the longer view reveals a deterministic historical trend toward greater equality. For example, in their book, *The Spirit Level: Why More Equal Societies Almost Always Do Better*, Kate Pickett and Richard Wilkinson argue that this trend "runs like a river of human progress" from the first constitutional limits on autocracy through to public education and healthcare.[58] And yet, successful policies to achieve progress on these accounts have been fraught.[59] Writing in 2018, ten years after the Commission on Social Determinants of Health, a public health physician observed that social injustice remains the leading cause of bad health.[60] Despite significant evidence that the best way to improve population health is through relatively low-cost public health measures and that restricting the use of some technologies keeps healthcare costs down, research funding is overwhelmingly directed toward biomedicine.[61] If education, housing, and transportation remain important for governments across the Global North, the percentage of GDP devoted to healthcare is increasing. As a rule,

---

[57] R. G. Wilkinson and K. E. Pickett, "Income Inequality and Population Health: A Review and Explanation of the Evidence," *Social Science and Medicine*, 62 (2006), 1768–84.

[58] Kate Pickett and Richard Wilkinson, *The Spirit Level: Why More Equal Societies Almost Always Do Better* (London: Allen Lane, 2009), pp. 267–68.

[59] Fran E. Baum, Monique Bégin, Tanja A. J. Houweling, and Sebastian Taylor, "Changes Not for the Fainthearted: Reorienting Health Care Systems Toward Health Equity through Action on the Social Determinants of Health," *American Journal of Public Health*, 99 (11) (2009), 1967–74. See also Kumanan Rasanathan and Theresa Diaz, "Research on Health Equity in the SDG Era: The Urgent Need for Greater Focus on Implementation," *International Journal for Equity in Health*, 15 (202) (2016), https://doi.org/10.1186/s12939-016-0493-7.

[60] Kumanan Rasanathan, "10 Years after the Commission on Social Determinants of Health: Social Injustice Is Still Killing on a Grand Scale," *The Lancet*, 392 (2018), 1176–77.

[61] Editorial, "UK Life Science Research: Time to Burst the Biomedical Bubble," *The Lancet*, 392 (2018): 1227–28. See also Jon L. Wardle, Fran E. Baum, and Matthew Fisher, "The Research Commercialisation Agenda: A Concerning Development for Public Health Research," *Australian and New Zealand Journal of Public Health*, 43 (5) (2019), 407–09 and Joseph E. Davis and Ana Marta Gonzalez, eds., *To Fix or to Heal: Patient Care, Public Health, and the Limits of Biomedicine* (New York: New York University Press, 2016).

physicians continue to treat patients as individuals with self-contained health problems, without reference to their life contexts, using what Rupa Marya and Raj Patel have termed colonial thinking.[62] As discussed in the previous chapter, the promoters of personalized/precision medicine have been challenged to explain and respond to the reality that zip codes are more predictive of health than genetic codes. At stake are differing views about what medical progress consists in and how to achieve it.

4.5 Progress as Justice: Critiques

Justice considerations for progress imply a significant recalibration of the goals of medicine. When medical progress is reframed as progress toward social justice, and based on a broad view of health that includes social factors, the repercussions are vast. Take, for example, diabetes. In its shorthand form, the research mission of the American Diabetes Association is "Science. Progress. Hope."[63] And yet, diabetes has long been a disease that reflects the anxieties and aspirations of specific historical moments, particularly with regard to race.[64] Appeals to, for example, population genetics as the crucial tool for understanding different rates of diabetes mask important factors such as poverty and racism. Making progress on diabetes, therefore, implies more than scientific understandings of different forms of the disease and their genetic origins; it also involves more than targeted campaigns to ensure better access to treatments and monitoring. Rather, progress requires understanding and addressing the racial, social, and economic factors that contribute to diabetes, including discrimination, lack of education, and limited access to nutritious food. In short, progress implies fostering social change in the name of health.

The desire to refashion societies using better health for all as a touchstone has been critiqued from various angles. First of all, it can be argued that policies designed to achieve medical progress lack precision if they attempt to address multiple social phenomena whose only

---

[62] Rupa Marya and Raj Patel, *Inflamed: Deep Medicine and the Anatomy of Injustice* (New York: Farrar, Straus and Giroux, 2021).
[63] Research Mission, American Diabetes Association, https://diabetes.org/research/research-foundation-mission-and-vision.
[64] See Arleen Marcia Tuchman, *Diabetes: A History of Race and Disease* (New Haven, CT: Yale University Press, 2020).

point in common is that they have negative effects on health. Medical personnel have no special expertise to redress economic, class, and racial inequalities, reduce violence, and so on. For this reason, a persistent critique of using the social determinants of health as a measure of health progress is that the latter has gone beyond its natural boundaries. Addressing broader health determinants for injuries and disease inevitably requires social and political engagement and priority setting.[65] Meanwhile, a fundamental question is whether health justice is better served by narrow interventions targeting groups of individuals or communities or by broader measures aiming to reallocate the societal resources that have such a profound influence on health. Some have sought to combine this policy agenda by presenting targeted interventions and social change not as opposing choices, but rather as harmonious complements to each other. Technical, curative, and preventative measures could – at least theoretically – be integrated with far-reaching measures to improve the living conditions of people at risk of poor health by inadequate policies.[66] For example, it is possible to argue that we do not yet have a good understanding of the diverse and deep-seated health effects of racism, yet need not worry about the fact that the net health effects of reducing the social problem of racism – or poverty, or housing – will be negative.[67] At the same time, the specific mechanisms and outcomes for health are variable and poorly understood, and it is difficult to understand what to prioritize.

Second, there is a persistent difficulty related to distinguishing between causes and correlations of progress. The social determinants of health can manifest as direct causes of ill health, for example with regard to how diet affects individual biology. They can also affect health in macrosocial ways, such as when the stress of disenfranchisement causes health problems. But they can also act as what are called the causes of causes.[68] Smoking, for example, is associated with both a lower socioeconomic status and a higher risk of certain diseases than

---

[65] Lawrence O. Gostin and Madison Powers, "What Does Social Justice Require for the Public's Health? Public Health Ethics & Policy Imperatives," *Health Affairs*, 25 (4) (2006), 1055.
[66] James Colgrove, "The McKeown Thesis," p. 729.
[67] Y. Paradies, J. Ben, N. Denson, et al. "Racism as a Determinant of Health: A Systematic Review and Meta-Analysis," *PLoS One*, 10 (2015), e0138511.
[68] Michael Marmot and Richard G. Wilkinson, eds., *Social Determinants of Health*, 2nd ed. (Oxford: Oxford University Press, 2006 [1999]), p. 2.

4 "Health for All": Medical Progress as Justice

not smoking.[69] Disadvantaged members of society and minorities are also more affected by substandard healthcare. But how to be sure these are not just correlations and actual causal relationships? As Marcia Angell notes, the fact that social advantage correlates so powerfully with health makes it extremely difficult to interpret research into the effects of one on the other.[70] For this reason, it can also be difficult to compare the net outcomes of policy measures. Philosopher Frances Kamm has pointed out that policy proposals designed to address social inequality and health must compare the health we gain by improving social equality with the health resulting from economic growth that itself is associated with social inequality.[71] The importance of recognizing and intervening in the causal chains through which socioeconomic conditions directly affect health and longevity is crucial, yet highly complex.

Third, by becoming involved with redistribution and the reorganization of society, medicine becomes highly politicized. As discussed in Chapter 3, there are many things we can do to promote health through diet, exercise, and so on. MD Sally Satel has criticized a view of progress as health justice by remarking that, taken to its extreme, personal responsibility for one's own health and care becomes a quaint and even suspect notion. And she argues that while it may be politically expedient to blame ill health on oppression, alienation, or other overwhelming factors, the reality is far more complicated.[72]

If medicine is perceived as a vehicle for infinite human progress, the allocation of resources to medicine is profoundly influenced by this belief. But there is no guarantee that market forces, or even human sensibilities, conform with the requirements of social justice.[73]

---

[69] See also Bruce G. Link, Jo Phelan, "Social Conditions as Fundamental Causes of Disease," *Journal of Health and Social Behaviour*, Special Issue: Forty Years of Medical Sociology: The State of the Art and Directions for the Future (1995), 80–94.
[70] Marcia Angell, "Pockets of Poverty," *The Boston Review*, 25 July 2014, https://bostonreview.net/forum_response/marcia-angell-pockets-poverty/
[71] Frances M. Kamm, "Health and Equality of Opportunity," *American Journal of Bioethics*, 1 (2001), 19.
[72] Sally Satel, *PC, M.D.: How Political Correctness Is Corrupting Medicine* (New York City: Basic Books, 2000), pp. 14, 232.
[73] For an argument that commonsense morality is consistent with moderate deontology, as opposed to for example consequentialism, which seeks to maximize the good for all, see Eyal Zamir, *Law, Psychology, and Morality:*

Providing care in a society involves hard choices about which illness conditions should be prioritized in research and funding. There are tensions between providing expensive medical care to one individual and ensuring that all benefit from equal medical care. Rare diseases, diseases with expensive, labor-intensive treatments, and interventions affecting elderly people with a limited life expectancy; all these are candidates for being rethought in a system that privileges a more socially oriented view of medical progress. Daniel Callahan has gone so far as to highlight a clash between biomedical progress and equity and to argue that the very success of scientific-technological progress in medicine is a menace to progress toward health justice.[74] Others have countered that this problem can be overcome by pursuing better health through technologies and addressing health inequalities simultaneously. But seen from a historical perspective, technologies aimed at improving health equity and democratizing healthcare access consistently fail to deliver on their creators' promises.[75] Rather, it seems more honest to acknowledge that sacrifices must be made in order to provide a socialized medicine.

Such tradeoffs are visible in tensions that arise between the goals of improving the health of the entire population, of distributing health benefits fairly, and reducing health inequities.[76] New interventions, even as they are beneficial to the health of individuals, often increase inequalities in health outcomes and may conflict with the principle of distributive justice.[77] Sometimes called the dilemma of social progress, similar dilemmas occur in numerous fields beyond medicine. They can be seen, for example, when inequality between groups increases alongside social progress – for example, an overall decline in child

---

The Role of Loss Aversion (Oxford: Oxford University Press, 2015), p. 177 e passim.

[74] Daniel Callahan, "How Much Medical Progress Can We Afford: Equity and the Cost of Health Care," *Journal of Molecular Biology*, 319 (2002), 886, 888.

[75] See, for example, Jeremy A. Greene, *The Doctor Who Wasn't There* (Chicago: University of Chicago Press, 2022).

[76] Norman Daniels, "Reconciling Two Ethics Goals of Public Health: Reducing Health Disparities and Improving Population Health," in *Oxford Handbook of Public Health Ethics*, eds. Anna C. Mastroianni, Jeffrey P. Kahn, and Nancy E. Kass (Oxford: Oxford University Press, 2019), pp. 290–300.

[77] Jo C. Phelan and Bruce G. Link, "Fundamental Cause Theory," *Medical Sociology on the Move: New Directions in Theory*, ed. William C. Cockerham (Dordrecht: Springer, 2013), p. 119.

mortality, though one that is distributed unevenly between different social groups. There is no easy solution to potential tensions between the fact that generalized social progress is important and the fact that all individuals within a society deserve equal respect and concern. By focusing too much on any one dimension of health – in this case, the social dimension – justice-driven visions of medical progress risk masking the conflicts between different dimensions of progress.

4.6 Medical Progress and COVID-19

COVID partout, justice nulle part

Graffiti seen in Montréal, Canada, 2020

As the critiques of progress-as-justice in medicine became more granular and articulated, this particular conception of progress took on a new urgency in the context of the COVID-19 pandemic.[78] Originating in China in 2019, severe acute respiratory syndrome coronavirus 2 (SARS-CoV-2), responsible for COVID-19, is a virus that primarily affects the respiratory system, though it can touch multiple organs, including the heart, kidneys, gut, and brain. This section discusses briefly how narratives of progress played out during the emergence of this global medical event. Beyond the disease, containment policies including lockdowns, quarantines, curfews, and the use of technologies to comply with physical distancing – for example by moving to online work and schooling – affected billions of people. More specifically, I consider the early stages of the pandemic in 2020–2021 and the heated debates it occasioned about medical progress. The pandemic allowed for unprecedented collaborative scientific efforts, expedited technological advances, and a race for vaccines that embodied the hope that scientific progress can act as a magic bullet for solving health problems. At the same time, by making visible the importance of social environments for disease generally, and the deployment of scientific advances in particular, it threw narrowly scientific models

---

[78] Histories of COVID-19 include Jacalyn Duffin, *COVID-19: A History* (Montreal: McGill-Queens University Press, 2022) and Richard Horton, *The COVID-19 Catastrophe: What's Gone Wrong and How to Stop It Happening Again* (Cambridge: Polity Press, 2020).

of medical progress into question.[79] The inequalities of the pandemic's effects within Western societies, and those of the vaccine rollout globally, brought the problems of the social dimensions of scientific progress into stark relief. I believe that these questions deserve analysis as a crucial moment for a clash of competing medical progress narratives, as well as shed renewed light on what medical progress as health justice entails.

Evidence from other epidemics confirms how disease outbreaks reveal preexisting problems. Epidemic disease has been called a "breaching experiment," in that it brings to light long-standing fractures and forms of suffering.[80] The COVID-19 pandemic revealed existing vulnerabilities in societies that thought of themselves as embodying a particular kind of cutting-edge, high-tech medical progress but had not invested similarly in disease prevention and public health. Particularly notable in the case of COVID-19 was the speed with which the disease destabilized and overwhelmed the healthcare systems of exceptionally wealthy and privileged societies. In doing so, it unsettled received assumptions about a particular kind of technology-intensive medicine as the locus of progress. Countries' successes in combatting the virus proceeded in a way that was to some extent decoupled from their per capita healthcare budgets and technological capacities.[81] Despite the importance of hospitals and intensive care units for treating severe cases, at times the sickest patients could not be helped by existing medical resources. Switzerland, for example, experienced the seventh highest rate of per capita deaths in November 2020 during the pandemic's second wave, as high as Iran, Russia,

---

[79] See Peter Strasser, "Paradoxien des medizinischen Fortschritts – kann es sein, dass die immer bessere Gesundheitsversorgung die Würde des Menschen mehr bedroht als stärkt?," *Neue Zürcher Zeitung*, June 22, 2020, www.nzz.ch/meinung/die-frage-der-wuerde-paradoxien-des-medizinischen-fortschritts-ld.1543009?reduced=true.

[80] See Luisa Enria and A. F. Tengbeh, "Ebola Wahala: Breaching Experiments in a Sierra Leonean Border Town," in *Feeling Disease: Experiencing Medicine and Illness in Modern History*, eds. R. Boddice and B. Hitzer (London: Bloomsbury, 2022), pp. 43–60 and Graham Scambler, "Covid-19 as a 'Breaching Experiment': Exposing the Fractured Society," *Health Sociology Review*, 29 (2) (2022), 140–48.

[81] Arusha Cooray, Krishna Chaitanya Vadlamannati, and Indra de Soysa, "Do Bigger Health Budgets Cushion Pandemics? An Empirical Test of COVID-19 Deaths across the World," *WIDER Working Paper*, 165 (2020), www.econstor.eu/bitstream/10419/229389/1/wp2020-165.pdf

4 *"Health for All": Medical Progress as Justice* 167

and Croatia.[82] Cuba was very successful at managing the early stages of the pandemic, as were Thailand and Vietnam.[83] While the United States is a global leader in biomedical science and technology, this failed to protect American society as a whole, and people at risk in particular, from COVID-19.

The pandemic also shed renewed light on the shortcomings of excessively one-dimensional forms of medical progress. For example, it revealed how illusory certain forms of progress have been because it exposed how unequally they have been shared. In particular, it put on display the extent to which inequitable social structures affect people's health both within and between different countries. US chief medical advisor Anthony Fauci referred to COVID-19 as having shone a bright light on American society's failings, in particular on the social determinants of health.[84] In a similar fashion, Michael Marmot asserted that COVID-19 had both divulged and amplified existing inequalities.[85] The virus drastically affected those whose health situation was already so precarious that illness – even a mild one – or disruption to their daily routines profoundly threatened their livelihood; elderly people living in precarious situations, people without housing or food security, and prisoners are all examples thereof.[86]

---

[82] See "Tracking Covid-19 Excess Deaths across Countries," *The Economist*, www.economist.com/graphic-detail/coronavirus-excess-deaths-tracker

[83] Talha Burki, "Behind Cuba's Successful Pandemic Response," *The Lancet Infectious Diseases*, 21 (4) (2021), 465–66. On Vietnam, see Tuyet-Anh T. Le et al., "Policy Responses to the COVID-19 Pandemic in Vietnam," *International Journal of Environmental Research and Public Health*, 18 (2) (2021), 559, https://doi.org/10.3390/ijerph18020559, and on Thailand Viroj Tangcharoensathien, Mary T. Bassett, Qingyue Meng, and Anne Mills, "Are Overwhelmed Health Systems an Inevitable Consequence of COVID-19? Experiences from China, Thailand, and New York State," *The BMJ*, 372 (2021), n83.

[84] "Fauci: 'Undeniable Effects of Racism' Have Worsened Covid for U.S. Minorities," *The Guardian Online*, May 16, 2021, www.theguardian.com/world/2021/may/16/fauci-racism-covid-us-black-hispanic-native-americans-emory-university-graduation.

[85] Michael Marmot, interviewed in Stewart Paterson, "Boris Johnson Didn't Get 'Big Decisions Right' on Covid, Says Leading Epidemiologist," *Glasgow Times*, June 21, 2022, www.glasgowtimes.co.uk/news/20224923.boris-johnson-didnt-get-big-decisions-right-covid-says-leading-epidemiologist/?ref=twtrec.

[86] See, for example, Paul Webster, "COVID-19 Highlights Canada's Care Home Crisis," *The Lancet*, 397 (10270) (2021), 183 and Léa Sanchez, "Les résidents d'Ehpad représentent 44% des morts du Covid-19," *Le Monde*, December 3,

National lockdowns designed to reduce physical interactions shed further light on the link between health and social justice considerations. For desk workers, this largely meant working from home and moving in-person activities online, effectively receiving an extra layer of protection. Other workers, for example in child care, transportation, public utilities, food and agriculture, slaughterhouses, garbage collection, and delivery services, were now identified by governments as "essential" and still required to be present in-person. Many essential jobs are poorly paid and done by people who are socioeconomically disadvantaged, including visible minorities, women, and migrants.[87] African-American and Latino communities in the United States, for example, were disproportionately affected by the disease in a striking manner, and in other OECD countries, the situation was similar.[88] Discussing why Montreal was the seventh deadliest city worldwide for COVID-19 in May 2020, a commentator noted that the reason lies in public health patterns that long predate the virus: Those infected already experience systematic inequality, poverty, and discrimination, and COVID-19 is merely making this situation more visible. In light of this reality, the idea that progress is shared in a democratic, nondiscriminatory way rings increasingly hollow.[89]

Occurring in the last year of Donald Trump's 2017–2021 presidency and directly related to the Black Lives Matter movements, one of the recurring impressions of the pandemic was that the health disparities between different social groups, and the underlying racist, classist, and sexist structures that determine those disparities, were being held up for all to see.[90] The traditional foci of medical progress

---

2020, www.lemonde.fr/les-decodeurs/article/2020/12/03/les-residents-d-ehpad-representent-44-des-morts-du-covid-19_6062084_4355770.html.

[87] See Editorial, "The Plight of Essential Workers during the COVID-19 Pandemic," *The Lancet*, 395 (10237) (2020), 1587.

[88] Isaac Chotiner, "The Interwoven Threads of Inequality and Health," *The New Yorker*, April 14, 2020, www.newyorker.com/news/q-and-a/the-coronavirus-and-the-interwoven-threads-of-inequality-and-health and Daniel Morales, "COVID 19 and Disparities Affecting Ethnic Minorities," *The Lancet*, 397 (10286) (2021), 1684–85.

[89] See Colleen M. Flood et al., eds., *Vulnerable: The Law, Policy & Ethics of COVID-19* (Ottawa: University of Ottawa Press, 2020).

[90] Clyde W. Yancy, "Academic Medicine and Black Lives Matter: Time for Deep Listening," *JAMA*, 324 (5) (2020), 435–36.

on improved technology and healthcare access seemed fundamentally incomplete in light of these lived realities. In their intervention *Pandémopolitique*, Gaudillière, Izambert, and Juven draw attention to what they call the systematic health triage that has socioeconomic origins and that precedes clinical triage for COVID-19 and call for prioritizing the common good over individual decisions in the medical context. In particular, they highlight the need to replace growth as the obligatory horizon of progress, in favor of a more radically democratic concept of progress in tune with collective needs.[91] Reflecting on the import of his previous work in the context of the pandemic, Michael Marmot contemplated an idea of progress whereby the aim is not simply to restore GDP growth but to create better societies, which have both better health and narrower health inequities. And such prescriptions regarding health do not relate to medicine narrowly conceived. Rather, they concern improving the lives of children, enhancing public education and working conditions, and ensuring that everybody has the minimum income necessary to pursue healthy and sustainable behaviors.[92]

While introducing research on the AIDS epidemic, and skeptical of the desire to draw simple, historical lessons from the unanticipated outbreak of a new, lethal disease, Barbara Rosenkrantz observed that we face the recurring temptation to "celebrate linear progress and reassuringly demonstrate how evil is overwhelmed by good."[93] In the era of COVID-19, the temptation to replace the uncertainties surrounding epidemics with a simple historical story – and linear, medical progress in particular – feels ill-advised. Philosopher Bruno Latour pinpointed COVID-19 as an event that profoundly threw into question the belief in a single path of progress. He highlights instead a new collective awareness, whereby we all began to understand that each item of our daily lives – drugs, food, clothing, and means of transport – is, in fact, the subject of ongoing negotiations, and it is, therefore, possible to

---

[91] Jean-Paul Gaudillière, Caroline Izambert, and Pierre-André Juven, *Pandémopolitique : Réinventer la santé en commun* (Paris: La Découverte, 2021), p. 14.

[92] Michael Marmot, "Society and the Slow Burn of Inequality," *The Lancet*, 395 (10234) (2020), 1413–14. See also Jennifer Prah Ruger, "Social Justice as a Foundation for Democracy and Health," *BMJ*, 371 (2020), 4049.

[93] Barbara Gutmann Rosenkrantz, "Case Histories – An Introduction," *Social Research*, 55 (3) (1988), 399.

change or reverse what previously seemed inevitable.[94] Against the background of climate change, and the flaws inherent in the argument that we are embarked on an irreversible path of progress, he argues that it is only by acknowledging the multidimensionality of progress that we can find a solution to the problems that face us.

4.7 Conclusion

While many people benefit from technological-scientific medical advances, disadvantaged members of society remain less well integrated into healthcare systems, less able to take advantage of their benefits because of discrimination and bias, and have poorer health when they do engage with medicine. To the extent that equity is acknowledged as a medical goal in a democratic society, it should be particularly apparent in medical priorities. The vision of medical progress as social justice has offered various scenarios, for example by emphasizing an effective and widely available – but more basic – array of medical services. Its advocates have also suggested that health and progress should be conceived much more broadly to encompass a person's roles as a family member, employee, political being, and so on. In such a view, medical progress is measured not so much by life expectancy, or survival rates, but rather in terms of the ability of persons to fulfill their various social roles and achieve their personal goals.[95] In short, progress would be measured by its impact on population health and not on individual health.

Such conceptions of progress have many real advantages for health. In Western societies where the basic health needs of different groups are not met – think, for example, of Indigenous populations in Canada – there is an urgent need to better address those who are harmed when the social dimension of medical progress gets left out. At the same time, such visions of progress are not immune to the utopianism inherent in one-dimensional views of medical progress. To the extent that they mask potential tensions between individual freedom, social justice, and scientific advances, they offer an illusory picture of a harmonious social life that would more accurately be described as a permanent compromise.

---

[94] Bruno Latour, "Le train du progrès n'emprunte pas qu'une seule voie," *Le Monde*, September 25, 2020, p. 29.
[95] Callahan, "How Much Medical Progress Can We Afford?," 885–90.

Epilogue
Medical Progress as Achieving Sustainability

[A]ll progress in capitalistic agriculture is a progress in the art, not only of robbing the labourer, but of robbing the soil; all progress in increasing the fertility of the soil for a given time, is a progress towards ruining the lasting sources of that fertility.

Karl Marx, Capital, vol. I, p. 329

By the early 2020s, when this book was written, the idea of medical progress had undergone various transformations and continued to hold different meanings simultaneously. Yet it is also possible to think that the concept's most significant metamorphoses may very well lie in the future. As we have seen, the idea of a single path of historical progress entered a crisis in the twentieth century because of increased awareness that history has no goal, just as there are no laws shaping the historical process. But another essential source of the critique of conventional ideas of progress was rooted in environmental concerns about the side effects of current forms of economic progress and the limits of the natural world. As depicted in Chapter 1, major strands of Enlightenment-era thought represented progress as human mastery over other species and over nature itself. Nature was largely conceived as facilitating growth at the service of progress; little thought was given to "The End of Nature," as the environmentalist Bill McKibben put it in 1989.[1]

In the course of the twentieth century, the shortcomings of this view, and the harms resulting from associated visions of progress, became increasingly evident. The Club of Rome published its landmark publication, *The Limits to Growth* (1972), with the intention of encouraging each reader to think through the consequences of continuing "to equate growth with progress."[2] In 1991, Christopher Lasch singled

---

[1] Bill McKibben, *The End of Nature* (New York: Random House, 1989).
[2] William Watts, "Foreword," in Donella H. Meadows et al. *The Limits to Growth: A Report for the Club of Rome's Project on the Predicament of Mankind* (New York: Universe Books, 1972), p. 12.

out the belated discovery that the earth's ecosystems cannot sustain the indefinite expansion of productive forces as dealing "the final blow to the belief in progress."[3] Meanwhile, different ideologies grappled with an increased awareness of the material limits to the ideas of progress and development around which they have traditionally been conceived. Liberalism, for example, even as it is sometimes portrayed as the "evil genius" behind the ecological crisis, sought to pull apart its conceptions of progress and economic growth.[4]

The ecological perspective that animated the critique of linear forms of progress was concerned first and foremost with making visible what such narratives left out, in the form of side effects and externalities, but also with articulating an alternative. And while some forms of progress were the objects of environmentalist ire, the notion was also reclaimed by green movements. The idea of progress – with its well-known political power – could be reinterpreted rather than rejected and integrated into innovative visions of development.[5] In a widely read book published in 1999, John Barry interprets all of green political theory as an immanent critique of the idea of progress, while simultaneously suggesting an alternative understanding of it underpinned by new social and environmental relationships.[6] The term progress easily retains the justice-oriented and emancipatory connotations of "progressive," while opening up to include a more holistic and ecological approach to social change.[7]

But perhaps most significant for the reappropriation of progress by environmental movements was its association with the notion of sustainable development, presented in its modern version in *Our Common Future* (1987) – also known as the *Brundtland Report* – as

---

[3] Christopher Lasch, "The Fragility of Liberalism," *Salmagundi*, 92 (1991), 8.
[4] Marcel Wissenburg, "Liberalism," in *Political Theory and the Ecological Challenge*, eds. Andrew Dobson and Robyn Eckersley (Cambridge: Cambridge University Press, 2006), pp. 20–21.
[5] Lucas Seghezzo, "The Five Dimensions of Sustainability," *Environmental Politics*, 18 (4) (2009), 544.
[6] John Barry, *Rethinking Green Politics: Nature, Virtue and Progress* (London, Thousand Oaks, CA, and New Delhi: Sage Publications, 1999), p. 9.
[7] See Robert Paehlke, "Environmentalism and the Future of Progressive Politics: An Update" in *Explorations in Environmental Political Theory: Thinking about What We Value*, ed. Joel Jay Kassiola (London and New York: Routledge, 2003), pp. 81–103 and Lara Monticelli, "On the Necessity of Prefigurative Politics," *Thesis Eleven*, 167 (1) (2021), 99–118.

development that "meets the needs of the present without compromising the ability of future generations to meet their own needs."[8] The notion of sustainability emerged as a particularly powerful form of collective obligation that could breathe fresh life into the notion of progress. As sustainability came to represent a kind of moral high ground for the twenty-first century, progress toward achieving sustainability was inherently part of how to overcome the lamentable aspects of the present situation.[9] The association between the terms is so strong that progress came to be a persistent ideological feature of sustainability, and the conceptualization of sustainability as progress became increasingly common.[10] Sustainable development can be defined precisely as the kind of development that allows human progress to continue indefinitely.[11]

The association between progress and sustainability replicates several well-worn thought processes. Historian Aurore Schwab refers to this conceptual linkage, as embodied in the UN's sustainability goals, as an emerging planetary religion, complete with a superhuman actor – planet Earth – as well as collective myths and rites.[12] Schwab's work asks us to reflect on the extent to which a quasi-religious belief in sustainability masks the value conflicts that are a persistent part of human life and offers its own form of eschatological salvation. With regard to the normative assumptions embedded in sustainable progress, many prominent suggestions regarding progress as sustainability come from economists, who are generally sympathetic to the notion

---

[8] *Report of the World Commission on Environment and Development of the United Nations: Our Common Future* (1987), p. 41, available at https://sustainabledevelopment.un.org/content/documents/5987our-common-future.pdf.

[9] Ming-Jui Yeh, "Discourse on the Idea of Sustainability: With Policy Implications for Health and Welfare Reform," *Medicine, Health Care and Philosophy*, 23 (2020), 155.

[10] Jacobus A. Du Pisani, "Sustainable Development: Historical Roots of the Concept," *Environmental Sciences*, 3 (2) (2006), 83–96.

[11] Alan Holland, "Sustainability," in *A Companion to Environmental Philosophy*, ed. Dale Jamieson (Malden, MA: Blackwell Publishers, 2001), p. 391. See also Benjamin Görgen and Björn Wendt, "Nachhaltigkeit als Fortschritt denken: Grundrisse einer soziologisch fundierten Nachhaltigkeitsforschung," *Soziologie und Nachhaltigkeit*, 1 (1) (2015), 3–21.

[12] See Schwab's ongoing research project, *The United Nations Sustainable Development Goals: An Emerging "Planetary Religion?,"* described at https://orcid.org/0000-0002-6940-4658, as well as N. D. van Egmond, H. J. M. de Vries, "Sustainability: The Search for the Integral Worldview," *Futures*, 43 (2011), 853–67.

of step-by-step progress. Contemporary sustainable development discourse has been characterized as a "collective capitalist project, based on a vision of continuous progress" overseen by Western scientists and economists in various international financial institutions.[13] However, abstract visions of continuous progress notwithstanding, conceptualizing progress as sustainability also suggests the possibility of new approaches to personhood and to health.

Environmental concerns, while fundamental for the critique of progress in its "classical" version, are not well developed with regard to medicine. That this material should feature in an epilogue, rather than a stand-alone chapter of this book, bears witness to some of the problems with associating medicine and the notion of sustainability. An extensive edited publication, *Sustainable Healthcare* (2013), opened by asking: "Should people working in the health sector be interested in sustainability?" and gave as an answer a resounding "yes." The authors, nevertheless, admit that despite their salience, ideas about sustainability have been slow to catch on in healthcare contexts.[14] As might be expected, I do think there is a potential case for reimagining medical progress as sustainability. In fact, the material presented here suggests that it may well be one further iteration of the idea of medical progress. It builds quite naturally on previous conceptual iterations of progress, though it differs from these in several important respects.

To start with the similarities, some of the most prominent voices calling for green medical progress explicitly refer back to other, preceding critiques of progress discussed in this book. Environmental historian Linda Nash blames the scientific narrative of medical progress, in particular, for obscuring the link between the environment and health.[15] In a landmark book written in 2004, *The Ethics of Environmentally Responsible Health Care*, Jessica Pierce, Andrew Jameton, and Canadan Boulder draw on Daniel Callahan's castigation

---

[13] John Harlow, Aaron Golub, Braden Allenby, "A Review of Utopian Themes in Sustainable Development Discourse," *Sustainable Development*, 21 (4) (2013), 276.

[14] Knut Schroeder, Trevor Thompson, Kathleen Frith, and David Pencheon, *Sustainable Healthcare* (Chichester, West Sussex: Wiley-Blackwell, 2013), pp. vii, 69, 238.

[15] Linda Nash, *Inescapable Ecologies: A History of Environment, Disease, and Knowledge* (Oakland: University of California Press, 2007), p. 6.

of economically unsustainable healthcare based on a misguided notion of "infinite progress." The authors further reference René Dubos (discussed in Chapter 2), observe that modern medicine embodies the dream of progress as increasing human material comfort and mastery over nature, and conclude that this dream is turning into a nightmare.[16] And they link Dubos's work on ecosystemic health to their own interests in environmentally responsible healthcare practices. In Pierce, Jameton, and Boulder's view, the work of Callahan et al. pioneered an approach to medicine that does not require constant progress toward unlimited future goals and drew attention to how the obsession with progress can be harmful to medicine and those it purports to serve. In essence, such arguments draw on previous critiques of progress to contend that a medical system designed to cater to potentially infinite health needs is not only conceptually and economically flawed but fundamentally incompatible with environmental scarcities.[17] A sustainable healthcare system, as the above authors and others have formulated it, is responsive to environmental limits and willing to change current healthcare priorities in order to achieve good human and ecological health.

While advocates of green medical progress see themselves as building on an existing body of work, they expand their approaches to personhood and health to include the natural environment. In addition to being fundamentally mortal and existing in a web of human relationships – points emphasized in previous chapters – this strand of thinking further emphasizes the relationships of persons with natural systems. Concepts of the human – as environmental philosopher Val Plumwood argues – must now be rethought together in ecological terms that recognize and respect human differences and continuities with nature and are attentive to how human life in general is embedded in the material, ecological world.[18] If modern biomedicine approaches

---

[16] Jessica Pierce, Andrew Jameton, and Canadan Boulder, *The Ethics of Environmentally Responsible Health Care* (Oxford: Oxford University Press, 2004), pp. 49–50.
[17] See also P. Tijmes, and R. Luijf, "The Sustainability of Our Common Future: An Inquiry into the Foundations of an Ideology," *Technology in Society*, 17 (3) (1995), 327–36.
[18] Val Plumwood, "Feminism," in *Political Theory and the Ecological Challenge*, eds. Andrew Dobson and Robyn Eckersley (Cambridge: Cambridge University Press, 2006), p. 55.

the body as a self-contained, mechanical system, the insight that bodies are permeable to their environment requires new approaches to illness.[19] Personhood, therefore, is not simply reconceived as part of a larger network of relationships and organisms that now includes nature; rather, human health has to be fundamentally reassessed in light of its dependence on nature.

As a rule, this shift seeks to correct existing, predominant views of human superiority to and separation from nature. But more integrated views of personhood, health, and nature also challenge head-on views of progress underpinned by such assumptions. For one, advocates for "green" medical progress argue that the conventional timescales we use to assess medical progress are too short by far. Adding an environmental perspective to health results in increased awareness of the time frame in which we measure progress; part of the difficulty inherent in defining what exactly should be sustained requires thinking critically about temporal categories and deciding whether progress should be measured in days, years, or centuries. Once the temporal framework becomes longer, progress easily loses its association with the success of a specific medical intervention or even how an intervention affects the course of a person's life. Instead, the concept of sustainability and green theory generally perceive events in human lives from a multigenerational perspective. Environmental processes such as climate change require that we temporally extend ideas about medical progress to safeguard the health of current and future generations.[20]

Second, green theories of medical progress tend to be critical of claims about the metaphysical status of progress. They note that progress is not linear but rather multifaceted, that technological advances do not always improve well-being, and that regression is a real possibility. Prominent precursors of this line of thinking include Jared Diamond's *Collapse: How Societies Choose to Fail or Succeed* (2005) and Ronald Wright's *A Short History of Progress* (2011). Wright refers to practices that drive environmentally unsustainable growth and that

---

[19] Nitin K. Ahuja, "The Body Is Not a Machine," *Aeon*, November 11, 2021, https://aeon.co/essays/how-ecological-thinking-fills-the-gaps-in-biomedicine

[20] See Kristine Belesova, Daivd L. Heymann, and Andy Haines, "Integrating Climate Action for Health into Covid-19 Recovery Plans," *BMJ*, 370 (2020), m3169. See also Itsuki C. Handoh and Toshitaka Hidaka, "On the Timescales of Sustainability and Futurability," *Futures*, 42 (7) (2010), 743–48.

are difficult to slow down or to stop once they have begun, as "progress traps."[21] In Wright's and Diamond's detailed analysis of such processes, they argue that the growth of a society, or its "progress," is tributary to its ability to exploit natural resources. The resultant progress may be rapid and accelerating, but once essential resources are depleted, a dramatic collapse occurs. These findings clash with established visions of progress because they posit a fundamental discontinuity between past growth and possible future trajectories. The notion of a progress trap reveals the rigidities and short-sightedness of existing ideas of medical progress. For instance, technological solutions to medical problems or individual freedom to maximize the pursuit of health may solve some health problems but can nevertheless contribute to catastrophic collective outcomes if due attention is not paid to their environmental consequences.

Finally, in terms of their ethics, green theories of medical progress build quite naturally on previous repudiations of a stereotypical liberal subject, an autonomous agent whose choice-making is inherently valuable. A vision of humans as ecological beings challenges single-minded devotion to the protection of individual rights, in favor of a more ecological or "ecozoic" perspective, that emphasizes the value of different forms of life. In related views of progress, excessive choices are portrayed as having a potentially detrimental relationship to human health (compare, for example, with personalized medicine) because they may threaten the life forms on which individual health ultimately depends.[22] In essence, the relationship between open-ended progress and health is fraught: New technologies with unpredictable consequences, increases in choice, and uncontrolled growth are not necessarily conducive to achieving health and well-being. Instead, humans have to use their creative powers to curb progress's most dangerous forms and preserve and protect the unique attributes of nature by placing a new value on limits.[23]

---

[21] Ronald Wright, *A Short History of Progress* (New York: Anansi Press, 2011), p. 30.
[22] On green theories where choice is given a more prominent role, see Karsten Gäbler, "Green Capitalism, Sustainability, and Everyday Practice," in *Global Sustainability*, eds. B. Werlen et al. (Cham: Springer, 2015), pp. 63–86.
[23] See Clinton E. Betts, "Progress, Epistemology and Human Health and Welfare: What Nurses Need to Know and Why," *Nursing Philosophy*, 6 (2005), 179.

All of these philosophical premises have the potential to underpin visions of medical progress that acknowledge the contingencies of any single historical moment and the multiple dimensions of progress. Yet many green health advocates posit a harmony whereby associating the notion of sustainability with medical progress would result in a single outcome: better health for both humans and the planet. Health and sustainable development, global health scholar Ilona Kickbusch has argued, are not only "interdependent, but they are reciprocal."[24] In a similar fashion, Pierce et al. state that the premise for their study of environmentally responsible healthcare is that human health is founded on healthy, stable ecosystems.[25] The ramifications of such assumptions for progress are clear: Progress in human health and in protecting nature are mutually reinforcing. Recent contributions argue that healthcare is "lucky" in this respect because almost everything that helps create a healthier planet has the "co-benefit" of making people both healthier and happier. More specifically, many interventions that improve individual health – such as fresh, local, and mainly plant-based food – are also good for the health of the planetary system – creating what have been termed "virtuous circles."[26] This inference was summarized succinctly in the title of a recent article: "Sustainable Medicine: Good for the Environment, Good for People."[27]

The "lucky" nature of health in terms of its consonance with the normative assumptions of sustainability has not gone unnoticed by multiple stakeholders, including several key industries. As a rule, the healthcare industry is portrayed as ideally positioned to benefit from the synergistic relationship between human and environmental health.[28] Advocates of renewable energies have been keen to

---

[24] Ilona Kickbusch, "Approaches to an Ecological Base for Public Health," *Health Promotion International*, 4 (4) (1989), 267.

[25] Pierce, Jameton, and Boulder, *The Ethics of Environmentally Responsible Health Care*, p. 1. See also Emily Farrow, "Embedding Sustainability into Clinical Medicine and Medical Education," *Health Management*, 17 (5) (2017), 369–71.

[26] Knut Schroeder et al., *Sustainable Healthcare*, pp. vii–viii, 69.

[27] Trevor Thompson and Tim Ballard, "Sustainable Medicine: Good for the Environment, Good for People," *British Journal of General Practice*, 61 (582) (2011), 3–4.

[28] M. J. Eckelman, Jodi D. Sherman, and Andrea J. MacNeill, "Life Cycle Environmental Emissions and Health Damages from the Canadian Healthcare System: An Economic-Environmental-Epidemiological Analysis," *PLoS Medicine*, 15 (7) (2018), e1002623, 14.

Epilogue: Medical Progress as Achieving Sustainability

emphasize the health aspects of their technologies, for example, the fact that they do not cause air pollution, produce no toxic wastes, and have relatively low water consumption.[29] Indeed, the health "co-benefits" of, for example, climate change mitigation have become a watchword and a crucial way of motivating individuals, businesses, and governments to make choices more aligned with climate goals.[30] An Intergovernmental Panel on Climate Change (IPCC) working group report went so far as to frame climate change as precisely that which interrupts a continuous path of medical progress, calling it an "impediment to continued health improvements in many parts of the world."[31] And an editorial published in 2021 in more than 200 health journals worldwide called for political leaders to take urgent action on climate change and thereby address the biggest threat to global public health today.[32] Other climate researchers emphasize important "win-win" benefits for short-term climate and human health brought about by specific, practical emission reductions. Better air quality alone, for example, is arguably enough to create health benefits that would offset the global costs of emission reductions.[33]

The notion of a symbiotic harmony between health and nature revives several long-established thought patterns. While "nature" has often been invoked in relation to medical progress, it has been

---

[29] See "Public Health Linkages with Sustainability: Workshop Summary" (Washington, DC: The National Academies Press, 2013), https://doi.org/10.17226/18375.

[30] See Marina Romanello et al., "The 2021 Report of the Lancet Countdown on Health and Climate Change: Code Red for a Healthy Future," *Lancet*, 398 (2021), 1619–62.

[31] Kirk R. Smith et al. "Human Health: Impacts, Adaptation, and Co-Benefits," in *Climate Change 2014: Impacts, Adaptation, and Vulnerability. Part A: Global and Sectoral Aspects. Contribution of Working Group II to the Fifth Assessment Report of the Intergovernmental Panel on Climate Change*, eds. C. B. Field et al. (Cambridge: Cambridge University Press, 2014), p. 713.

[32] L. Atwoli et al., "Call for Emergency Action to Limit Global Temperature Increases, Restore Biodiversity, and Protect Health," *BMJ*, (2021), 374, and "More than 200 health journals call for urgent action on climate crisis," *The Guardian*, September 6, 2021, www.theguardian.com/environment/2021/sep/06/more-than-200-health-journals-call-for-urgent-action-on-climate-crisis.

[33] Anil Markandya et al., "Health Co-Benefits from Air Pollution and Mitigation Costs of the Paris Agreement: A Modelling Study," *The Lancet Planetary Health*, 2 (3) (2018), 126–33 and N. Watts et al., "The Lancet Countdown: Tracking Progress on Health and Climate Change," *The Lancet*, 389 (2017), 1151–64.

constructed differently and associated with various therapies. As depicted in Chapter 1, the Hippocratic school adhered to a broadly ecological understanding of ill health, seeing it as the result of an imbalance between external forces and those within the sick person, and advocated acting in harmony with nature as a way to foster health.[34] In general, Hippocratic–Galenic humoral medicine perceived nature as a powerful agent of recovery and healer of disease.[35] Assigning nature a key role in health promotion continued through Rousseau, the Romantics and, as of the nineteenth century, the popularity of naturopathic healing practices and spa retreats, mud-bathing and vegetarianism, are but some examples of heterogeneous but increasingly popular forms of "nature therapy."[36] As a rule, references to the notion that nature is crucial for human health and well-being are often framed in explicitly historical terms, whereby progress is conceived as a return to nature.[37] Appeals to a more natural, organic, premodern past are precisely the point: If modern society, by its very existence, limits contact between people, plants, animals, and natural rhythms, and creates historically unfamiliar surroundings, there is a net loss to health.

While the health–nature connection is longstanding, it became the focus of sustained scientific attention relatively recently. Today, research across a range of fields emphasizes the extent to which proximity and access to natural settings have beneficial health effects for individuals and communities. The health benefits of nature contact range from increased prosocial behavior to improved mental health, postoperative recovery, and birth outcomes.[38] Researchers from the

---

[34] See Brigitte Lohff, "Self-Healing Forces and Concepts of Health and Disease. A Historical Discourse," *Theoretical Medicine and Bioethics*, 22 (2001), 543–64.

[35] See Max Neuburger, "An Historical Survey of the Concept of Nature from a Medical View Point," *Isis*, 35 (1) (1944), 16–28, and Hannah Newton, "'Nature Concocts and Expels': Defeating Disease," in *Misery to Mirth: Recovery from Illness in Early Modern England* (Oxford: Oxford University Press, 2018), pp. 33–64.

[36] See Samantha Walton, *Everybody Needs Beauty: In Search of the Nature Cure* (London: Bloomsbury, 2021).

[37] See Cecily Maller et al., "Healthy Nature Healthy People: 'Contact with Nature' as an Upstream Health Promotion Intervention for Populations," *Health Promotion International*, 21 (1) (2005), 52.

[38] Howard Frumkin et al., "Nature Contact and Human Health: A Research Agenda," *Environmental Health Perspectives*, 125 (7) (2017), https://doi.org/10.1289/EHP1663.

University of Exeter quantified this to conclude that spending at least two hours a week in nature is associated with better health and well-being.[39] Time spent in nature was portrayed both as one of the unfortunate victims of COVID-19 lockdowns and as a health-promoting countermeasure to the pandemic.[40] Increased attention has also been paid to the extent to which natural products such as medicinal herbs and spices have shaped human history; this also involves (re)acknowledging the role of such products for progress.[41] Contact with animals, the consumption of organic foods, free-range grass-fed livestock, and the Paleo Diet – based on consuming foods similar to what may have been consumed in the Paleolithic era – have all been invoked because of the ways in which their "natural qualities" contribute to health and the potential for redefining "progress" in a way that takes into account environmental aspects of well-being. Sadly, writes Loren Cordain in their study advocating the Paleo Diet, "with all of our progress, we have strayed from the path designed for us by nature."[42]

In addition to lauding the health benefits of "naturalness," advocates of medical progress as sustainability emphasize the extent to which current medical practices harm human health. Implicit in this argument is that disparities between past and present ways of living and practicing medicine have themselves contributed to the emergence of serious diseases. In doing so, critics highlight the relatively well-known instances of how environmental degradation – dirty water, lack of sanitation, and air pollution – is bad for health. Air pollution has long been identified as a leading cause of morbidity and mortality globally, and climate change, as mentioned above, has been labeled the single greatest public health threat of the twenty-first century. But

---

[39] Matthew P. White et al., "Spending At Least 120 Minutes a Week in Nature Is Associated with Good Health and Wellbeing," *Scientific Reports*, 9 (7730) (2019), https://doi.org/10.1038/s41598-019-44097-3.

[40] A government flyer delivered to private residences in Montréal, Canada, in 2020 advised citizens: "allez dans la nature et respirez profondément et tranquillement." Gouvernement du Québec, "Aller mieux en contexte de pandémie COVID-19," 2020, www.quebec.ca/sante/problemes-de-sante/a-z/coronavirus-2019/aller-mieux-en-contexte-de-pandemie-covid-19/.

[41] Afroz Alam, "Spices: The Hoard of Natural Remedies," *Annals of Phytomedicine*, 8 (2) (2019), 7.

[42] Loren Cordain, *The Paleo Diet Revised: Lose Weight and Get Healthy by Eating the Foods You Were Designed to Eat*, revised edition (Hoboken, NJ: John Wiley & Sons, 2011), pp. 10, 43 e passim.

they also go beyond this to emphasize the paradoxical fact that some of the most widely recognized symbols of progress in modern medicine, resource-intensive curative treatments, for example, come at the expense of environmental pollutants that damage human health.[43]

Healthcare services range between 1 percent and 5 percent of total global environmental impacts, depending on which indicator is considered, and more than 5 percent for some countries.[44] These include wasteful practices (unnecessary plastics and single-use items), pollution (greenhouse gas emissions, for example, from healthcare-related transport and inhaled anesthetics), and energy-intensive hospital activities.[45] A number of studies of the negative environmental impacts of healthcare for individual countries exist, and the problem has been acknowledged by major international organizations.[46] In the American context, for example, a 2018 report noted that healthcare organizations are very far from embracing sustainable practices; the industry produces 7,000 tons of waste daily.[47] Furthermore, the amount of medical waste produced per person per day worldwide grew significantly as a result of COVID-19.[48] This led to a number of observations that there is an urgent need to address the public health

---

[43] Among the extensive literature on this topic, see Jodi D. Sherman et al., "The Green Print: Advancement of Environmental Sustainability in Healthcare," *Resources, Conservation & Recycling*, 161 (2020), https://doi.org/10.1016/j.resconrec.2020.104882.

[44] Manfred Lezen et al., "The Environmental Footprint of Health Care: A Global Assessment," *Lancet Planetary Health*, 4 (2020), e271–79.

[45] Matthias Meili, "Die Ökobilanz der Spitäler," *Neue Zürcher Zeitung*, October 3, 2021. See also *Health Care without Harm*, https://noharm-global.org/.

[46] On the English case, see *Greener NHS: National Ambition*, NHS England, www.england.nhs.uk/greenernhs/national-ambition/, Arunima Malik et al., "The Carbon Footprint of Australian Health Care," *Lancet Planetary Health*, 2 (1) (2018), e27–e35, Matthew J. Eckelman and Jodi D. Sherman, "Environmental Impacts of the US Health Care System and Effects on Public Health," *PLoS One*, 11 (6) (2016), e0157014, M. J. Eckelman, Jodi D. Sherman, and Andrea J. MacNeill, "Life Cycle Environmental Emissions and Health Damages from the Canadian Healthcare System: An Economic-Environmental-Epidemiological Analysis," *PLoS Medicine*, 15 (7) (2018), e1002623.

[47] Carrie R. Rich, J. Knox Singleton, and Seema S. Wadhwa, *Sustainability for Healthcare Management: A Leadership Imperative* (Abingdon, Oxon: Routledge, 2018), p. 60.

[48] World Health Organization, *Global Analysis of Healthcare Waste in the context of COVID-19: Status, Impacts and Recommendations* (Geneva: World Health Organization, 2022).

crisis arising from misplaced commitments to medical progress, mainly by promoting the rise of "healthcare sustainability" and green healthcare. A crucial point of connection between these arguments is that fundamentally misguided definitions of medical progress are actively harming health.[49]

Health. Nature. Sustainability. Progress. In the overview presented above, these are repeatedly described as self-reinforcing and good for health. But we have seen in previous chapters that attempts to paint different dimensions of progress as harmonious inevitably fall back onto flawed assumptions about what the health of a holistic entity such as a person requires. Meanwhile, appeals to specific kinds of health/medical progress are inevitably political and underpinned by visions of how to govern and improve human societies. Just as health is not fixed, there is no true "nature" that can be grasped separately from human culture and politics. The idea of medical progress as sustainability is, therefore, a set of political ideas about a particular kind of health and society and reveals various dilemmas and conflicts, not least between some widely accepted social and medical goals.

While the advocates of medical progress as sustainability have focused on the largely positive health effects of our contacts with nature, that is not the only way to read human beings' entanglement with nature. It is possible to understand health services and aspirations for progress as consistently trying to mitigate the potential dangers nature poses to human health. From a health perspective, the natural environment has traditionally been viewed with ambivalence. While clean air, water, and nutritious food are crucial for health, infectious diseases, weather, and geological events regularly sicken, injure, and kill people, often in large numbers. The contact with animals lauded above has an equally long history of being blamed for ill health, from Edward Jenner's pioneering work on the *variolae vaccinae*, or cowpox, to animal sources of COVID-19 contagion. Urban environments can provide improved access to healthcare, physical security, and comparative health advantages.[50] A traditionally recurring assumption of the idea of progress is the validity of the struggle against

---

[49] See Cécile M. Bensimon and Solomon Benatar, "Developing Sustainability: A New Metaphor for Progress," *Theoretical Medicine and Bioethics*, 27 (1) (2006), 59–79.

[50] Christopher Dye, "Health and Urban Living," *Science*, 319 (5864) (2008), 766–69.

humans' vulnerability and finitude in their natural environment. If we fundamentally question the association between medical progress and the struggle against death, we are left with the observation that sickness and death are "natural," and it is better for the environment and the planet to accept this and act accordingly. As one disillusioned friend told me when we discussed the issue, the only coherent response to the climate crisis is suicide.

Humans and other species rely on natural cycles, and the consequences of disturbing those cycles are increasingly acknowledged. But exactly how humans experience "nature," and the benefits they derive from this, depends on a great deal of factors, including the meanings ascribed to natural conditions, a human environment, and how the links between them are conceived. "Nature" is an umbrella term that is used colloquially to denote the very different experiences of, for example, an urban park, a mountain view shaped by hundreds of years of human residence, or a mosquito-filled swamp where humans rarely go. A natural environment and the animals and insects that flourish there can be threatening, inhospitable, and inconducive to the health of individuals, while remaining a healthy and thriving ecosystem on its own terms, and thereby furthering the health of the human species. Eating local, organic meat can be a health choice more in tune with humans' traditional diet but have high CO_2 emissions and is at odds with veganism, a different vision of a more "natural" path to health.

At the political level, the desire for better health and the wish to protect nature have no single, predictable outcome. Historically speaking, ecologism has been associated with both nationalistic movements and fascist sentiments, as well as left-wing political ideologies. Many have pointed out that current ecological imperatives call for drastic, unpopular measures, the full benefits of which will only become clear in the long run. Progress toward sustainable healthcare in Western countries may be in tension with equity if environmental costs are transferred to people living in poverty, to future generations, or to other countries.[51] Politically, the lack of a substantive basis within democracy to support sustainability issues has been well canvassed. Democracy is a reflection of the short-term preferences of human persons, and it therefore struggles to incorporate the notion of rights and obligations to

---

[51] Delia Paul, "Merging the Poverty and Environment Agendas," Brief #11, *IISD Earth Negotiations Bulletin*, (2021), 1–9.

subsequent generations, and the value of nature in and of itself. Some observers describe what they call an "intrinsic tension" between the concepts of sustainability and democracy.[52] The problem that democracy poses for ideas of medical progress as sustainability is that it must take into account diverse, often conflicting, interests, preferences, and values beyond environmental ones. The incrementalism and localism associated with democratic procedures may simply be insufficient to deal with large-scale global problems.

Finally, taking an earth-centric approach to health seriously might mean rejecting both the concepts of sustainability and conventional approaches to progress. Activist-scholar Leanne Betasamosake Simpson reflects on how the teachings of her Indigenous ancestors reveal that the concept of sustainability is exactly backward. "You don't develop as much as Mother Earth can handle. [...] You think about how much you can give up to promote more life."[53] Betasamosake Simpson further outlines how her rejection of the idea of progress is based on her ancestors' nonlinear, expansive linking of cycles, in a way that challenges progressive, temporal logic. She describes the present moment as collapsing into the past and the future simultaneously and thereby generating an ongoing conversation with both time spans.[54] If the future and the past can be seen in the present, this offers not a progressive view of history, but rather evidence of multiple worlds coexisting simultaneously and rich possibilities for imagining different forms of nonlinear progress.

***

In a post-post-modern world, the value of health seems to be one normative good on which we can agree. But perhaps the biggest problem relating to the shared agreement about health is that it underpins an inflationary view of medical progress. By inflationary I mean that claims on behalf of medical progress rely on the assumption that the

---

[52] Ming-Jui Yeh, "Discourse on the Idea of Sustainability," p. 161.
[53] Cited in Naomi Klein, "Dancing the World into Being: A Conversation with Idle No More's Leanne Simpson," *Yes! Magazine*, March 6, 2013, www.yesmagazine.org/peace-justice/dancing-the-world-into-being-a-conversation-with-idle-no-more-leanne-simpson.
[54] Robyn Maynard et al., "Every Day We Must Get Up and Relearn the World: An Interview with Robyn Maynard and Leanne Betasamosake Simpson," *Interfere: Journal for Critical Thought and Radical Politics*, 2 (2021), 154.

consensus around health is larger than whatever that consensus actually is. Past medical successes, the commodification of medicine, and the persistent idea that we "know" what health is and can achieve it unequivocally, blended together with the hope of overcoming the existential fears and uncertainties of patients, all drive the belief in medical progress. But as an inflationary concept, progress in medicine easily grafts onto the normative high ground of a particular moment, such as the Cold War commitment to progress via science or the heightened environmental sensibilities of today. By uncovering the assumptions about health and personhood that inform a particular vision of medical progress, we lay bare its political nature and the way in which it is used by different actors to galvanize resources that benefit them. In doing so, we are better able to see who profits when medical progress is associated with particular kinds of knowledge, who gets left out, and who is harmed by a particular narrative of progress.

There is a multidimensionality to health and medical problems that makes a notion of progress too closely aligned with any one dimension of health unstable and particularly liable to be affiliated with the interests of a particular set of actors. Medical progress that refers to increases in knowledge, freedom, justice, or sustainability is insufficient on its own and must be incorporated into a more systems-based approach, alive to potential tensions between the different dimensions of health and the difficulty of gaining knowledge of a holistic entity like a person. But such a multidimensional view of progress is not without its own internal contradictions. There are tensions between providing expensive medical care to one individual and ensuring equal care for all, as well as between the technical advances of modern medicine and healthy ecosystems. Faced with different views of medical progress, which all have some claim to validity, there is no way to discover what the definitive view of medical progress should be. Rather, a multidimensional concept of medical progress reveals the shortcomings of utopian visions that discount the tensions between different dimensions of progress.

While it might seem that changing from a vague agreement about medical progress to a more precise disagreement is counterproductive, this is not the case. Better understanding the choices and trade-offs implied by a particular vision of progress can itself be described as progress. Creating a more complex, but more realistic conceptual framework to approach the idea of progress in medicine reveals the contingencies of some of our current ways of thinking. This is particularly important given the huge political and economic capital that comes from being on the side of medical progress. Meanwhile, the notion of progress in medicine has changed in the past and will undoubtedly change again in the future. Political theorist Terence Ball observes that concepts lose their previous meanings and acquire new ones through a process of external challenge and immanent critique; in this way, internal tensions and contradictions within belief systems are exposed, and the arguments that support them are countered.[55] Because of its vagueness, frequent use, and ability to give actions meaning, progress may be even more malleable and capable of reinvention than other concepts. Progress in medicine may once have referred to energy-intensive and wasteful practices that improve the health and life of the few; in the future, it may well come to refer to measures that limit those same practices and promote the life and health of the many.

---

[55] Terence Ball, "Democracy," in *Political Theory and the Ecological Challenge*, eds. Andrew Dobson and Robyn Eckersley (Cambridge: Cambridge University Press, 2006), pp. 135–36.

Bibliography

Ackerknecht, Erwin H., *A Short History of Medicine* (Baltimore: Johns Hopkins University Press, 2016 [1955])
Aday, Lu Ann and Ronald M. Andersen, "Equity of Access to Medical Care: A Conceptual and Empirical Overview," *Medical Care*, 12 (19) (1981), 4–27
Adorno, Theodor, *Minima Moralia: Reflections from Damaged Life*, trans. E. F. N. Jephcott (Frankfurt: Suhrkamp, 1951)
Agar, Nicholas, *The Sceptical Optimist* (Oxford: Oxford University Press, 2015)
Ahuja, Nitin K., "The Body Is Not a Machine," *Aeon*, November 11, 2021, https://aeon.co/essays/how-ecological-thinking-fills-the-gaps-in-biomedicine
Alam, Afroz, "Spices: The Hoard of Natural Remedies," *Annals of Phytomedicine*, 8 (2) (2019), 7–18
Allen, Amy, "How Not to Critique the Critique of Progress: A Reply to Payrow Shabani," *Journal of Value Inquiry*, 51 (2017), 681–87
Allen, Amy, *The End of Progress: Decolonizing the Normative Foundations of Critical Theory* (New York: Columbia University Press, 2016)
Allen, Arthur, "How the Anti-Vaccine Movement Crept into the GOP Mainstream," *Politico*, May 27, 2019, www.politico.com/story/2019/05/27/anti-vaccine-republican-mainstream-1344955
Altini, Carlo, *Le maschere del progresso: Ascesa e caduto di un'idea moderna* (Bologna: Marietti, 2018)
Altwicker, Tilmann and Olivier Diggelmann, "How Is Progress Constructed in International Legal Theory," *The European Journal of International Law*, 25 (2) (2014), 425–44
"AMA President Applauds Members Moving Medicine Forward," *AMA Press Release*, June 8, 2019, www.ama-assn.org/press-center/press-releases/ama-president-applauds-members-moving-medicine-forward
"America Speaks: Polling Data Reflecting the Views of Americans on Medical, Health and Scientific Research," *Research!America: An Alliance for Discoveries in Health*, 14 (2022), 2–20
Anderson, Joel, "Regimes of Autonomy," *Ethical Theory and Moral Practice*, 17 (3) (2014), 355–68
Anderson, Margaret and K. Kimberly McCleary, "From Passengers to Co-Pilots: Patient Roles Expand," *Science Translational Medicine*, 7 (291) (2015), 291fs25

Angell, Marcia, "Pockets of Poverty: Response to Social Justice Is Good for Our Health," *Boston Review*, July 25, 2014, www.bostonreview.net/forum/social-justice-good-our-health/marcia-angell-pockets-poverty

Annas, George, "The Songs of Spring: Quest Myths, Metaphors, and Medical Progress," in *Ethics and the Arts*, ed. Paul Macneil (Dordrecht: Springer, 2014), pp. 225–34

Ariffin, Yohan, *Généalogie de l'idée de progrès. Histoire d'une philosophie cruelle sous un nom consolant* (Paris: Editions du Félin, 2012)

Aristotle, *Politics*, trans. H. Rackham, Loeb Classical Library (Cambridge, MA: Harvard University Press, 1932)

Arnold, Gary, "ADA Legacy Tour: Get on the Bus!," Abilities.com, The Resource for the Disability Community, www.abilities.com/community/ada-bus-tour.html

Atwoli, Lukoye et al., "Call for Emergency Action to Limit Global Temperature Increases, Restore Biodiversity, and Protect Health," *BMJ*, 374 (8305) (2021), n1734

Augustine, *The City of God against the Pagans*, vol. 4, book 15, XXII, Loeb Classical Library 414, trans. Philip Levine (Cambridge, MA: Harvard University Press, 1966)

Baccarini, Elvio, "Personalized Medicine, Justice and Equality," in *Personalized Medicine in Health Care Systems*, eds. Nada Bodiroga-Vukobrat et al. (Switzerland: Springer Nature, 2019), pp. 137–47

Bacon, Francis, *New Atlantis* (New York: P. F. Collier & Son, 1901 [1626]), www.marxists.org/reference/archive/bacon/1626/new-atlantis/index.htm

Bacon, Francis, *Novum Organum, or True Suggestions for the Interpretation of Nature*, ed. Joseph Devey (New York: P. F. Collier & Son, 1902)

Bacon, Francis, "Preface to the Instauratio Magna," in *Prefaces and Prologues*, vol. 39, Harvard Classics, ed. Charles W. Eliot (New York: P. F. Collier & Son, 1909–1914), www.bartleby.com/39/20.html

Bacon, Francis, *The Advancement of Learning*, ed. William Aldis Wright (Oxford: Clarendon Press, 1869 [1605])

Baillie, John, *The Belief in Progress* (London: Oxford University Press, 1950)

Ball, Terence, "Democracy," in *Political Theory and the Ecological Challenge*, eds. Andrew Dobson and Robyn Eckersley (Cambridge: Cambridge University Press, 2006), pp. 131–47

Banerjee, Abhijit and Esther Duflo, *Poor Economics: A Radical Rethinking of the Way to Fight Global Poverty* (New York: PublicAffairs, 2012)

Baril, Alexandre, *Undoing Suicidism: A Trans, Queer, Crip Approach to Rethinking (Assisted) Suicide* (Philadelphia: Temple University Press, 2023)

Barrett, William, *Death of the Soul. Philosophical Thought from Descartes to the Computer* (Oxford: Oxford University Press, 1987)

Barry, John, *Rethinking Green Politics: Nature, Virtue and Progress* (London, Thousand Oaks, CA, and New Delhi: Sage Publications, 1999)

Battista, Renaldo N., "Practice Guidelines for Preventative Care: The Canadian Experience," *British Journal of General Practice*, 43 (1993), 301–4

Baum, Fran E., Monique Bégin, Tanja A. J. Houweling, and Sebastian Taylor, "Changes Not for the Fainthearted: Reorienting Health Care Systems toward Health Equity through Action on the Social Determinants of Health," *American Journal of Public Health*, 99 (11) (2009), 1967–74

Baumgartner, Renate et al., "Fair and Equitable AI in Biomedical Research and Healthcare: Social Science Perspectives," *Artificial Intelligence in Medicine*, 144 (2023), https://doi.org/10.1016/j.artmed.2023.102658

Baylis, Françoise, Nuala P. Kenny, and Susan Sherwin, "A Relational Account of Public Health Ethics," *Public Health Ethics*, 1 (3) (2008), 196–209

Beauchamp, Dan E., "Public Health as Social Justice," in *New Ethics for the Public's Health*, eds. Dan E. Beauchamp and Bonnie Steinbock (Oxford: Oxford University Press, 1999), pp. 101–09

Beauchamp, Tom and James F. Childress, *Principles of Biomedical Ethics*, 7th ed. (Oxford: Oxford University, 2013)

Beaudry, Jonas-Sébastien, "Somatic Oppression and Relational Autonomy: Revisiting Medical Aid in Dying through a Feminist Lens," *UBC Law Review*, 2 (53) (2020), 241–98

Beaujouan, Guy, "Histoire des sciences et philosophie au moyen âge: L'émergence médiévale de l'idée du progrès," *Bulletin de philosophie médiévale*, 30 (1988), 20–36

Beck, Birgit, "Infantilisation through Technology," in *Technology, Anthropology, and Dimensions of Responsibility*, eds. Birgit Beck and Michael Kühler (Stuttgart: J. B. Metzler, 2020), pp. 33–44

Becker, Marshall H., "A Medical Sociologist Looks at Health Promotion," *Journal of Health and Social Behaviour*, 34 (1993), 1–6

Beeson, Paul B., "Changes in Medical Therapy during the Past Half Century," *Medicine*, 59 (2) (1980), 79–99

Belesova, Kristine, Daivd L. Heymann, and Andy Haines, "Integrating Climate Action for Health into COVID-19 Recovery Plans," *BMJ*, 370 (2020), m3169

Benjamin, Walter, "Theses on the Philosophy of History," in *Illuminations*, ed. and intro. Hannah Arendt, trans. Harry Zohn (New York: Schocken Books, 1969), pp. 253–64

Bensimon, Cécile M. and Solomon Benatar, "Developing Sustainability: A New Metaphor for Progress," *Theoretical Medicine and Bioethics*, 27 (1) (2006), 59–79

Bergdolt, Klaus, *Das Gewissen der Medizin: Ärztliche Moral von der Antike bis Heute* (Munich: C. H. Beck, 2004)

Bergdolt, Klaus, *Well-Being: A Cultural History of Healthy Living* (Cambridge: Polity Press, 2009)

Berlin, Isaiah, "Two Concepts of Liberty" (1958), in *Liberty: Incorporating Four Essays on Liberty*, ed. Henry Hardy (Oxford: Oxford University Press, 2002), pp. 166–217

Bertolaso, Marta and Bernhard Strauss, "The Search for Progress and a New Theory Framework in Cancer Research," in *Rethinking Cancer: A New Paradigm for the Postgenomics Era*, eds. Bernhard Strauss et al. (Cambridge, MA: The MIT Press, 2021), pp. 13–40

Betts, Clinton E., "Progress, Epistemology and Human Health and Welfare: What Nurses Need to Know and Why," *Nursing Philosophy*, 6 (2005), 174–88

Biggs, Hermann, "Public Health Is Purchasable," *Monthly Bulletin of the Department of Health of the City of New York*, 1 (10) (1911), 225–26

Bird, Alexander, *Knowing Science* (Oxford: Oxford University Press, 2022)

Birn, Anne-Emmanuelle, "Making It Politic(al): Closing the Gap in a Generation: Health Equity through Action on the Social Determinants of Health," *Social Medicine*, 4 (3) (2009), 166–82

Blasimme, Alessandro and Effy Vayena, "Becoming Partners, Retaining Autonomy: Ethical Considerations on the Development of Precision Medicine," *BMC Medical Ethics*, 67 (2016) 1–8

Boddice, Rob, "Vaccination, Fear and Historical Relevance," *History Compass*, 14 (2) (2016), 71–78

Bok, Sissela, "Rethinking the WHO Definition of Health," in *International Encyclopedia of Public Health*, ed. Harald Kristian Heggenhougen (Amsterdam: Elsevier, 2008), pp. 590–97

Bolton, Derek and Grant Gillett, *The Biopsychosocial Model of Health and Disease: New Philosophical and Scientific Developments* (Cham, Switzerland: Palgrave Pivot, 2020)

Bourke, Joanna, "Pain Sensitivity: An Unnatural History from 1800 to 1965," *Journal of Medical Humanities*, 35 (3) (2014), 301–19

Boyer, Paul, *By the Bomb's Early Light: American Thought and Culture at the Dawn of the Atomic Age* (Chapel Hill & London: University of North Carolina Press, 1985)

Bozok, Nihan, From Modern to Postmodern Medicine: The Case of Organ Transplants, unpublished PhD thesis, Middle East Technical University, Ankara, 2015

Breczko, Anetta, "' Interest of the Individual' versus 'Common Good' and 'Public Interest' in the Context of Technological Progress in Medicine," *Journal of the Polish Section of IVR*, 3 (2020), 41–52

Brey, Philip, "Human Enhancement and Personal Identity," in *New Waves in Philosophy of Technology*, eds. Jan Kyrre Berg Olsen, Evan Selinger, and Søren Riis (New York: Palgrave Macmillan, 2008), pp. 169–85

Brody, Howard, "Autonomy Revisited: Progress in Medical Ethics: Discussion Paper," *Journal of the Royal Society of Medicine*, 78 (1985), 380–87

Brooks, James Lee, "Postmodern Medicine; Review of *PC, MD: How Political Correctness Is Corrupting Medicine*, by Sally Satel," *The Atlas Society*, (2010 [2001]), www.atlassociety.org/post/postmodern-medicine

Brooks, Rodney, *Flesh and Machines: How Robots Will Change Us* (New York: Pantheon, 2002)

Brown, Donald, *Human Universals* (New York: McGraw Hill, 1991)

Broyard, Anatole, *Intoxicated by My Illness: And Other Writings on Life and Death* (New York: Random House, 1993)

Brynjolfsson, Erik and Andrew McAfee, *The Second Machine Age: Work, Progress, and Prosperity in a Time of Brilliant Machines* (New York: W. W. Norton, 2014)

Buchanan, Allen, Dan W. Brock, Norman Daniels, and Daniel Winkler, *From Chance to Choice: Genetics and Justice* (Cambridge: Cambridge University Press, 2000)

Buchanan, Allen and Russell Powell, *The Evolution of Moral Progress: A Biocultural Theory* (Oxford: Oxford University Press, 2018)

Burkeman, Oliver, "Is the World Really Better Than Ever?," *The Guardian*, the Long Read, July 28, 2017, www.theguardian.com/news/2017/jul/28/is-the-world-really-better-than-ever-the-new-optimists

Burkert, W., "Impact and Limits of the Idea of Progress in Antiquity," in *The Idea of Progress*, eds. Arnold Burgen, Peter McLaughlin, and Jürgen Mittelstrass (Berlin, New York: De Gruyter, 1997), pp. 19–46

Burki, Talha, "Behind Cuba's Successful Pandemic Response," *The Lancet Infectious Diseases*, 21 (4) (2021), 465–66

Bury, John Bagnell, *The Idea of Progress: An Inquiry into Its Origin and Growth* (London: Macmillan & Co., 1920)

Bush, Vannevar, "Science, the Endless Frontier," A Report to the President by Vannevar Bush, Director of the Office of Scientific Research and Development, 1945, *U.S. National Science Foundation*, www.nsf.gov/about/history/nsf50/vbush1945.jsp

Butterfield, Herbert, *The Whig Interpretation of History* (London: G. Bell and Sons, 1931)

Bynum, William, *The History of Medicine: A Very Short Introduction* (Oxford: Oxford University Press, 2008)

Callahan, Daniel, "Finite Lives and Unlimited Medical Aspirations," in *The Contingent Nature of Life: Bioethics and the Limits of Human Existence*, eds. Marcus Düwell, Christoph Rehmann-Sutter, and Dietmar Mieth (New York: Springer, 2008), pp. 159–67

Callahan, Daniel, "How Much Medical Progress Can We Afford? Equity and the Cost of Health Care," *Journal of Molecular Biology*, 319 (4), 885–90

Callahan, Daniel, "Modernizing Mortality: Medical Progress and the Good Society," *The Hastings Center Report*, 20 (1) (1990), 28–32

Callahan, Daniel, *What Kind of Life? The Limits of Medical Progress* (Washington, DC: Georgetown University Press, 1990)

Campbell, Louise, "Kant, Autonomy and Bioethics," *Ethics, Medicine and Public Health*, 3 (3) (2017), 381–92

Canguilhem, Georges, *On the Normal and the Pathological*, trans. Carolyn R. Fawcett, intro. Michel Foucault (Dordrecht: D. Reidel Publishing Co., 1978)

Carr, Nicholas, *Utopia Is Creepy and Other Provocations* (New York: W. W. Norton & Company, 2016)

Casassus, Philippe, "Les idées de Jean-Jacques Rousseau sur la médecine," *Médecine*, 13 (7) (2017), 330–34

Cassell, Eric, "Pain, Suffering, and the Goals of Medicine," in *The Goals of Medicine: The Forgotten Issues in Health Care Reform*, eds. Mark J. Hanson and Daniel Callahan (Washington, DC: Georgetown University Press, 1999), pp. 101–17

Cassell, Eric, *The Nature of Healing: The Modern Practice of Medicine* (Oxford: Oxford University Press, 2013)

Cassell, Eric, *The Nature of Suffering and the Goals of Medicine* (New York and Oxford: Oxford University Press, 2004)

Chandler, Jennifer A., "'Obligatory Technologies' and the Autonomy of Patients in Biomedical Ethics," *Griffith Law Review*, 20 (4) (2011), 905–30

Chapman, Allan, *Physicians, Plagues and Progress: The History of Western Medicine from Antiquity to Antibiotics* (Oxford: Lion Books, 2018)

Charlton, Bruce, "Medicine and Post-Modernity," *Journal of the Royal Society of Medicine*, 86 (1993), 497–99

Chokshi, Dave A. and Louise Cohen, "Progress in Primary Care – From Alma-Ata to Astana," *Journal of the American Medical Association*, 320 (19) (2018), 1965–66

Chotiner, Isaac, "The Interwoven Threads of Inequality and Health," *The New Yorker*, April 14, 2020, www.newyorker.com/news/q-and-a/the-coronavirus-and-the-interwoven-threads-of-inequality-and-health

Christiansen, John B. and Irene Leigh, *Cochlear Implants in Children: Ethics and Choices* (Washington, DC: Gallaudet University Press, 2002)

Cleghorn, Elinor, *Unwell Women: Misdiagnosis and Myth in a Man-Made World* (London: Penguin, 2022)

Cognition and Fact: Materials on Ludwik Fleck eds. Robert S. Cohen and Thomas Schnelle, Boston Studies in the Philosophy of Science, 87 (Dordrecht: Springer, 1986)

Cohen, Esther, *The Modulated Scream: Pain in Late Medieval Culture* (Chicago: University of Chicago Press, 2010)

Colgrave, James, "The McKeown Thesis: A Historical Controversy and Its Enduring Influence," *American Journal of Public Health*, 92 (5) (2002), 725–29

Collins, Francis, *The Language of Life: DNA and the Revolution in Personalized Medicine* (New York: Harper Perrenial, 2011)

Colton, F. Barrows, "Your New World of Tomorrow," *National Geographic Magazine*, 88 (4) (1945), 385–410

Commission on Social Determinants of Health, *Closing the Gap in a Generation: Health Equity through Action on the Social Determinants of Health*, Final Report (Geneva: World Health Organization, 2008)

Compton, Karl Taylor, "Science on the March," *Popular Mechanics*, 97 (1) (1952), 120–25

Condorcet, Marquis de, *Esquisse d'un tableau historique des progrès de l'esprit humain* (Paris: Masson et Fils, 1822 [1795])

Conis, Elena, "Beyond Silent Spring: An Alternate History of DDT," *Distillations* (Science History Institute, 2017), www.sciencehistory.org/distillations/beyond-silent-spring-an-alternate-history-of-ddt

Conley, Brandon and Shane Glackin, "How to Be a Naturalist and a Social Constructivist about Diseases," *Philosophy of Medicine*, 2 (2021), 1–21

"Constitution of the World Health Organization," in *Basic Documents*, 49th ed. (Geneva: World Health Organization, 2020), https://apps.who.int/gb/bd/PDF/bd47/EN/constitution-en.pdf?ua=1

Cooper, Amelia, "Hear Me Out: Hearing Each Other for the First Time: The Implications of Cochlear Implant Activation," *Missouri Medicine*, 116 (6) (2019), 469–71

Cooper Owens, Deirdre, *Medical Bondage: Race, Gender and the Origins of American Gynecology* (Atlanta: University of Georgia Press, 2017)

Cooray, Arusha, Krishna Chaitanya Vadlamannati, and Indra de Soysa, "Do Bigger Health Budgets Cushion Pandemics? An Empirical Test of COVID-19 Deaths across the World," *WIDER Working Paper*, 165 (2020), www.econstor.eu/bitstream/10419/229389/1/wp2020-165.pdf

Cooter, Roger, "Medicine and the Goodness of War," *Canadian Bulletin of Medical History*, 7 (1990), 147–59

Cordain, Loren, *The Paleo Diet Revised: Lose Weight and Get Healthy by Eating the Foods You Were Designed to Eat* (Hoboken, NJ: John Wiley & Sons, 2011, revised ed.)

Cortesi, Giacomo, "Hans Jonas, il progresso medico e le verità della scienza," *Humana.Mente* 7 (2008), 107–20

Coulter, A., "Paternalism or Partnership: Patients Have Grown Up – and There's No Going Back," *British Medical Journal*, 319 (7212) (1999), 719–20

Craik, Elizabeth M., "Teleology in Hippocratic Texts: Clues to the Future?," in *Teleology in the Ancient World: Philosophical and Medical Approaches*, ed. Julius Rocca (Cambridge: Cambridge University Press, 2017), pp. 203–16

Crawford, Robert, "You Are 'Dangerous to Your Health': The Ideology and Politics of Victim Blaming," *International Journal of Health*, 7 (4) (1977), 663–80

Crisciani, Chiara, "History, Novelty and Progress in Scholastic Medicine," *Osiris*, 6 (1990), 118–39

Crombie, Alistair C., "Some Attitudes to Scientific Progress: Ancient, Medieval and Early Modern," *History of Science*, 1975 (13), 213–30

d'Angour, Armand, *The Greeks and the New: Novelty in Ancient Greek Imagination and Experience* (Cambridge: Cambridge University Press, 2011)

Dance, Amber, "Survival of the Littlest: The Long-Term Impacts of Being Born Extremely Early," *Nature*, 582 (2020), 20–23

Daniels, Norman, *Just Health Care* (Cambridge: Cambridge University Press, 1985)

Daniels, Norman, *Just Health: Meeting Health Needs Fairly* (Cambridge: Cambridge University Press, 2007)

Daniels, Norman, "Justice, Health, and Health Care," in *Medicine and Social Justice: Essays on the Distribution of Health Care*, eds. Rosamond Rhodes, Margaret Pabst Battin, and Anita Silvers (New York: Oxford University Press, 2002), pp. 6–23

Daniels, Norman, "Reconciling Two Ethics Goals of Public Health: Reducing Health Disparities and Improving Population Health," in *Oxford Handbook of Public Health Ethics*, eds. Anna C. Mastroianni, Jeffrey P. Kahn, and Nancy E. Kass (Oxford: Oxford University Press, 2019), pp. 290–300

Daniels, Norman, Bruce P. Kennedy, and Ichiro Kawachi, "Why Justice Is Good for Our Health: The Social Determinants of Health Inequalities," *Daedalus*, 128 (4) (1999), 215–51

Darwin, Charles, *On the Origin of Species* (Minneapolis, MN: Lerner, 2008 [1859])

Darwin, Charles, *The Descent of Man*, vol. 1 (New York: American Home Library, 1902 [1871])

Daschuk, James, *Clearing the Plains: Disease, Politics of Starvation, and the Loss of Indigenous Life* (Regina: University of Regina Press, 2014)

Daston, Lorraine, "The History of Science and the History of Knowledge," *Know: A Journal on the Formation of Knowledge*, 1 (1) (2017), 131–54

Davey Smith, George and Jerry Morris, "Increasing Inequalities in the Health of the Nation," *BMJ*, 309 (1994), 1453

Davis, Joseph E., *Chemically Imbalanced: Everyday Suffering, Medication, and Our Troubled Quest for Self-Mastery* (Chicago: University of Chicago Press, 2020)

Davis, Joseph E., "Ivan Illich and Irving Kenneth Zola: Disabling Medicalisation," in *The Palgrave Handbook of Social Theory in Health, Illness and Medicine*, ed. Fran Collyer (London: Palgrave Macmillan, 2015), pp. 306–23

Davis, Joseph E. and Ana Marta Gonzalez, eds., *To Fix or to Heal: Patient Care, Public Health, and the Limits of Biomedicine* (New York: New York University Press, 2016)

Davis, Lennard J., "Constructing Normalcy: The Bell Curve, the Novel, and the Invention of the Disabled Body in the Nineteenth Century," in *The Disabilities Studies Reader*, ed. Lennard J. Davis (New York: Routledge, 1997), pp. 3–16

de Vreese, Leen, "Evidence-Based Medicine and Progress in the Medical Sciences," *Journal of Evaluation in Clinical Practice*, 17 (2011), 852–56

de Wert, Guido et al., "Opportunistic Genomic Screening. Recommendations of the European Society of Human Genetics," *European Journal of Human Genetics*, 29 (2021), 365–77

"Declaration of Alma-Ata," International Conference on Primary Health Care, Alma-Ata, USSR, September 6–12, 1978, available at *World Health Organization*, www.who.int/teams/social-determinants-of-health/declaration-of-alma-ata

Delamothe, Tony, "Social Inequalities in Health," *BMJ*, 303 (1991), 1046–50

Delgado, Janet, "Re-thinking Relational Autonomy: Challenging the Triumph of Autonomy through Vulnerability," *Bioethics Update*, 5 (2019), 50–65

Dellsén, Finnur, "Scientific Progress: Knowledge versus Understanding," *Studies in the History and Philosophy of Science*, 56 (2016), 72–83

Descartes, *Discours de la méthode pour bien conduire sa raison et chercher la vérité dans les sciences* (Paris: Librairie Hachette, 1876 [1637])

Descartes and Medicine: Problems, Responses and Survival of a Cartesian Discipline, ed. Fabrizio Baldassarri (Turnhout, Belgium: Brepols, 2023)

Devisch, Ignass, "Progress in Medicine: Autonomy, Oughtonomy and Nudging," *Journal of Evaluation in Clinical Practice* 17 (2011), 857–61

Devisch, Ignass and Stuart J. Murray, "'We Hold These Truths to be Self-Evident': Deconstructing 'Evidence-Based' Medical Practice," *Journal of Evaluation in Clinical Practice*, 15 (2009), 950–54

Diamond, Jared, *Collapse: How Societies Choose to Fail or Succeed* (New York: Viking Press, 2005)
Dickenson, Donna, *Me Medicine vs. We Medicine: Reclaiming Biotechnology for the Common Good* (New York: Columbia University Press, 2013)
Dienstag, Joshua Foa, *Pessimism: Philosophy, Spirit, Ethic* (Princeton, NJ: Princeton University Press, 2009)
Disability Rights Education & Defense Fund, "Road to Freedom," https://dredf.org/2006/11/15/road-to-freedom/
Djulbegovic, Benjamin and Gordon H. Guyatt, "Progress in Evidence-Based Medicine: A Quarter Century On," *Lancet*, 390 (2017), 415–23
Djulbegovic, Benjamin, Gordon H. Guyatt, and Richard E. Ashcroft, "Epistomologic Inquiries in Evidence-Based Medicine," *Cancer Control*, 16 (2) (2009), 158–68
Dodds, Eric Robertson, *The Ancient Concept of Progress and Other Essays on Greek Literature and Belief* (Oxford: Clarendon Press, 1973)
Douglas, James William Bruce, "Social Class Differences in Health and Survival during the First Two Years of Life; the Results of a National Survey," *Population Studies*, 5 (1) (1951), 35–58
Du Pisani, Jacobus A. "Sustainable Development: Historical Roots of the Concept," *Environmental Sciences*, 3 (2) (2006), 83–96
Dubos, René, "Medical Utopias," *Daedalus*, 88 (3) (1959), 410–24
Dubos, René, *Mirage of Health: Utopias, Progress and Biological Change* (New York: Harper, 1959)
Dubos, René, "The Conflict between Progress and Safety," *Archives of Environmental Health: An International Journal*, 6 (4) (1963), 449–52
Dubos, René, "The Evolution of Infectious Diseases in the Course of History," *The Canadian Medical Association Journal*, 79 (6) (1958), 445–51
Duffin, Jacalyn, *COVID-19: A History* (Montreal: McGill-Queens University Press, 2022)
Duffin, Jacalyn, *Lovers and Livers: Disease Concepts in History* (Toronto: University of Toronto Press, 2005)
Dumit, Joseph, "Illnesses You Have to Fight to Get: Facts as Forces in Uncertain, Emergent Illnesses," *Social Science & Medicine*, 62 (2006), 577–90
Dye, Christopher, "Health and Urban Living," *Science*, 319 (5864) (2008), 766–69
Eckelman, Matthew J. and Jodi D. Sherman, "Environmental Impacts of the US Health Care System and Effects on Public Health," *PLoS One*, 11 (6) (2016), e0157014
Eckelman, Matthew J., Jodi D. Sherman, and Andrea J. MacNeill, "Life Cycle Environmental Emissions and Health Damages from the Canadian

Healthcare System: An Economic-Environmental-Epidemiological Analysis," *PLoS Medicine*, 15 (7) (2018), e1002623

Edelstein, Ludwig, *The Idea of Progress in Classical Antiquity* (Baltimore: Johns Hopkins Press, 1967)

Editorial, "The Plight of Essential Workers during the COVID-19 Pandemic," *The Lancet*, 395 (10237) (2020), 1587

Editorial, "UK Life Science Research: Time to Burst the Biomedical Bubble," *The Lancet*, 392 (2018), 1227–28

Eisenberg, Leon, "Medicine and the Idea of Progress," in *Progress: Fact or Illusion*, eds. Leo Marx and Bruce Mazlish (Ann Arbor, MI: University of Michigan Press, 1998 [1996]), pp. 45–64

Elkana, Yehuda, "The Emergence of Second-Order Thinking in Classical Greece," in *The Origins and Diversity of Axial Age Civilizations*, ed. Shmuel N. Eisenstadt (Albany, NY: State University of Albany Press, 1986), pp. 40–65

Ells, Carolyn, Matthew R. Hunt, and Jane Chambers-Evans, "Relational Autonomy as an Essential Component of Patient-Centered Care," *International Journal of Feminist Approaches to Bioethics*, 4 (2) (2011), 79–101

Embodiment: A History, ed. Justin E. H. Smith (Oxford: Oxford University Press, 2017).

Engel, George, "The Need for a New Medical Model: A Challenge for Biomedicine," *Science*, 196 (4286), 129–36

Engels, Frederick, *The Condition of the Working Class in England in 1844*, trans. Florence Kelley Wischnewetzky (London: Swan Sonnenschein & Co., 1892 [1845])

Enria, Luisa and Angus Tengbeh, "Ebola Wahala: Breaching Experiments in a Sierra Leonean Border Town," in *Feeling Disease: Experiencing Medicine and Illness in Modern History*, eds. Rob Boddice and Bettina Hitzer (London: Bloomsbury, 2022), pp. 43–60

Eubanks, Virginia, *Automating Inequality: How High-Tech Tools Profile, Police, and Punish the Poor* (New York: St Martin's, 2018)

Everything4Everyone, ""Covid Partout, Justice Nulle Part": Graffiti in Montreal," April 27, 2020, www.reddit.com/r/Quebec/comments/g97t7q/covid_partout_justice_nulle_part_graffiti_in/

Evidence-Based Medicine Working Group, "Evidence-Based Medicine: A New Approach to Teaching the Practice of Medicine," *Journal of the American Medical Association*, 268 (17) (1992), 2420–25

Faden, Ruth, Thomas Beauchamp, and Nancy King, *A History and Theory of Informed Consent* (New York: Oxford University Press, 1986)

Fallah, Mosoka P., & S. Harris Ali, "When Maximizing Profit Endangers Our Humanity: Vaccines and the Enduring Legacy of Colonialism during the COVID-19 Pandemic," *Studies in Political Economy*, 103 (1) (2022), 94–10

Fang, Fang, *Wuhan Diary: Dispatches from a Quarantined City*, trans. Michael Berry (New York: Harper, 2020)

Farrow, Emily, "Embedding Sustainability into Clinical Medicine and Medical Education," *Health Management*, 17 (5) (2017), 369–71

Fattori, Marta, "*Prolongatio Vitae* and *Euthanasia* in Francis Bacon," in *Francis Bacon on Motion and Power*, eds. Guido Giglioni, et al. (Cham, Switzerland: Springer, 2016), pp. 115–32

"Fauci: 'Undeniable Effects of Racism' Have Worsened Covid for U.S. Minorities," *The Guardian Online*, May 16, 2021, www.theguardian.com/world/2021/may/16/fauci-racism-covid-us-black-hispanic-native-americans-emory-university-graduation

Faulkner, Robert K., *Francis Bacon and the Project of Progress* (Lanham, MD: Rowman & Littlefield, 1993)

Fendall, Neville R., "Auxiliaries and Primary Medical Care," *Bulletin of the New York Academy of Medicine*, 48 (10) (1972), 1291–300

Ferngren, Gary B., *Medicine and Health Care in Early Christianity* (Baltimore: Johns Hopkins University Press, 2009)

Feyerabend, Paul, *Against Method: Outline of an Anarchistic Theory of Knowledge* (London: New Left Books, 1975)

Fioretti, Chiara et al., "Research Studies on Patients' Illness Experience Using the Narrative Medicine Approach: A Systematic Review," *BMJ Open*, 6 (2016), e011220

Firestein, Stuart, *Failure* (Oxford: Oxford University Press, 2015)

Fissell, Mary E., *Patients, Power, and the Poor in Eighteenth-Century Bristol* (Cambridge: Cambridge University Press, 1991)

Fissell, Mary E., "The Disappearance of the Patient's Narrative and the Invention of Hospital Medicine," *British Medicine in an Age of Reform*, eds. Andrew Wear and Roger French (London: Routledge, 1991), pp. 92–109

Fleurbaey, Marc et al., *A Manifesto for Social Progress: Ideas for a Better Society* (Cambridge: Cambridge University Press, 2018)

Flexner, Abraham, *Medical Education in the United States and Canada*, intro. Henry S. Pritchett (New York: Carnegie Foundation for the Advancement of Teaching, 1910)

Flood, Colleen M. et al., eds., *Vulnerable: The Law, Policy & Ethics of COVID-19* (Ottawa: University of Ottawa Press, 2020)

Folbre, Nancy et al., "The Multiple Directions of Social Progress: Ways Forward," in *Rethinking Society for the 21st Century*, ed. International Panel on Social Progress, vol. 2 (Cambridge: University of Cambridge Press, 2018), pp. 815–46

Folbre, Nancy et al., *Rethinking Society for the 21st Century: Report of the International Panel on Social Progress*, vol. 3 (Cambridge: Cambridge University Press, 2018)

Follman, Joseph F., *Medical Care and Health Insurance: A Study in Social Progress* (Homewood, IL: R. D. Irwin, 1963)

Forst, Rainer, "The Justification of Progress and the Progress of Justification," in *Justification and Emancipation: The Critical Theory of Rainer Forst*, eds. Amy Allen and Eduardo Mendieta (State College, PA: Penn State University Press, 2019), pp. 17–37

Forst, Rainer, "Zum Begriff des Fortschritts," in *Vielfalt der Moderne – Ansichten der Moderne*, ed. Hans Joas (Frankfurt am Main: Fischer, 2012), pp. 41–52

Forte, Maximilian C., "Progress, Progressivism, and Progressives," *Zero Anthropology*, February 28, 2018, https://zeroanthropology.net/2018/02/28/progress-progressivism-and-progressives/

Fortier, Suzanne, "Message to the McGill Community Regarding COVID-19," via email to all McGill staff and students, April 29, 2020

Foster, Charles, "Autonomy Should Chair Not Rule," *The Lancet*, 375 (2010), 368–69

Foucault, Michel, *History of Sexuality*, vol. I, An Introduction (New York: Pantheon, 1978)

Foucault, Michel, "The Crisis of Medicine or the Crisis of Antimedicine," *Foucault Studies*, 1 (2004 [1974])), 5–19

Fox, Ellen, "Rethinking DoctorThink: Reforming Medical Education by Nurturing Neglected Goals," in *The Goals of Medicine*, eds. Mark J. Hanson and Daniel Callahan (Washington, DC: Georgetown University Press, 1999), pp. 186–87

Fox, Renée C., "The Evolution of American Bioethics: A Sociological Perspective," in *Social Science Perspectives on Medical Ethics*, ed. George Weisz (Dordrecht: Kluwer Academic Publishers, 1990), pp. 201–17

Frampton, Sally, *Belly-Rippers, Surgical Innovation and the Ovariotomy Controversy* (Cham: Palgrave Macmillan, 2018)

Frank, Arthur W., *The Wounded Storyteller: Body, Illness, and Ethics* (Chicago: University of Chicago Press, 1995)

Frankel, Charles, "Progress, Idea of," in *Encyclopedia of Philosophy*, 2nd ed., ed. Donald M. Borchert (Detroit: Thomson Gale, 2006), www.encyclopedia.com/humanities/encyclopedias-almanacs-transcripts-and-maps/progress-idea

Frankel, Charles, *The Faith of Reason: The Idea of Progress in the French Enlightenment* (New York: Columbia University Press, 1948)

Fredriksen, Ståle, "Tragedy, Utopia and Medical Progress," *Journal of Medical Ethics*, 32 (2006), 450–53

Freeden, Michael, *The New Liberalism: An Ideology of Social Reform* (Oxford: Clarendon Press, 1986 [1978])

Freeman, Bill, "Healthcare Futurist: Evolving Technologies "Re-alter the Fabric of Humanity," *World Health Net*, (2006), www.worldhealth.net/news/healthcare_futurist_evolving_technologie/

Fried, Charles, "Equality and Rights in Medical Care," *Hastings Center Report*, 6 (1) (1976), 29–34

Friend, John, *The History of Physic from the Time of Galen to the Beginning of the Sixteenth Century* (London: J. Walthoe, 1725)

"From Benjamin Franklin to Joseph Priestley, 8 February 1780," *Founders Online*, National Archives, https://founders.archives.gov/documents/Franklin/01-31-02-0325

Frumkin, Howard et al., "Nature Contact and Human Health: A Research Agenda," *Environmental Health Perspectives*, 125 (7) (2017), https://doi.org/10.1289/EHP1663

Fuller, Jonathan, "Epidemiological Evidence: Use at Your "Own Risk"?" *Philosophy of Science*, 87 (5) (2020), 1119–29

Fuller, Steve, *Knowledge: The Philosophical Quest in History* (London: Routledge, 2015)

Gäbler, Karsten "Green Capitalism, Sustainability, and Everyday Practice," in *Global Sustainability*, eds. Benno Werlen et al. (Cham: Springer, 2015), pp. 63–86

Galea, Sandro, *Well: What We Need to Talk about When We Talk about Health* (Oxford: Oxford University Press, 2019)

Ganz, Cheryl R., *The 1933 Chicago World's Fair: A Century of Progress* (Urbana, Chicago and Springfield: University of Illinois Press, 2008)

Garcia, Tamara and Ronald Sandler, "Enhancing Justice?," *Ethics and Emerging Technologies*, ed. Ronald Sandler (London: Palgrave Macmillan, 2014), pp. 252–66

Garland-Thomson, Rosemarie, "Welcoming the Unexpected," in *Human Flourishing in an Age of Gene Editing*, eds. Erik Parens and Josephine Johnston (Oxford: Oxford University Press, 2019), pp. 15–28

Gaudillière, Jean-Paul, Caroline Izambert, and Pierre-André Juven, *Pandémopolitique : Réinventer la santé en commun* (Paris: La Découverte, 2021)

Gawande, Atul, *Complications: A Surgeon's Notes on an Imperfect Science* (London: Profile Books, 2002)

Gawdat, Mo, *Scary Smart: The Future of Artificial Intelligence and How You Can Save Our World* (London: Pan Macmillan, 2021)

Gay, Peter, *Enlightenment: An Interpretation*, vol. 2, *The Science of Freedom* (New York: Alfred A. Knopf, 1969)

Geddes, Gary, *Medicine Unbundled: A Journey through the Minefields of Indigenous Health Care* (Victoria: Heritage House, 2017)

George, Tobias, "From Reading to Understanding: Profectus in Abelard and Origen," in *Progress in Origen and the Origenian Tradition*, eds. Gaetano Lettieri, Maria Fallica, and Anders-Christian Jacobsen (Berlin: Peter Lang, 2020), pp. 127–39

Getz, Faye, *Medicine in the English Middle Ages* (Princeton, NJ: Princeton University Press, 1999)

Getz, Faye, "Roger Bacon and Medicine: The Paradox of the Forbidden Fruit and the Secrets of Long Life," in *Roger Bacon and the Sciences: Commemorative Essays*, ed. Jeremiah Hackett (Leiden and New York: Brill, 1997), pp. 337–64

Gillies, Donald, "Hempelian and Kuhnian Approaches in the Philosophy of Medicine: The Semmelweis Case," *Studies in the History and Philosophy of Biological and Biomedical Sciences*, 36 (2015), 159–81

Gluckman, Peter et al., *Principles of Evolutionary Medicine* (Oxford: Oxford University Press, 2016)

Goldenberg, Maya J., *Vaccine Hesitancy: Public Trust, Expertise, and the War on Science* (Pittsburgh, PA: Pittsburgh University Press, 2021)

Goodman, Melody, cited in "Zip Code Better Predictor of Health Than Genetic Code," News, Harvard T. H. Chan School of Public Health, August 4, 2014, www.hsph.harvard.edu/news/features/zip-code-better-predictor-of-health-than-genetic-code/

Goodwin, William, "Revolution and Progress in Medicine," *Theoretical Medicine and Bioethics*, 36 (2015), 25–39

Gordon, Deborah R., "Tenacious Assumptions in Western Medicine," in *Biomedicine Examined*, eds. Margaret Lock and Deborah R. Gordon (Dordrecht: Kluwer Academic Publishers, 1988), pp. 19–56

Görgen, Benjamin and Björn Wendt, "Nachhaltigkeit als Fortschritt denken: Grundrisse einer soziologisch fundierten Nachhaltigkeitsforschung," *Soziologie und Nachhaltigkeit*, 1 (1) (2015), 3–21

Gostin, Lawrence O., "Public Health, Ethics, and Human Rights: A Tribute to the Late Jonathan Mann," *Journal of Law, Medicine & Ethics*, 29 (2001), 121–30

Gostin, Lawrence O. and Madison Powers, "What Does Social Justice Require for the Public's Health? Public Health Ethics & Policy Imperatives," *Health Affairs*, 25 (4) (2006), 1053–60

Gouvernement du Québec, "Aller mieux en contexte de pandémie COVID-19," 2020, www.quebec.ca/sante/problemes-de-sante/a-z/coronavirus-2019/aller-mieux-en-contexte-de-pandemie-covid-19/

Gracia, Diego, "What Kind of Values? A Historical Perspective on the Ends of Medicine," in *The Goals of Medicine: The Forgotten Issues in Health Care Reform*, eds. Mark J. Hanson and Daniel Callahan (Washington, DC: Georgetown University Press, 1999), pp. 88–100

Gray, John, "An Illusion with a Future," *Daedalus*, 133 (3) (2004), 10–17

Gray, John, "Cats Can Teach Us about the Meaning of Life," *JSTOR Daily*, December 6, 2020, https://daily.jstor.org/john-gray-cats-can-teach-us-about-the-meaning-of-life/

Gray, John, *Heresies: Against Progress and Other Illusions* (London: Granata Books, 2015)

Gray, John, *The Silence of Animals: On Progress and Other Modern Myths* (London: Penguin, 2013)

Green, Stefanie, *This Is Assisted Dying: A Doctor's Story of Empowering Patients at the End of Life* (New York: Scribner, 2022)

Greene, Jeremy A., *The Doctor Who Wasn't There* (Chicago: University of Chicago Press, 2022)

Greener NHS: National Ambition, NHS England, www.england.nhs.uk/greenernhs/national-ambition/

Griffiths, Simon, "What Was Progressive in "Progressive Conservatism"?," *Political Studies Review*, 12 (2014), 29–40

Grob, Gerald N., *Aging Bones: A Short History of Osteoporosis* (Baltimore: Johns Hopkins University Press, 2014)

Grob, Gerald N. and Allan V. Horwitz, *Diagnosis, Therapy, and Evidence: Conundrums in Modern American Medicine* (New Brunswick, NJ: Rutgers University Press, 2010)

Gunter, Jen, "Mother of 3, Parent of 2. Reflections on the Saddest Sorority," July 7, 2017, https://drjengunter.com/2017/07/07/mother-of-3-parent-of-2-reflections-on-the-saddest-sorority/

Habermas, Jürgen, *The Future of Human Nature* (Cambridge: Polity Press, 2001)

Handoh, Itsuki C. and Toshitaka Hidaka, "On the Timescales of Sustainability and Futurability," *Futures*, 42 (7) (2010), 743–48

Hanemaayer, Ariane, ed., *Artificial Intelligence and Its Discontents: Critiques from the Social Sciences and Humanities* (Cham, Switzerland: Palgrave Macmillan, 2022)

Hansen, Bert, *Picturing Medical Progress from Pasteur to Polio: A History of Mass Media Images and Popular Attitudes in America* (Newark, NJ: Rutgers University Press, 2009)

Hanson, Mark J., "The Idea of Progress and the Goals of Medicine," in *The Goals of Medicine: The Forgotten Issues in Health Care Reform*, eds. Mark J. Hanson and Daniel Callahan (Washington, DC: Georgetown University Press, 1999), pp. 137–51

Harding, Sandra, *The Science Question in Feminism* (Ithaca, NY: Cornell University Press, 1986)

Harding, Sandra, *Whose Science? Whose Knowledge?: Thinking from Women's Lives* (Ithaca, NY: Cornell University Press, 1991)

Harper, Douglas, "Etymology of progress," *Online Etymology Dictionary*, www.etymonline.com/word/progress

Harrington, Anne, *The Cure Within: A History of Mind-Body Medicine* (New York: W. W. Norton, 2008)

Harrington, John A., "The Idea of Progress in Medicine and the Common Law," *Social & Legal Studies*, 11 (2) (2002), 211–32

Harris, John, *Enhancing Evolution: The Ethical Case for Making Better People* (Princeton, NJ: Princeton University Press, 2011)

Harlow, John, Aaron Golub, and Braden Allenby, "A Review of Utopian Themes in Sustainable Development Discourse," *Sustainable Development*, 21 (4) (2013), 270–80

Hayes, Jeanne and Elizabeth "Lisa" M. Hannold, "The Road to Empowerment: A Historical Perspective on the Medicalization of Disability," *Journal of Health and Human Services Administration*, 30 (3) (2007), 352–77

Hayles, N. Katherine and Todd Gannon, "Mood Swings: The Aesthetics of Ambient Emergence," in *The Mourning After: Attending the Wake of Postmodernism*, eds. Neil Brooks and Josh Toth (Amsterdam & New York: Rodopi, 2007), pp. 99–142

Hawkins, Anne Hunsaker, *Reconstructing Illness: Studies in Pathography* (West Lafayette, IN: Purdue University, 1993)

Health Care Without Harm, https://noharm-global.org/

Healthy Scepticism, www.healthyscepticism.com

Heilinger, Jan-Christoph, ed. and intro. *Philip Kitcher: Moral Progress*, (Oxford: Oxford University Press, 2021)

Heilinger, Jan-Christoph and Katja Crone, "Human Freedom and Enhancement," *Medicine Health Care and Philosophy*, 17 (1) (2014), 13–21

Hippocrates, *Ancient Medicine*, ed. and trans. Paul Potter, Loeb Classical Library 147 (Cambridge, MA: Harvard University Press, 2022)

Hippocrates, *The Art*, ed. and trans. Paul Potter, Loeb Classical Library 148 (Cambridge, MA: Harvard University Press, 2022)

Ho, Dien, *A Philosopher Goes to the Doctor: A Critical Look at Philosophical Assumptions in Medicine* (New York: Routledge, 2019)

Hodgkin, Paul, "Medicine, Postmodernism, and the End of Certainty," *BMJ*, 313 (1996), 1568–69

Holland, Alan, "Sustainability," in *A Companion to Environmental Philosophy*, ed. Dale Jamieson (Malden, MA: Blackwell Publishers, 2001), pp. 390–401

Honneth, Axel, "How to Envision Social Progress Today," *Social Imaginaries*, 1 (2018), 157–69
Honneth, Axel, "The Irreducibility of Progress: Kant's Account of the Relationship between Morality and History," *Critical Horizons*, 8 (1) (2007), 1–17
Honneth, Axel and Felix Koch, "The Normativity of Ethical Life," *Philosophy and Social Criticism*, 40 (8) (2014)
Hôpitaux Universitaires Genève, Recherche & Innovation, www.hug.ch/recherche-innovation-0
Horn, Werner, "AI in Medicine on Its Way from Knowledge-Intensive to Data-Intensive Systems," *Artificial Intelligence in Medicine*, 23 (2001), 5–12
Horton, Richard, "Marx and Medicine," *The Lancet*, 390 (2017), 2026
Horton, Richard, "Offline: Rebelling against the Dictatorship of Reason," *The Lancet*, 381 (9869) (2013), 790
Horton, Richard, *The COVID-19 Catastrophe: What's Gone Wrong and How to Stop It Happening Again* (Cambridge: Polity Press, 2020)
Hrubec, Zdenek, "The Association of Health and Social Welfare Problems in Individuals and Their Families," *Milbank Memorial Fund Quarterly*, 37 (3) (1959), 251–76
Huber, Jakob, "Looking Back, Looking Forward: Progress, Hope, and History," *Constellations*, 28 (2021), 126–39
Hughes, H. Stuart, *Consciousness and Society: The Reorientation of European Social Thought, 1890–1930*, intro. Stanley Hoffman (New York: Routledge, 2017 [1958])
Huisman, Frank, "Shaping the Medical Market: On the Construction of Quackery and Folk Medicine in Dutch Historiography," *Medical History*, 43 (1999), 359–75
Humphrey, Hubert H., *The United States and the World Health Organization: Teamwork for Mankind's Well-Being. Report of Senator Hubert H. Humphrey* (Washington, DC: Government Printing Office, 1959)
Hussain, Azhar et al., "The Anti-Vaccination Movement: A Regression in Modern Medicine," *Cureus*, 10 (7) (2018), e2919
Ignatieff, Michael, "Modern Dying: The Soul Returns to the Sick Bed," *The New Republic* (26 December 1988), 28–33
Illich, Ivan, *Disabling Professions* (London: Marion Boyars, 1977)
Illich, Ivan, *Medical Nemesis: The Expropriation of Health* (London: Marion Boyars, 1975)
Inequalities in Health: The Black Report (1980) available at *Socialist Health Association*, https://sochealth.co.uk/national-health-service/public-health-and-wellbeing/poverty-and-inequality/the-black-report-1980/black-report-material/

Irwin, Alec and Elena Scali, "Action on the Social Determinants of Health: A Historical Perspective," *Global Public Health*, 2 (3) (2007), 235–56

Isidorus (Isidore of Seville), *Sententiae*, 2, 5, *Monumenta*, http://monumenta.ch/latein/text.php?tabelle=Isidorus&rumpfid=Isidorus,%20Sententiae,%202,%20%20%20%205&level=4&domain=&lang=1&links=1&inframe=1&hide_apparatus=1

Itay, Anat, "Conceptions of Progress: How Is Progress Perceived? Mainstream versus Alternative Conceptions of Progress," *Social Indicators Research*, 92 (2009), 529–50

Jaeger, Werner, "Aristotle's Use of Medicine as Model of Method in His Ethics," *The Journal of Hellenic Studies*, 77 (1) (1957), 54–61

Jaeggi, Rahel, *Fortschritt und Regression* (Berlin: Suhrkamp, 2023)

Jaki, Stanley L., "Medieval Christianity: Its Inventiveness in Technology and Science," in *Technology in the Western Political Tradition*, eds. Arthur M. Melzer, Jerry Weinberger, and M. Richard Zinman (Ithaca, NY and London: Cornell University Press, 1993), pp. 46–69

James, Robert, *A Medicinal Dictionary Including Physic, Surgery, Anatomy, Chemistry and Botany in All Their Branches Relative to Medicine* (London: T. Osborne, 1743)

Jaspers, Karl, *The Origin and Goal of History* (London and New York: Routledge, 2021 [1949])

Jauss, Hans Robert, "Ursprung und Bedeutung der Fortschrittsidee in der 'Querelle des Anciens et des Modernes,'" in *Die Philosophie und die Frage nach dem Fortschritt*, eds. Helmut Kuhn and Franz Wiedmann (Munich: Anton Pustet, 1964), pp. 51–72

Jonas, Hans, "Philosophical Reflections on Experimenting with Human Subjects," *Daedalus*, 98 (2) (1969), 219–47

Jonas, Hans, "Reflections on Technology, Progress, and Utopia," *Social Research*, 48 (3) (1981), 411–55

Jonas, Hans, *The Imperative of Responsibility: In Search of an Ethics for the Technological Age* (Chicago: University of Chicago Press, 1984)

Jonsen, Albert R., *The Birth of Bioethics* (Oxford: Oxford University Press, 2003)

Jordanova, Ludmilla, "Reflections on Medical Reform: Cabanis' Coup d'Oeuil," in *Medicine in the Enlightenment*, ed. Roy Porter (Amsterdam: Rodopi, 1995), pp. 166–80

joski65, June 3, 2014, 12:25, comment to "The Case for Eating Steak and Cream: Why Everything You Heard about Fat Is Wrong," review of Nina Teicholz, *The Big Fat Surprise: Why Butter, Meat and Cheese Belong in a Healthy Diet*, May 31, 2014, *The Economist*, www.economist.com/news/books-and-arts/21602984-why-everything-you-heard-about-fat-wrong-case-eating-steak-and-cream?zid=318&ah=ac379c09c1c3fb67e0e8fd1964d5247f

Juengst, Eric, Michael A. Flatt, and Richard A. Settersten, Jr., "Personalized Genomic Medicine and the Rhetoric of Empowerment," *Hastings Center Report*, 42 (5) (2012), 34–40

Jutel, Annemarie, *Putting a Name to It: Diagnosis in Contemporary Society* (Baltimore: Johns Hopkins University Press, 2011)

Kalanithi, Paul, *When Breath Becomes Air* (New York: Random House, 2016)

Kamm, Frances M., "Health and Equality of Opportunity," *American Journal of Bioethics*, 1 (2001), 17–19

Kant, Immanuel, "An Old Question Raised Again: Is the Human Race Constantly Progressing," in *Religion and Rational Theology*, trans. and eds. Allen W. Wood and George di Giovanni (Cambridge: Cambridge University Press, 2012), pp. 297–309

Kant, Immanuel, "On the Common Saying: 'This May Be True in Theory, but It Does Not Apply in Practice,'" in *Kant, Political Writings*, ed. and intro. Hans Reiss, trans. H. B. Nisbet (Cambridge: Cambridge University Press, 1991 [1970]), 2nd enlarged ed., pp. 61–92

Kaplan, Abraham, "Social Ethics and the Sanctity of Life: A Summary," in *Life or Death: Ethics and Options*, eds. Edward Shils and Daniel H. Labby (Portland, OR: Reed College, 1968), pp. 152–67

Kekes, John, *The Morality of Pluralism* (Princeton, NJ: Princeton University Press, 1993)

Kelly, Michael P. et al., "The Importance of Values in Evidence-Based Medicine," *BMC Medical Ethics*, 16 (69) (2015), doi 10.1186/s12910-015-0063-3

Kelvin, William, "Electrical Units of Measurement," May 3, 1883, *Popular Lectures and Addresses*, ed. Sir William Thomson, vol. 1 (London: Macmillan and Co., 1889), pp. 73–136

Kennedy, Ian, *The Unmasking of Medicine* (London: George Allen and Unwin, 1981)

Keohane, Nannerl O., "The Enlightenment Idea of Progress Revisited," in *Progress and Its Discontents*, eds. Gabriel A. Almond, Marvin Chodorow, and Roy Harvey Pearce (Berkeley: University of California Press, 1982), pp. 21–40

Kerridge, Ian and Michael Lowe, "Bloodletting: The Story of a Therapeutic Technique," *Medical Journal of Australia*, 163 (4) (1995), 631–33

Kickbusch, Ilona, "Approaches to an Ecological Base for Public Health," *Health Promotion International*, 4 (4) (1989), 265–68

Kinzig, Wolfram, *Novitas Christiana. Die Idee des Fortschritts in der Alten Kirche bis Eusebius* (Göttingen: Vandenhoeck & Ruprecht, 1994)

Kitcher, Philip, "On Progress," in *Performance and Progress: Essays on Capitalism, Business, and Society*, ed. Subramanian Rangan (Oxford: Oxford University Press, 2015), pp. 115–33

Kitcher, Philip, "Pragmatism and Progress," *Transactions of the Charles S. Peirce Society: A Quarterly Journal in American Philosophy*, 51 (4) (2015), 475–94

Klein, Naomi, "Dancing the World into Being: A Conversation with Idle No More's Leanne Simpson," *Yes! Magazine*, March 6, 2013, www.yesmagazine.org/peace-justice/dancing-the-world-into-being-a-conversation-with-idle-no-more-leanne-simpson

Kleingeld, Pauline, "Kant, History and the Idea of Moral Development," *History of Philosophy Quarterly*, 16 (1) 1999, 59–80

Kleinman, Arthur, *The Illness Narratives: Suffering, Healing, and the Human Condition* (New York: Basic Books, 1988)

Kolata, Gina, "Advances Elusive in the Drive to Cure Cancer," *The New York Times*, April 24, 2009, www.nytimes.com/2009/04/24/health/policy/24cancer.html

Korinek, Anton and Joseph E. Stiglitz, "Artificial Intelligence and Its Implications for Income Distribution and Unemployment," in *The Economics of Artificial Intelligence: An Agenda*, eds. Ajay Agrawal, Joshua Gans, and Avi Goldfarb (Chicago: University of Chicago Press, 2019), pp. 349–90

Körtner, Ulrich, "The Challenge of Genetic Engineering to Medical Anthropology and Ethics," *Human Reproduction and Genetic Ethics*, 7 (1) (2001), 21–25

Koselleck, Reinhart and Christian Meier, "Fortschritt," in *Geschichtliche Grundbegriffe*, Historisches Lexikon zur politisch-sozialen Sprache in Deutschland, eds. Otto Brunner, Wilhelm Conze, and Reinhart Koselleck (Stuttgart: Klett-Cotta, 1977), vol. 2, pp. 351–423

Kuhn, Thomas, *The Essential Tension: Selected Studies in Scientific Tradition and Change* (Chicago & London, University of Chicago Press, 1977)

Kuhn, Thomas, *The Structure of Scientific Revolutions*, 2nd ed. (Chicago: University of Chicago Press, 1970 [1962])

Lasch, Christopher, "The Fragility of Liberalism," *Salmagundi*, 92 (1991), 5–18

Lasch, Christopher, *The True and Only Heaven: A History of Progress and Its Critics* (New York: W. W. Norton & Company, 1991)

Latour, Bruno, "Le train du progrès n'emprunte pas qu'une seule voie," *Le Monde*, September 25, 2020, p. 29

Laudan, Larry, *Progress and Its Problems: Towards a Theory of Scientific Growth* (Oakland: University of California Press, 1977)

Layne, Linda L., "'How's the Baby Doing?' Struggling with Narratives of Progress in a Neonatal Intensive Care Unit," *Medical Anthropology Quarterly*, 10 (4) (1996), 624–56

Lazar, Philippe, "The Idea of Progress and Human Health," in *The Idea of Progress*, eds. Jürgen Mittelstrass, Peter McLaughlin, and Arnold S. V. Burgen (New York: W. de Gruyter, 1997), pp. 219–29

Le, Tuyet-Anh T. et al., "Policy Responses to the COVID-19 Pandemic in Vietnam," *International Journal of Environmental Research and Public Health*, 18 (2) (2021), 559, https://doi.org/10.3390/ijerph18020559

Le Clerc, Daniel, *Histoire de la médecine, où l'on voit l'origine et les progrès de cet art, de siècle en siècle* (The Hague: Isaac van der Kloot, 1729)

Ledford, Heidi, "Millions of Black People Affected by Racial Bias in Health-Care Algorithms," *Nature*, 574 (2019), 608–9

Leibniz, *Monadology* (1714) in Lloyd Strickland, *Leibniz's Monadology: A New Translation and Guide* (Edinburgh: Edinburgh University Press, 2014)

Lengwiler, Martin and Jeannette Madarász, "Präventionsgeschichte als Kulturgeschichte der Gesundheitspolitik," in *Das präventive Selbst: Eine Kulturgeschichte moderner Gesundheitspolitik*, eds. Martin Lengwiler and Jeannette Madarász (Bielefeld: Transcript, 2010), pp. 11–28

Leonard, Eileen B., *Women, Technology, and the Myth of Progress* (Upper Saddle River, NJ: Prentice Hall, 2003)

Lesher, James H., *Xenophanes of Colophon: Fragments* (Toronto: University of Toronto Press, 1992)

Lezen, Manfred et al., "The Environmental Footprint of Health Care: A Global Assessment," *Lancet Planetary Health*, 4 (2020), e271–79

Lima, Meiriany Arruda and Camilo Manchola-Castillo, "Bioethics, Palliative Care and Liberation: A Contribution to 'Dying Well'," *Revista Bioética*, 29 (2) (2021), 268–78

Lindeboom, Gerrit Arie, *Descartes and Medicine* (Amsterdam: Rodopi, 1979)

Link, Bruce G. and Jo Phelan, "Social Conditions as Fundamental Causes of Disease," *Journal of Health and Social Behaviour*, Special Issue: Forty Years of Medical Sociology: The State of the Art and Directions for the Future (1995), 80–94

Liu, Xiaoxuan, Pearse A. Keane, and Alastair K. Denniston, "Time to Regenerate: The Doctor in the Age of Artificial Intelligence," *Journal of the Royal Society of Medicine*, 111 (4) (2018), 113–16

Lohff, Brigitte, "Fortschritt mit der Wissenschaft: Wissenschaft ist Fortschritt. Der Wandel der Fortschrittsidee in der deutschen Medizin im 19. Jahrhundert," *Wissenschaftstheorien in der Medizin*, eds. Wolfgang Deppert, Hartmut Kliemt, Brigitte Lohff and Jochen Schäfer (Berlin and Boston: De Gruyter, 2015), pp. 327–54

Lohff, Brigitte, "Self-Healing Forces and Concepts of Health and Disease. A Historical Discourse," *Theoretical Medicine and Bioethics*, 22 (2001), 543–64

Lomasky, Loren E., "Medical Progress and National Health Care," *Philosophy & Public Affairs*, 10 (1) (1981), 65–88
Losee, John, *Theories of Scientific Progress: An Introduction* (London: Psychology Press, 2004)
Löwith, Karl, *Meaning and History: The Theological Implications of the Philosophy of History* (Chicago: University of Chicago Press, 1957)
Löwy, Ilana, ed., "Medicine and Change," in *Innovations in Health and Medicine. Diffusion and Resistance in the Twentieth Century* (London: Routledge, 2002), pp. 1–15
Lu, Catherine, "Progress, Decolonization and Global Justice: A Tragic View," *International Affairs*, 99 (1) (2023), 141–59
Lupton, Deborah, *Medicine as Culture: Illness, Disease and the Body* (Los Angeles: SAGE, 2012 [1994])
Lupton, Deborah, "The Digitally Engaged Patient: Self-Monitoring and Self-Care in the Digital Health Era," *Social Theory and Health*, 11 (3) (2013), 256–70
Lyotard, Jean-François, *La condition postmoderne: rapport sur le savoir* (Paris: Minuit, 1979)
MacDonald, Noni E., SAGE Working Group on Vaccine Hesitancy, "Vaccine Hesitancy: Definition, Scope and Determinants," *Vaccine*, 33 (34) (2015), 4161–64
Mackenzie, Catriona and Natalie Stoljar, eds. *Relational Autonomy: Feminist Perspectives on Autonomy, Agency, and the Social Self* (New York: Oxford University Press, 2000)
Macklin, Ruth, "Moral Progress," *Ethics*, 87 (4) (1977), 370–82
Magalhães, Susana, "Looking behind the Veil: Why Narrative Medicine Matters in Times of Uncertainties," in *Health Humanities for Quality of Care in Times of COVID-19*, eds. Maria Giulia Marini and Jonathan McFarland (Cham: Springer, 2022), pp. 25–36
Mahler, Halfdan, "The Meaning of 'Health for All by the Year 2000'," *World Health Forum*, 2 (1) (1981), excerpted in "Voices from the Past," *American Journal of Public Health*, 106 (1) (2016), 36–38
Malik, Arunima et al., "The Carbon Footprint of Australian Health Care," *Lancet Planetary Health*, 2 (1) (2018), e27–e35
Maller, Cecily et al., "Healthy Nature Healthy People: 'Contact with Nature' as an Upstream Health Promotion Intervention for Populations," *Health Promotion International*, 21 (1) (2005), 45–54
Maller, Cecily et al., "Healthy Parks, Healthy People: The Health Benefits of Contact with Nature in a Park Context," *The George Wright Forum*, 26 (2) (2009), 51–83
Man and His Future: A Ciba Foundation Volume, ed. Gordon Wolstenholme (London: J. & A. Churchill Ltd, 1963)

Manciaux, Michel and Theodor M. Fliedner, "World Health: A Mobilizing Utopia?," in *Understanding the Global Dimensions of Health*, eds. Sisvan W. A. Gunn et al., (Boston: Springer, 2005), pp. 69–82

Markandya, Anil et al., "Health Co-Benefits from Air Pollution and Mitigation Costs of the Paris Agreement: A Modelling Study," *The Lancet Planetary Health*, 2 (3) (2018), 126–33

Marmor, Theodore R., Morris L. Barer, and Robert G. Evans, "The Determinants of a Population's Health: What Can Be Done to Improve a Democratic Nation's Health Status?," in *Why Are Some People Healthy and Others Not? The Determinants of the Health of Populations*, eds. Robert G. Evans, Morris L. Barer, and Theodore R. Marmor (London and New York: Routledge, 1994), pp. 217–30

Marmot, Michael, "Global Action on Social Determinants of Health," *Bulletin of the World Health Organization*, 89 (2011), 702

Marmot, Michael, "Society and the Slow Burn of Inequality," *The Lancet*, 395 (10234) (2020), 1413–14

Marmot, Michael, Geoffrey Rose, Martin Shipley, and Patrick J. Hamilton, "Employment Grade and Coronary Heart Disease in British Civil Servants," *Journal of Epidemiology and Community Health*, 32 (4) (1978), 244–49

Marmot, Michael and Richard Wilkinson, eds., *Social Determinants of Health* (Oxford: Oxford University Press, 2005)

Marmot, Michael and Ruth Bell, "Fair Society, Healthy Lives," *Public Health*, 126 (2012), 4–10

Marmot, Michael et al., "Closing the Gap in a Generation: Health Equity through Action on the Social Determinants of Health," *The Lancet*, 372 (2008), 1661–69

Marmot, Michael et al. "Health Inequalities among British Civil Servants: The Whitehall II Study," *The Lancet*, 337 (8754) (1991), 1387–93

Martin, Adrienne, *How We Hope: A Moral Psychology* (Princeton, NJ: Princeton University Press, 2013)

Marya, Rupa and Raj Patel, *Inflamed: Deep Medicine and the Anatomy of Injustice* (New York: Farrar, Straus and Giroux, 2021)

Marx, Karl, *Capital: A Critique of Political Economy*, vol. 1, (Moscow: Progress Publishers, first English edition of 1887 [1867])

Maynard, Robyn et al., "Every Day We Must Get Up and Relearn the World: An Interview with Robyn Maynard and Leanne Betasamosake Simpson," *Interfere: Journal for Critical Thought and Radical Politics*, 2 (2021), 140–65

McGregor, Gordon, "Social Determinants of Health Practices," *American Journal of Public Health and the Nation's Health*, 51 (11) (1961), 1709–14

McKeown, Thomas, *The Role of Medicine: Dream, Mirage, or Nemesis?* (Princeton, NJ: Princeton University Press, 1980)

McKibben, Bill, *The End of Nature* (New York: Random House, 1989)

McKinlay, John B. "A Case for Refocusing Upstream: The Political Economy of Illness," *Interdisciplinary Association for Population Health Science Occasional Classics*, 1 (2019 [1975]), 1–10

McVeigh, Tracy, "Interview: Nathan was born at 23 weeks. If I'd known then what I do now, I'd have wanted him to die in my arms," *The Guardian*, March 20, 2011, www.theguardian.com/society/2011/mar/20/nathan-born-premature-life-death

Medical Innovations in Historical Perspective, ed. John V. Pickstone (New York: St Martin's Press, 1992)

Medically Unexplained Symptoms, Somatisation and Bodily Distress: Developing Better Clinical Services, eds. Francis Creed, Peter Henningsen, and Per Fink (Cambridge: Cambridge University Press, 2011)

"Medizin Nach Mass: Mit Personalisierter Medizin zur Gesundheit von Morgen," *ETH Zürich Globe*, 1 (2018), 1–52

Mehta, Neeta, "Mind-Body Dualism: A Critique from a Health Perspective," *Mens Sana Monographs*, 9 (1) (2011), 202–9

Meier, Christian, "Ein antikes Äquivalent des Fortschrittsgedankens: das "Könnens-Bewusstsein" des 5. Jahrhunderts v. Chr.," *Historische Zeitschrift*, 226 (1) (1978), 265–316

Meili, Matthias, "Die Ökobilanz der Spitäler," *Neue Zürcher Zeitung*, October 3, 2021

Melzer, Arthur M., "The Problem with the 'Problem of Technology,'" in *Technology in the Western Political Tradition*, eds. Arthur M. Melzer, Jerry Weinberger, and M. Richard Zinman (Ithaca, NY: Cornell University Press, 1993), pp. 287–321

Merton, Robert K., *On the Shoulders of Giants: The Post-Italianate Edition* (Chicago: University of Chicago Press, 1993 [1965])

Moberg, Carol, "René Dubos: A Harbinger of Microbial Resistance to Antibiotics," *Microbial Drug Resistance*, 2 (3) (1996), 287–97

Molland, A. George, "Medieval Ideas of Scientific Progress," *Journal of the History of Ideas*, 39 (1978), 561–77

Møller, Sofie, "Kant on Non-Linear Progress," *Ethics & Politics*, 23 (2), 127–47

Momigliano, Arnaldo, "Time in Ancient Historiography," *History and Theory*, 6 (1966), 1–23

Mommsen, Theodor E., "St Augustine and the Christian Idea of Progress: The Background of the City of God," *Journal of the History of Ideas*, 2 (3) (1951), 346–74

Monticelli, Lara, "On the Necessity of Prefigurative politics," *Thesis Eleven*, 167 (1) (2021), 99–118

Morales, Daniel, "COVID 19 and Disparities Affecting Ethnic Minorities," *The Lancet*, 397 (10286) (2021), 1684–85

Morange, Michel, *The Black Box of Biology: A History of the Molecular Revolution*, trans. M. Cobb (Cambridge, MA: Harvard University Press, 2020)

"More than 200 Health Journals Call for Urgent Action on Climate Crisis," *The Guardian*, September 6, 2021, www.theguardian.com/environment/2021/sep/06/more-than-200-health-journals-call-for-urgent-action-on-climate-crisis

Moscucci, Ornella, *The Science of Woman: Gynaecology and Gender in England, 1800–1929* (Cambridge: Cambridge University Press, 1990)

Moskop, John C., "Rawlsian Justice and Human Right to Health Care," *Journal of Medicine and Philosophy*, 8 (1983), 329–38

Mouzakitis, Angelos, "Modernity and the Idea of Progress," *Frontiers in Sociology*, 2 (3) (2017), 1–11

Mukherjee, Siddhartha, "A.I. Versus M.D.: What Happens When Diagnosis Is Automated?," *The New Yorker*, March 27, 2017, www.newyorker.com/magazine/2017/04/03/ai-versus-md

Musschenga, A. W. and G. Meynen, eds., "Moral Progress: Special Issue," *Ethical Theory and Moral Practice*, 20 (1) (2017), 1–183

Nadin, Mihai, "Aiming AI at a Moving Target: Health (or Disease)," *AI & Society*, https://doi.org/10.1007/s00146-020-00943-x

Nam, Ramez, *More Than Human: Embracing the Promise of Biological Enhancement* (New York: Broadway Books, 2005)

Narrative Ethics: The Role of Stories in Bioethics, special report, ed. Martha Montello, *Hastings Center Report*, 44 (1) (2014), 2–44

Nash, Linda, *Inescapable Ecologies: A History of Environment, Disease, and Knowledge* (Oakland: University of California Press, 2007)

National Institutes of Health and National Human Genome Research Institute, Advancing Genomic Medicine Research Exploratory/Developmental Grant, https://grants.nih.gov/grants/guide/rfa-files/RFA-HG-20-037.html

Nelson, Richard R. et al., "How Medical Know-How Progresses," *Research Policy*, 40 (2011), 1339–44

Nemeth, Thomas, "Positivism in Late Tsarist Russia: Its Introduction, Penetration and Diffusion," in *The Worlds of Positivism: A Global Intellectual History, 1770–1930*, eds. Johannes Feichtinger, Franz L. Fillafer, and Jan Surman (Cham, Switzerland: Springer, 2018), pp. 273–91

Neuburger, Max, "An Historical Survey of the Concept of Nature from a Medical View Point," *Isis*, 35 (1) (1944), 16–28

Newell, Kenneth W., "Selective Primary Health Care: The Counter Revolution," *Social Science and Medicine*, 26 (9) (1988), 903–6

Newton, Hannah, ed., "'Nature Concocts and Expels': Defeating Disease," in *Misery to Mirth: Recovery from Illness in Early Modern England* (Oxford: Oxford University Press, 2018), pp. 33–64

Newton, Warren, "Rationalism and Empiricism in Modern Medicine," *Law and Contemporary Problems*, 64 (4) (2001), 299–316

NHS Forest Project, Centre for Sustainable Healthcare, https://nhsforest.org/

Nietzsche, Friedrich, *The Birth of Tragedy*, trans. and intro. Douglas Smith (Oxford: Oxford University Press, 2008 [1872])

Niiniluoto, Ilkka, "Scientific Progress as Increasing Verisimilitude," *Studies in the History and Philosophy of Science*, 46 (2014), 73–77

Nisbet, Robert A., *History of the Idea of Progress* (New Brunswick & London: Transaction Publishers, 1980)

Nisbet, Robert A., "Idea of Progress: A Bibliographical Essay," *Literature of Liberty*, 2 (1) (1979), 7–47

Nisbet, Robert A., "Turgot and the Contexts of Progress," *Proceedings of the American Philosophical Society*, 119 (3) (1975), 214–22

Noble, Safiya Umoja, *Algorithms of Oppression: How Search Engines Reinforce Racism* (New York: New York University Press, 2018)

Noll, Peter, *In the Face of Death*, trans. Hans Noll (New York: Viking, 1989 [1984])

Norberg, Johan, *Progress: Ten Reasons to Look Forward to the Future* (New York City: Simon and Schuster, 2016)

Norgaard, Richard, *Development Betrayed: The End of Progress and a Co-Evolutionary Revisioning of the Future* (London: Routledge, 1994)

Numbers, Ronald L., "The Third Party: Health Insurance in America," in *The Therapeutic Revolution: Essays in the Social History of American Medicine*, eds. Morris J. Vogel and Charles E. Rosenberg (Philadelphia: University of Pennsylvania Press, 2017), pp. 177–200

Nussbaum, Martha, ed., "Review of Allen Buchanan, Dan W. Brock, Norman Daniels, and Daniel Winkler, *From Chance to Choice* (2000)," in *Philosophical Interventions: Reviews 1986–2011* (Oxford: Oxford University Press, 2012), pp. 234–45

Nutton, Vivian, "The Fatal Embrace: Galen and the History of Ancient Medicine," *Science in Context*, 18 (1) (2005), 111–21

Olby, Robert, "The Molecular Revolution in Biology," in *Companion to the History of Modern Science*, eds. Geoffrey N. Cantor et al. (London: Routledge, 1996), pp. 503–20

Oliver, Mike, "The Social Model of Disability: Thirty Years On," *Disability & Society*, 28 (2013), 1024–26

"Opening Assembly: Selections from the Addresses and Panel Discussions of the Convocation, The Dartmouth Convocation on Great Issues of Conscience in Modern Medicine, September 8–10, 1960," *Dartmouth Alumni Magazine* (1960), https://archive.dartmouthalumnimagazine.com/article/1960/11/1/opening-assembly

Oreskes, Naomi, "Why I Am a Presentist?," *Science in Context*, 26 (4) (2013), 595–609

Orth, Matthias et al., "Redefining the Role of the Physician in Laboratory Medicine in the Context of Emerging Technologies, Personalised Medicine and Patient Autonomy ('4P Medicine')," *Journal of Clinical Pathology*, 72 (3) (2019), 191–97

Osler, William, *The Evolution of Modern Medicine: A Series of Lectures Delivered at Yale University on the Silliman Foundation in April* (Champagne, IL: Project Gutenberg, 1998 [1913])

"Our Founding Mission," *The Economist*, www.economistgroup.com/businesses/the-economist

Outka, Gene, "Social Justice and Equal Access to Health Care," *The Journal of Religious Ethics*, 2 (1) (1974), 11–32

Paehlke, Robert, "Environmentalism and the Future of Progressive Politics: An Update" in *Explorations in Environmental Political Theory: Thinking about What We Value*, ed. Joel Jay Kassiola (London and New York: Routledge, 2003), pp. 81–103

Paradies, Yin, Jehonathan Ben, Nida Denson, et al. "Racism as a Determinant of Health: A Systematic Review and Meta-Analysis," *PLoS One*, 10 (2015), e0138511

Parsons, Talcott, *The Structure of Social Action: A Study in Social Theory with Special Reference to a Group of Recent European Writers* (Glencoe, IL: The Free Press, 1949)

Paterson, Stewart, "Boris Johnson Didn't Get 'Big decisions Right' on COVID, says Leading Epidemiologist," *Glasgow Times*, June 21, 2022, www.glasgowtimes.co.uk/news/20224923.boris-johnson-didnt-get-big-decisions-right-covid-says-leading-epidemiologist/?ref=twtrec

Paul, Delia, "Merging the Poverty and Environment Agendas," Brief #11, *IISD Earth Negotiations Bulletin*, (2021), 1–9

Peabody, Francis, "The Care of the Patient," *The Journal of the American Medical Association*, 88 (12) (1927), 877–82

Peitzman, Steven J., "When Did Medicine Become Beneficial? The Perspective from Internal Medicine," *Caduceus*, 12 (3) (1996), 39–44

Pelka, Fred, *What We Have Done: An Oral History of the Disability Rights Movement* (Boston: University of Massachusetts Press, 2012)

Pernick, Martin A., *A Calculus of Suffering: Pain, Professionalism and Anesthesia in Nineteenth-Century America* (New York: Columbia University Press, 1985)

Pernick, Mark S., "Bioethics and History," in *The Cambridge World History of Medical Ethics*, eds. Robert Baker and Laurence B. McCullough (New York: Cambridge University Press, 2009), pp. 16–20

Phelan, Jo C. and Bruce G. Link, "Fundamental Cause Theory," in *Medical Sociology on the Move: New Directions in Theory*, ed. William C. Cockerham (Dordrecht: Springer, 2013), pp. 105–26

Philippi, Cristian Larroulet, "There Is Cause to Randomize," *Philosophy of Science*, 89 (2022), 152–70

Pickering, Mary, *Auguste Comte: An Intellectual Biography*, vol. 3 (Cambridge: Cambridge University Press, 2009)

Pickett, Kate and Richard Wilkinson, *The Spirit Level: Why More Equal Societies Almost Always Do Better* (London: Allen Lane, 2009)

Pickover, Clifford A., *The Medical Book: From Witch Doctors to Robot Surgeons, 250 Milestones in the History of Medicine* (New York: Union Square, 2012)

Pickstone, John V., ed., *Medical Innovations in Historical Perspective* (Houndmills: Macmillan, 1992)

Pielke, Roger Jr., "A 'Sedative' for Science Policy," *Issues in Science and Technology*, 36 (1) (2020), https://issues.org/endless-frontier-sedative-for-science-policy-pielke/

Pierce, Jessica, Andrew Jameton, and Canadan Boulder, *The Ethics of Environmentally Responsible Health Care* (Oxford: Oxford University Press, 2004)

Pinker, Steven, *The Better Angels of Our Nature* (London: Penguin, 2011)

Plumwood, Val, "Feminism," in *Political Theory and the Ecological Challenge*, eds. Andrew Dobson and Robyn Eckersley (Cambridge: Cambridge University Press, 2006), 51–74

Poirier, Jean-Pierre, *Turgot: Laissez-faire et progrès social* (Paris: Perrin, 1999)

Pollard, Sidney, *The Idea of Progress* (London: C. A. Watts, 1986)

Poole, Randall, "Conceptions of Humanity in Health Humanities," presentation at the International Health Humanities Conference, McGovern Center for Humanities and Ethics, University of Texas Health Sciences Center at Houston, March 2017

Popper, Karl, *The Logic of Scientific Discovery* (London: Hutchison, 1959)

Porter, Roy, "The Patient's View: Doing Medical History from Below," *Theory and Society*, 14 (1985), 175–98

Porter, Roy and Dorothy Porter, *In Sickness and in Health: The British Experience, 1650–1850* (New York: Basil Blackwell, 1988)

Potter, Van Rensselaer, *Bioethics: Bridge to the Future* (Englewood Cliffs, NJ: Prentice-Hall, 1971)

Prainsack, Barbara, *Personalized Medicine: Empowered Patients in the 21st Century?* (New York: New York University Press, 2017)

"President Donald J. Trump's State of the Union Address," The White House, January 30, 2018, www.whitehouse.gov/briefings-statements/president-donald-j-trumps-state-union-address/

Prioreschi, Plinio, "The Idea of Scientific Progress in Antiquity and in the Middle Ages," *Vesalius*, 8 (1) (2002), 34–45

Pritchett, H. S., "The Medical School and the State," *Journal of the American Medical Association*, 63 (8) (1914), 648–51

"Profit, n.," *Oxford English Dictionary*, Oxford University Press, March 2024, https://doi.org/10.1093/OED/6630322299

"Progress, n.," *Oxford English Dictionary*, March 2024, https://doi.org/10.1093/OED/3034306464

"Progress, Change, Development: Special Issue," *International Journal of Postcolonial Studies*, 19 (5) (2017), 599–705

"Public Health Linkages with Sustainability: Workshop Summary" (Washington, DC: The National Academies Press, 2013), https://doi.org/10.17226/18375

Rabinow, Paul, *Making PCR: A Story of Biotechnology* (Chicago: University of Chicago Press, 1996)

Ramsey, Paul, *The Patient as Person: Explorations in Medical Ethics* (New Haven, CT: Yale University Press, 1970)

Rapp, Friedrich, *Fortschritt: Entwicklung und Sinngehalt einer philosophischen Idee* (Darmstadt: Wissenschaftliche Buchgesellschaft, 1992)

Rasanathan, Kumanan, "10 Years after the Commission on Social Determinants of Health: Social Injustice Is Still Killing on a Grand Scale," *The Lancet*, 392 (2018), 1176–77

Rasanathan, Kumanan and Theresa Diaz, "Research on Health Equity in the SDG Era: The Urgent Need for Greater Focus on Implementation," *International Journal for Equity in Health*, 15 (202) (2016), https://doi.org/10.1186/s12939-016-0493-7

Rawls, John, *A Theory of Justice* (Cambridge, MA: Belknap Press, 1971)

Rawls, John, *Justice as Fairness: A Restatement* (Cambridge, MA: Belknap Press, 2001)

Rawls, John, *Political Liberalism*, Expanded edn (New York: Columbia University Press, 1996)

Regalado, Antonio, "Engineering the Perfect Baby," *MIT Technology Review*, 118 (3) (2015), 26–33

"Remarks made by the President, Tony Blair, Francis Collins, and Craig Venter," The White House, Office of the Press Secretary, June 26, 2000, www.genome.gov/10001356

Report of the World Commission on Environment and Development of the United Nations: Our Common Future (1987), https://sustainabledevelopment.un.org/content/documents/5987our-common-future.pdf

Research Mission, American Diabetes Association, https://diabetes.org/research/research-foundation-mission-and-vision

Rich, Carrie R., J. Knox Singleton, and Seema S. Wadhwa, *Sustainability for Healthcare Management: A Leadership Imperative* (New York: Routledge, 2018)

Riddle, John M., "Theory and Practice in Medieval Medicine," (1974) in *Viator: Medieval and Renaissance Studies*, vol. 5 (Berkeley: University of California Press, 2020), pp. 158–85

Rifkin, Susan B., "Alma Ata after 40 Years: Primary Health Care and Health for All – from Consensus to Complexity," *BMJ Global Health*, 2018, 3 (3), e001188

Robinson, Walter M., "The Narrative of Rescue in Pediatric Practice," in *Stories Matter: The Role of Narrative in Medical Ethics*, eds. Rita Charon and Martha Montello (New York, London: Routledge, 2002), pp. 100–12

Rolleston, John D., "Voltaire and Medicine," *Proceedings of the Royal Society of Medicine*, 19 (1926), 17–28

Romanello, Marina et al., "The 2021 Report of the Lancet Countdown on Health and Climate Change: Code Red for a Healthy Future," *The Lancet*, 398 (2021), 1619–62

Roosevelt, Franklin D., "President Roosevelt's Letter to Vannevar Bush," 1945, *U. S. National Science Foundation*, www.nsf.gov/about/history/nsf50/vbush1945_roosevelt_letter.jsp

Rose, Nikolas, "The Politics of Life Itself," *Theory, Culture & Society*, 18 (6) (2001), 1–30

Rosenberg, Charles E., "The Therapeutic Revolution: Medicine, Meaning, and Social Change in Nineteenth-Century America," in *The Therapeutic Revolution: Essays in the Social History of American Medicine*, eds. Morris J. Voegel and Charles E. Rosenberg (Philadelphia: University of Pennsylvania Press, 1979), pp. 3–23

Rosenberg, Lawrence, "Disintermediation," Presentation given at *Workshop: Medicine without Doctors? Disintermediation and Patient Agency*, 4th Workshop on the Impact of Technological Change on the Surgical Profession, May 8, 2019, Jewish General Hospital, Montréal

Rosenkrantz, Barbara Gutmann, "Case Histories – An Introduction," *Social Research*, 55 (3) (1988), 397–99

Rosner, David, "Tempest in a Test Tube: Medical History and the Historian," *Radical History Review*, 26 (1982), 166–71

Ross, Lauren N., "The Doctrine of Specific Etiology," *Biology & Philosophy*, 33 (37) (2018), https://doi.org/10.1007/s10539-018-9647-x

Roth, Amanda, "Ethical Progress as Problem-Resolving," *The Journal of Political Philosophy*, 20 (4) (2012), 384–406

Rothman, Juliet C., "The Challenge of Disability and Access: Reconceptualizing the Role of the Medical Model," *Journal of Social Work in Disability & Rehabilitation*, 9 (2010), 194–222

Rousseau, J. J., *Discours sur l'inégalité parmi les hommes; Contrat social; Discours sur l'économie politique; Projet de paix perpétuelle* (Amsterdam: Marc-Michel Rey, 1776)

Rowbottom, Darrell, *Scientific Progress* (Cambridge: Cambridge University Press, 2023)
Ruger, Jennifer Prah, "Social Justice as a Foundation for Democracy and Health," *BMJ*, 371 (2020), 4049
Rütten, Thomas, "Hippocrates and the Construction of 'Progress' in Sixteenth- and Seventeenth-Century Medicine," in *Reinventing Hippocrates*, ed. David Cantor (London and New York: Routledge, 2001), pp. 37–58
Saad, Toni C., "The History of Autonomy in Medicine from Antiquity to Principlism," *Medicine Health Care and Philosophy*, 21 (2018), 125–37
Saatsi, Juha, "What Is Theoretical Progress in Science," *Synthese*, 196 (2019), 611–31
Sackett, David L. et al., "Evidence Based Medicine: What It Is and What It Isn't," *BMJ*, 312 (1996), 71–72
Sadowsky, Jonathan, *Electroconvulsive Therapy in America: The Anatomy of a Medical Controversy* (New York and London: Routledge, 2017)
Salander, Pär and Clare Moynihan, "Facilitating Patients' Hope Work through Relationship: A Critique of the Discourse of Autonomy," in *Configuring Health Consumers: Health Work and the Imperative of Responsibility*, eds. Roma Harris, Nadine Wathen, and Sally Wyatt (London: Palgrave Macmillan, 2010), pp. 113–25
Salma, Asem, Letter: "Neurosurgery in the Post-Postmodernism Era: On the Upcoming Discourse of Medicine," *World Neurosurgery*, 82 (1/2) (2014), 395–96
Sanchez, Léa, "Les résidents d'Ehpad représentent 44% des morts du Covid-19," *Le Monde*, December 3, 2020, www.lemonde.fr/les-decodeurs/article/2020/12/03/les-residents-d-ehpad-representent-44-des-morts-du-covid-19_6062084_4355770.html
Sand, René, *Health and Human Progress: An Essay in Sociological Medicine* (New York: Macmillan, 1936)
Sandweiss, Donald A., "Letter Response to Varieties of Healing 1 & 2," *Annals of Internal Medicine*, 137 (2002), 217–18
Sarasin, Philipp, "Was ist Wissensgeschichte?," *Internationales Archiv für Sozialgeschichte der deutschen Literatur*, 36 (1) (2011), 159–72
Sarewitz, Daniel, *Frontiers of Illusion: Science, Technology, and the Politics of Progress* (Philadelphia: Temple University Press, 1996)
Sartea, Claudio, "Il passato dell'idea di progresso ed il futuro della bioetica," *Medicina e Morale*, 69 (3) (2020), 293–310
Sarton, Georges, *The Study of the History of Science* (Cambridge, MA: Harvard University Press, 1936)
Satel, Sally, *PC, MD. How Political Correctness Is Corrupting Medicine* (New York: Basic Books, 2000)

Sauer, Hanno et al., "Moral Progress: Recent Developments," *Philosophy Compass*, 16 (10) (2021), e12769

Saunders, Cicely, *Living with Dying: The Management of Terminal Disease* (Oxford: Oxford University Press, 1967)

Savransky, Martin and Craig Lundy, eds. *After Progress* (Thousand Oaks, CA: Sage, 2022)

Scambler, Graham, "Covid-19 as a 'Breaching Experiment': Exposing the Fractured Society," *Health Sociology Review*, 29 (2) (2022), 140–48

Schlich, Thomas, *Palgrave Companion to the History of Surgery* (New York: Palgrave Macmillan, 2018)

Schmidt, Hans-Joachim ed., *Tradition, Innovation, Invention: Fortschrittsverweigerung und Fortschrittsbewusstsein im Mittelalter* (Berlin: Walter de Gruyter, 2005)

Schramme, Thomas, "Health as Complete Well-Being: The WHO Definition and Beyond," *Public Health Ethics*, 16 (3) (2023), 210–18

Schroeder, Knut, Trevor Thompson, Kathleen Frith, and David Pencheon, *Sustainable Healthcare* (Chichester, West Sussex: Wiley-Blackwell, 2013)

Schwab, Aurore, Ongoing Research Project, *The United Nations Sustainable Development Goals: An Emerging "Planetary Religion?,"* https://orcid.org/0000-0002-6940-4658

Scotch, Richard K., "Politics and Policy in the History of the Disability Rights Movement," *The Milbank Quarterly*, 67 (2) (1989), 380–400

Scull, Andrew, *Desperate Remedies: Psychiatry's Turbulent Quest to Cure Mental Illness* (Cambridge, MA: Harvard University Press, 2022)

Segall, Shlomi, "Is Health Care (Still) Special?," *The Journal of Political Philosophy*, 15 (3) (2007), 342–61

Seghezzo, Lucas, "The Five Dimensions of Sustainability," *Environmental Politics*, 18 (4) (2009), 539–56

Seigel, Jerrold, *The Idea of the Self: Thought and Experience in Western Europe since the Seventeenth Century* (New York: Cambridge University Press, 2005)

Sen, Amartya, "Why Health Equity?," *Health Economics*, 11 (2002), 659–66

Sève, Lucien, *Pour une critique de la raison bioéthique* (Paris: Odile Jacob, 1994)

Shaheen-Hussein, Samir, *Fighting for a Hand to Hold: Confronting Medical Colonialism against Indigenous Children in Canada* (Montreal: McGill-Queen's University Press, 2020)

Shakespeare, Tom, "The Social Model of Disability," in *The Disability Studies Reader*, ed. Lennard J. Davis, 5th ed. (New York and London: Routledge, 2017), pp. 195–203

Shan, Yafeng, "A New Functional Approach to Scientific Progress," *Philosophy of Science*, 86 (2019), 739–58

Shapin, Steven, "Possessed by the Idols," *London Review of Books*, 28 (3) (2006), 31–33

Sharon, Rita, *Narrative Medicine: Honoring the Stories of Illness* (Oxford: Oxford University Press, 2006)

Sharon, Tamar, "Self-Tracking for Health and the Quantified Self: Re-articulating Autonomy, Solidarity, and Authenticity in an Age of Personalized Healthcare," *Philosophy of Technology*, 30 (2017), 93–121

Sheridan, Desmond J. and Desmond G. Julian, "Achievements and Limitations of Evidence-Based Medicine," *Journal of the American College of Cardiology*, 68 (2) (2016), 204–13

Sherman, Jodi D. et al., "The Green Print: Advancement of Environmental Sustainability in Healthcare," *Resources, Conservation & Recycling*, 161 (2020), https://doi.org/10.1016/j.resconrec.2020.104882

Shermer, Michael, *The Moral Arc: How Science Leads Humanity toward Truth, Justice, and Freedom* (New York: Henry Holt and Co., 2015)

Shindell, Drew et al., "Simultaneously Mitigating Near-Term Climate Change and Improving Human Health and Food Security," *Science*, 335 (6065) (2012), 183–89

Sicard, Didier, "Réflexions sur le progrès en médecine," *Médecine & Hygiène*, 2491 (2004), 1535–38

Siegel, Rebbeca L., Angela N. Giaquinto, and Ahmedin Jemal, "Cancer Statistics, 2024," *CA: A Cancer Journal for Clinicians*, 74 (1) (2024), 12–49

Siegler, Mark, "The Progression of Medicine: From Physician Paternalism to Patient Autonomy to Bureaucratic Parsimony," *Archives of Internal Medicine*, 145 (1985), 713–15

Sigerist, Henry E., *Civilization and Disease* (Chicago: University of Chicago Press, 1970 [1943])

Sigerist, Henry E., *Medicine and Human Welfare: The Terry Lectures* (New Haven, CT: Yale University Press, 1941)

Sigerist, Henry E., "The Development of Medicine and Its Trends in the United States, 1636–1936," *The New England Journal of Medicine*, 218 (8) (1938), 325–28

Simon, Jeremy R., "How to Make Real Constructive Progress in Medicine," *Journal of Evaluation in Clinical Practice*, 17 (5) (2011), 845–51

Simpkin, Arabella and Richard Schwartzstein, "Tolerating Uncertainty – The Next Medical Revolution?," *New England Journal of Medicine*, 375 (18) (2016), 1713–15

Skouteris, Thomas, *The Notion of Progress in International Law Discourse* (The Hague: TMC Asser Press, 2010)

Slaboch, Matthew, *A Road to Nowhere: The Idea of Progress and Its Critics* (Philadelphia: University of Pennsylvania Press, 2017)

Smith, Adam, *An Inquiry into the Nature and Causes of the Wealth of Nations*, ed. Sálvio M. Soares (Amsterdam: MetaLibri, 2007 [1776])
Smith, Christian, *What Is a Person?: Rethinking Humanity, Social Life, and the Moral Good from the Person Up* (Chicago: University of Chicago Press, 2010)
Smith, Kirk R. et al. "Human Health: Impacts, Adaptation, and Co-Benefits," in *Climate Change 2014: Impacts, Adaptation, and Vulnerability. Part A: Global and Sectoral Aspects. Contribution of Working Group II to the Fifth Assessment Report of the Intergovernmental Panel on Climate Change*, eds. Christopher B. Field et al. (Cambridge: Cambridge University Press, 2014), pp. 709–54
Smith, Michael L., "Recourse of Empire: Landscapes of Progress in Technological America," in *Does Technology Drive History? The Dilemma of Technological Determinism*, eds. Merritt Roe Smith and Leo Marx (Cambridge, MA: MIT Press, 1994), pp. 37–52
Smith, Robert C., *Society and Social Pathology: A Framework for Progress* (Cham, Switzerland: Palgrave Macmillan, 2017)
Solomon, Miriam, *Making Medical Knowledge* (Oxford: Oxford University Press, 2016)
Sorel, Georges, *Réflexions sur la Violence* (Paris: Marcel Rivière et Cie, 1908)
Spadafora, David, *The Idea of Progress in Eighteenth-Century Britain* (New Haven, CT: Yale University Press, 1995)
Sparrow, Robert, "Better than Men? Sex and the Therapy/Enhancement Distinction," *Kennedy Institute of Ethics Journal*, 20 (2) (2010), 115–44
Spencer, Herbert, "Progress: Its Law and Cause," in *Essays: Scientific, Political and Speculative* (London: Williams and Norgate, 1891), vol. 1, pp. 8–62
Stahnisch, Frank W., "The Tertium Comparationis of the Elementa Physiologiae: Johann Gottfried von Herder's Conception of 'Tears' as Mediators between the Sublime and the Actual Bodily Physiology," in *Blood, Sweat and Tears: The Changing Concepts of Physiology from Antiquity into Early Modern Europe*, eds. Manfred Horstmanshoff, Helen King, and Claus Zittel, Intersections – Interdisciplinary Studies in Early Modern Culture, vol. 25 (Leiden and Boston, MA: Brill, 2012), pp. 595–626
Starfield, Barbara, "Are Social Determinants of Health the Same as Societal Determinants of Health?," *Health Promotion Journal of Australia*, 17 (3) (2006), 170–73
Starr, Paul, *The Social Transformation of American Medicine* (New York: Basic Books, 1982)
Stegenga, Jacob, "Is Meta-Analysis the Platinum Standard of Evidence?," *Studies in the History and Philosophy of Biology and Biomedical Sciences*, 42 (4) 2011, 497–507

Stegenga, Jacob, *Medical Nihilism* (Oxford: Oxford University Press, 2018)

Stirling, Andy, "Pluralising Progress: From Integrative Transitions to Transformative Diversity," *Environmental Innovation and Societal Transitions*, 1 (1) (2011), 82–88

Strasser, Peter, "Paradoxien des medizinischen Fortschritts – kann es sein, dass die immer bessere Gesundheitsversorgung die Würde des Menschen mehr bedroht als stärkt?," *Neue Zürcher Zeitung*, June 22, 2020, www.nzz.ch/meinung/die-frage-der-wuerde-paradoxien-des-medizinischen-fortschritts-ld.1543009?reduced=true

Streeck, Nina, *Jedem seinen eigenen Tod: Authentizität als ethisches Ideal am Lebensende* (Frankfurt, NY: Campus, 2020)

Sullivan, Mark, "The New Subjective Medicine: Taking the Patient's Point of View on Health Care and Health," *Social Science & Medicine*, 56 (2003), 1595–1604

Swan, Melanie, "Health 2050: The Realization of Personalized Medicine through Crowdsourcing, the Quantified Self, and the Participatory Biocitizen," *Journal of Personalized Medicine*, 2 (2012), 93–118

Sweeney, Peter, "The Pendulum of Progress," *Experfy* (August 14, 2018), https://resources.experfy.com/ai-ml/the-pendulum-of-progress/

Swiss National Science Foundation, *The SNSF's Model of Excellence*, www.snf.ch/en/theSNSF/research-policies/model-of-excellence/Pages/default.aspx#Question

Szreter, Simon, "The Importance of Social Intervention in Britain's Mortality Decline c. 1850–1914: A Re-Interpretation of the Role of Public Health," *Society for the Social History of Medicine*, 1 (1988), 1–37

Sztompka, Piotr, "Agency and Progress: The Idea of Progress and Changing Theories of Change," in *Rethinking Progress: Movements, Forces, and Ideas at the End of the Twentieth Century*, eds. Jeffrey C. Alexander and Piotr Sztompka (London: Routledge, 1990), pp. 247–65.

Tangcharoensathien, Viroj et al., "Are Overwhelmed Health Systems an Inevitable Consequence of COVID-19? Experiences from China, Thailand, and New York State," *The BMJ*, 372 (2021), n83

Tauber, Alfred I., "Historical and Philosophical Reflections on Patient Autonomy," *Health Care Analysis*, 9 (2001), 299–319

Taylor, Charles, *Modern Social Imaginaries* (Durham, NC: Duke University Press, 2004)

Taylor, Charles, "What's Wrong with Negative Liberty," in *The Idea of Freedom: Essays in Honour of Isaiah Berlin*, ed. Alan Ryan (Oxford: Oxford University Press, 1979), pp. 175–93

Teggart, Frederick J., "The Argument of Hesiod's Works and Days," *Journal of the History of Ideas*, 8 (1) (1947), 45–77

The Didascalicon of Hugh St Victor: A Medieval Guide to the Arts, trans. and intro. Jerome Taylor (New York and London: Columbia University Press, 1961)

The Goals of Medicine: The Forgotten Issues in Health Care Reform, eds. Mark J. Hanson and Daniel Callahan (Washington, DC: Georgetown University Press, 1999)

The Precision Medicine Initiative, The White House, President Barack Obama, https://obamawhitehouse.archives.gov/precision-medicine

The White House, "Highlighting a Year of Progress: The Biden-Harris Cancer Cabinet Takes Action to End Cancer as We Know It," March 8, 2024, https://bidenwhitehouse.archives.gov/ostp/news-updates/2024/03/08/highlighting-a-year-of-progress-the-biden-harris-cancer-cabinet-takes-action-to-end-cancer-as-we-know-it/

Thériault, Serge, *Jean-Jacques Rousseau et la médecine naturelle* (Montreal: Les Editions Univers, 1979)

Thomas, Keith, *Religion and the Decline of Magic: Studies in Popular Beliefs in Sixteenth and Seventeenth Century England* (New York: Penguin Books, 1982)

Thomas, Jean-Paul, "La médecine progresse-t-elle ?," *Raison présente*, 189 (2014), 31–41

Thomas, S. Joshua, "Does Evidence-Based Health Care Have Room for the Self?," *Journal of Evaluation in Clinical Practice*, 22 (2016), 502–8

Thompson, Trevor and Tim Ballard, "Sustainable Medicine: Good for the Environment, Good for People," *British Journal of General Practice*, 61 (582) (2011), 3–4

Tijmes, Pieter and Reginald Luijf, "The Sustainability of Our Common Future: An Inquiry into the Foundations of an Ideology," *Technology in Society*, 17 (3) (1995), 327–36

Topol, Eric et al., *The Topol Review. Preparing the Healthcare Workforce to Deliver the Digital Future: An Independent Report on Behalf of the Secretary of State for Health and Social Care*, NHS Health Education England, February 2019

"Tracking Covid-19 Excess Deaths across Countries," *The Economist*, www.economist.com/graphic-detail/coronavirus-excess-deaths-tracker

Tracy, Theodore James, *Physiological Theory and the Doctrine of the Mean in Plato and Aristotle* (Berlin and Boston: De Gruyter, 2014 [1969])

Tsanoff, Radoslav A., *Civilization and Progress* (Lexington: University Press of Kentucky, 2021)

Tuchman, Arleen Marcia, *Diabetes: A History of Race and Disease* (New Haven, CT: Yale University Press, 2020)

Tulin, Alexander, "Xenophanes Fr. 18 D.-K. and the Origins of the Idea of Progress," *Hermes*, 121 (2) (1993), 129–38

Turgot, *Discours sur les progrès successifs de l'esprit humain*, (1750), *Institut Coppet*, www.institutcoppet.org/turgot-discours-sur-les-progres-successifs-de-lesprit-humain-1750/

Tuveson, Ernest Lee, *Millennium and Utopia: A Study in the Background of the Idea of Progress* (Berkeley and Los Angeles: University of California Press, 1949)

Unschuld, Paul U., *Medicine in China: A History of Ideas* (Oakland: University of California Press, 1985)

Unzicker, Rae, "On My Own: A Personal Journey through Madness and Re-Emergence," *Psychosocial Rehabilitation Journal*, 13 (1) (1989), 71–77

Vagueness in Psychiatry, eds. Geert Keil, Lara Keuck, and Rico Hauswald (Oxford: Oxford University Press, 2017)

Valles, Sean A., *Philosophy of Population Health: Philosophy for a New Public Health Era* (London and New York: Routledge, 2018)

van der Eijk, Philip J., *Medicine and Philosophy in Classical Antiquity: Doctors and Philosophers on Nature, Soul, Health and Disease* (Cambridge: Cambridge University Press, 2005)

Van Doren, Charles Lincoln, *The Idea of Progress* (New York: F. A. Praeger, 1967)

van Egmond, N. D. (Klaas) and H. J. M. (Bert) de Vries, "Sustainability: The Search for the Integral Worldview," *Futures*, 43 (2011), 853–67

Vandenbroeck, Philippe, Jo Goossens, and Marshall Clemens, "Tackling Obesities: Future Choices – Building the Obesity System Map," *Foresight Programme, UK Government Office for Science*, 2007, p. 14, https://assets.publishing.service.gov.uk/government/uploads/system/uploads/attachment_data/file/295154/07-1179-obesity-building-system-map.pdf

Varga, Somogy, *Science, Medicine, and the Aims of Inquiry* (Cambridge: Cambridge University Press, 2024)

Varga, Somogy, "The Aim of Medicine. Sanocentricity and the Autonomy Thesis," *Pacific Philosophical Quarterly*, 104 (4) (2023), 720–45

Vaux, Kenneth, *Who Shall Live: Medicine, Technology, Ethics: Houston Conference on Ethics in Medicine and Technology* (1968) (Philadelphia: Fortress Press, 1970)

Veatch, Robert M., "Autonomy's Temporary Triumph," *The Hastings Center Report*, 5 (14) (1984), 38–40

Venkatapuram, Sridhar, *Health Justice: An Argument from the Capabilities Approach* (Cambridge: Polity Press, 2011)

Verkerk, Marian A., "The Care Perspective and Autonomy," *Medicine, Health Care and Philosophy*, 4 (2001), 289–94

Versions of History from Antiquity to the Enlightenment, ed. Donald R. Kelley (New Haven, CT: Yale University Press, 2008)

Virchow, Rudolf, *Collected Essays on Public Health and Epidemiology* (Cambridge: Science History Publications, 1985 [1848])
Virchow, Rudolf, "Lernen und Forschen: Rede beim Antritt des Rectorats an der Friedrich-Wilhelms-Universität zu Berlin," 15 October 1892 (Berlin: Angust Hirschwald, 1892)
Virchow, Rudolf, "Was die 'medicinische Reform' will," *Medicinische Reform*, 1 (1848) reproduced in *Gesammelte Abhandlungen aus dem Gebiete der öffentlichen Medicin und der Seuchenlehre*, vol. 1 (Berlin: August Hirschwald, 1879), pp. 3–5
Vollmann, Jochen, Verena Sandow, Sebastian Wäscher, and Jan Schildmann, eds., *The Ethics of Personalised Medicine: Critical Perspectives* (Farnham: Ashgate, 2015)
von Gunten, Charles F., "Prevent and Relieve Suffering: Professional Palliative Care," *Cancer Investigation*, 21 (6) (2003), 963–64
Vyverberg, Henry, *Historical Pessimism in the French Enlightenment* (Cambridge, MA: Harvard University Press, 1958)
Wagar, W. Warren, *Good Tidings: The Belief in Progress from Darwin to Marcuse* (Bloomington: Indiana University Press, 1972)
Wagner, Peter, *Progress: A Reconstruction* (Cambridge: Polity Press, 2016)
Wagner, Peter, "Progress and Modernity: The Problem with Autonomy," *Sociología Histórica*, 7 (2017), 71–94
Walton, Samantha, *Everybody Needs Beauty: In Search of the Nature Cure* (London: Bloomsbury, 2021)
Wang, Fei, Lawrence Peter Casalino, and Dhruv Khullar, "Deep Learning in Medicine – Promise, Progress, and Challenges," *JAMA Internal medicine*, 179 (3) (2018), 293–94
Wardle, Jon L., Fran E. Baum, and Matthew Fisher, "The Research Commercialisation Agenda: A Concerning Development for Public Health Research," *Australian and New Zealand Journal of Public Health*, 43 (5) (2019), 407–9
Wardrope, Alistair, "Relational Autonomy and the Ethics of Health Promotion," *Public Health Ethics*, 8 (1) (2015), 50–62
Warner, John Harley, *The Therapeutic Perspective: Medical Practice, Knowledge, and Identity in America, 1820–1885* (Princeton, NJ: Princeton University Press, 1997 [1986])
Watts, Nick et al., "The Lancet Countdown: Tracking Progress on Health and Climate Change," *The Lancet*, 389 (2017), 1151–64
Watts, William, "Foreword," in *The Limits to Growth: A Report for the Club of Rome's Project on the Predicament of Mankind*, ed. Donella H. Meadows et al. (New York: Universe Books, 1972), pp. 9–12
Waugh, Patricia, ed., *Postmodernism: A Reader* (London: Hodder Arnold, 1992)

Weber, Max, ed., "Wissenschaft als Beruf," in *Gesammelte Aufsätze zur Wissenschaftslehre* (Tübingen: J. C. B Mohr, 1922), pp. 524–55

Webster, Paul, "COVID-19 Highlights Canada's Care Home Crisis," *The Lancet*, 397 (10270) (2021), 183

Weinberg, Robert A., "Coming Full Circle – From Endless Complexity to Simplicity and Back Again," *Cell*, 157 (1) (2014), 267–71

Weinstock, Daniel, "'What Is Evidence?' A Philosophical Perspective," Presentation at 2007 National Collaborating Centres for Public Health Summer Institute *Making Sense of It All*, August 20–23, 2007

Weisser, Olivia, *Ill Composed: Sickness, Gender and Belief in Early Modern England* (New Haven, CT: Yale University Press, 2015)

White, Lynn Jr., "Science and the Sense of Self: The Medieval Background of a Modern Confrontation," *Daedalus*, 107 (2) (1978), 47–59

White, Matthew P. et al., "Spending At Least 120 Minutes a Week in Nature Is Associated with Good Health and Wellbeing," *Scientific Reports*, 9 (7730) (2019), https://doi.org/10.1038/s41598-019-44097-3

Whitehead, Cynthia, *The Good Doctor in Medical Education 1910–2010: A Critical Discourse Analysis*, unpublished PhD Thesis, University of Toronto, 2011

Whitehead, Cynthia R., Zubin Austin, and Brian D. Hodge, "Flower Power: The Armoured Expert in the CanMEDS Competency Framework?," *Advances in Health Sciences Education*, 16 (2011), 681–94

Wiens, Jenna, Melissa Creary, and Michael W. Sjoding, "AI Models in Health Care Are Not Colour Blind and We Should Not Be Either," *The Lancet: Digital Health*, 4 (6) (2022), 399–400

Wieringa, Sietse et al., "Has Evidence-Based Medicine Ever Been Modern? A Latour-Inspired Understanding of a Changing EBM," *Journal of Evaluation in Clinical Practice*, 23 (5) (2017), 964–70

Wiesemann, Claudia, "Das Recht auf Selbstbestimmung und das Arzt-Patient-Verhältnis aus sozialgeschichtlicher Perspektive," in *Geschichte und Ethik in der Medizin. Von den Schwierigkeiten einer Kooperation*, eds. Richard Toellner and Urban Wiesing (Stuttgart: Gustav Fischer, 1997), pp. 67–89

Wilkinson, Richard G., "Income Distribution and Life Expectancy," *BMJ*, 34 (1992), 165–68

Wilkinson, Richard G. and Kate E. Pickett, "Income Inequality and Population Health: A Review and Explanation of the Evidence," *Social Science and Medicine*, 62 (2006), 1768–84

Williams, Bernard, ed., "The Idea of Equality," in *Problems of the Self: Philosophical Papers, 1956–1972* (Cambridge: Cambridge University Press, 1973), pp. 230–49

Williams, Robert A., *Savage Anxieties: The Invention of Western Civilization* (New York: Palgrave, 2012)

Willis, Evan, "Talcott Parsons: His Legacy and the Sociology of Health and Illness," in *The Palgrave Handbook of Social Theory in Health, Illness and Medicine*, ed. Fran Collyer (London: Palgrave Macmillan, 2015), pp. 207–21

Wilson, Bobby M., "Social Justice and Neoliberal Discourse," *Southeastern Geographer*, 47 (1) (2007), 97–100

Wilson, Leonard, "Medical History without Medicine," *Journal of the History of Medicine*, 35 (1) (1980), 5–7

Wiltshire, John, "Pathography? Medical Progress and Medical Experience from the Viewpoint of the Patient," *Southerly*, 66 (1) (2006), 22–36

Wingert, Lutz, "Knowing the Whole. A Note on 'Integrated Knowledge' (*Zusammenhangwissen*)," unpublished article, April 2017

Winslow, Charles-Edward A., "The Untilled Fields of Public Health," *Science*, 51 (1306) (1920), 23–33

Winters, Joseph R., *Hope Draped in Black: Race, Melancholy and the Agony of Progress* (Durham, NC: Duke University Press, 2016)

Wissenburg, Marcel, "Liberalism," in *Political Theory and the Ecological Challenge*, eds. Andrew Dobson and Robyn Eckersley (Cambridge: Cambridge University Press, 2006), pp. 20–34

Wolfe, Audra J., *Freedom's Laboratory: The Cold War Struggle for the Soul of Science* (Baltimore: Johns Hopkins University Press, 2018)

Wootton, David, *Bad Medicine: Doctors Doing Harm Since Hippocrates* (Oxford: Oxford University Press, 2007)

Wootton, David, Letter "Understanding the History of Medicine," *BMJ*, 334 (7597) (2007), 762

Worboys, Michael, *Spreading Germs: Disease Theories and Medical Practice in Britain, 1865–1900* (Cambridge: Cambridge University Press, 2000)

World Health Organization, *Global Analysis of Healthcare Waste in the Context of COVID-19: Status, Impacts and Recommendations* (Geneva: World Health Organization, 2022)

World Health Organization, "Ten Threats to Global Health in 2019," www.who.int/emergencies/ten-threats-to-global-health-in-2019

World Health Organization Executive Board, *Organizational Study on "Methods of Promoting the Development of Basic Health Services,"* Report of the Working Group (Geneva: World Health Organization, 1973)

"World Health: Ten Years of Progress," *The UNESCO Courier: A Window Open on the World*, 11 (5) (1099) (1958), 4–32

Worrall, John, "Evidence in Medicine and Evidence-Based Medicine," *Philosophy Compass*, 2 (6) (2007), 981–1022

Worrall, John, "*What* Evidence in Evidence-Based Medicine?," *Philosophy of Science*, 69 (3) (2002), 316–30

Wright, Ronald, *A Short History of Progress* (New York: Anansi Press, 2011)
Wu, John, Letter: "Could Evidence-Based Medicine Be a Danger to Progress?," *The Lancet*, 366 (2005), 122
Yancy, Clyde W., "Academic Medicine and Black Lives Matter: Time for Deep Listening," *JAMA*, 324 (5) (2020), 435–36
Yeh, Ming-Jui, "Discourse on the Idea of Sustainability: With Policy Implications for Health and Welfare Reform," *Medicine, Health Care and Philosophy*, 23 (2020), 155–63
Zames Fleischer, Doris and Frieda Zames, *The Disability Rights Movement: From Charity to Confrontation* (Philadelphia: Temple University Press, 2011)
Zamir, Eyal, *Law, Psychology, and Morality: The Role of Loss Aversion* (Oxford: Oxford University Press, 2015)
Zhmud, Leonid, *The Origin of the History of Science in Classical Antiquity*, trans. Alexander Chernoglazov (New York: De Gruyter, 2006)
Zierler, Sally and Nancy Krieger, "Reframing Women's Risk: Social Inequalities and HIV Infection," *Annual Review of Public Health*, 18 (1997), 401–36
Zuckerberg, Mark, "Can We Cure All Diseases in Our Children's Lifetime?," September 21, 2016, *The Chan Zuckerberg Initiative*, https://chanzuckerberg.com/newsroom/can-we-cure-all-diseases-in-our-childrens-lifetime/
Zurn, Christopher F., "Political Progress: Piecemeal, Pragmatic, and Processual," in *Debating Critical Theory: Engagements with Axel Honneth*, eds. Julia Christ et al. (Rowman & Littlefield: Lanham, 2020), pp. 269–86
Zylberman, Patrick, "Fewer Parallels than Antitheses: René Sand and Andrija Stampar on Social Medicine, 1919–1955," *Social History of Medicine*, 17 (1) (2004), 77–92

Index

Abelard, Peter, 42
agents, moral, 52–53, 110, 121
AIDS, 116, 154, 169
   narratives, 116
air pollution, 181
Alma-Ata conference, 150
ancient Greece, 11, 36–37, 41,
   43, 114
Angell, Marcia, 163
antibiotics, 19, 28, 30, 88, 134
anti-psychiatry movements, 125
antiquity, 30, 36, 46, 49
Arabic, 40, 43, 45
Aristotle, 39, 77
artificial intelligence (AI), 4, 31, 97,
   100–1
assisted dying, 123–25
attention-deficit hyperactivity disorder
   (ADHD), 20
Augustine of Hippo, 40–41
Australia, 148
autonomy, 11, 105–6, 112–14,
   118–19, 121, 129, 131
   individual, 111, 114, 157
   Kantian, 53, 105, 109–10
   medicine's era of, 114
   of patients, 105, 110–11, 118, 134
   relational, 115, 117–20, 141

Bacon, Francis, 46–48
Bacon, Roger, 45
Ball, Terence, 187
Barry, John, 172
Beauchamp, Thomas, 106
Begriffsgeschichte, 30
Benjamin, Walter, 64
Bergdolt, Klaus, 47
Berlin, Isaiah, 77
Betasamosake Simpson, Leanne, 185
Biggs, Hermann M., 63

bioethics, 7, 107–9, 111, 113, 120,
   139–40
biomedicine, 7, 14, 30, 87–88, 102,
   129, 160, 167
Black Report, the, 153
Blair, Tony, 134
Bookchin, Murray, 73
Boulder, Canadan, 174
Britain, 58
   National Health Service (NHS), 132,
   153
Brody, Howard, 112
Brooks, Rodney, 11–12
Broyard, Anatole, 124
Brundtland Report, 172
Bush, Vannevar, 67–68, 142
Butterfield, Herbert, 2
Byzantium, 43

Callahan, Daniel, 35, 164, 174–75
Canada, 6, 61, 148, 165, 170
cancer, 70, 84, 88, 91–92, 134
Candau, Marcolino G., 70
Canguilhem, Georges, 15
capabilities approach, 158
capitalism, 24, 62, 144, 159
Carson, Rachel, 73
Cassell, Eric, 12, 110
Chamberlin, Judith, 128
Chan Zuckerberg Foundation, 88
Charlton, Bruce, 90
Charon, Rita, 116
Chartres, Bernard of, 44
China, 165
Christianity, 40–44, 48, 51, 54
   medieval, 42, 48
climate change, 2, 19, 170, 176,
   179, 181
Clinton, Bill, 134
cochlear implants, 125, 127

Index

Cold War, 68, 108, 146, 186
Collins, Francis, 134
Commission on Social Determinants of Health, 142, 160
Compton, Karl Taylor, 68
Comte, Auguste, 56–59, 63
Condorcet, Marquis de, 50–51, 54
Cooter, Roger, 69
Copernicus, 45, 115
Cordain, Loren, 181
COVID-19 pandemic, 104, 129, 143, 165–69, 181–83
Croatia, 167
Cuba, 167

Daniels, Norman, 148–49, 159
Dart Jr, Justin, 126
Darwin, 57. *See also* Social Darwinism
Daumier, Honoré, 60
DDT, chemical, 69
de Vreese, Leen, 96
deafness, 127
death, 1, 35, 40, 53, 80, 88, 119, 125, 184
   acceptance of, 43
   and cancer, 92
   elimination of, 51, 70, 184
   and freedom, 122–25
   good, 20, 124
   in hospital, 122
   and inequality, 145, 156
   premature, 113, 138
   and progress, 108
   rates, 63, 122, 145
democracy, 24, 107, 184–85
Descartes, René, 47, 54, 145
determinism, historical, 160
Devisch, Ignaas, 94
diabetes, 161
Diamond, Jared, 176
Diderot, Denis, 51
diet, 84, 162–63
disability, 15, 19, 125–26, 156
   Disabilities Act, 126
   medical, 127
   psychiatric, 127
   rights, 112, 125–27
   social model of, 15
disease
   infectious, 59, 72, 183

   rare, 9, 164
Djulbegovic, Benjamin, 94
DNA, 1, 134
Douglas, J. W. B., 146
Dubos, René, 71–74, 175
Dumit, Joseph, 90

Edelstein, Ludwig, 36–37
Eisenberg, Leon, 69
Eisenhower, Dwight, 70
Engel, George L., 14
Engels, Friedrich, 16, 62
enhancement, 121, 137–41
Enlightenment, 18, 49–51, 53–56, 66, 79, 87, 106, 141, 171
   medical, 53
ETH Zürich, 136
evidence-based medicine (EBM), 31, 93–96

Faber, Knud, 59
Faden, Ruth, 106
Fauci, Anthony, 167
Fendall, N. R. E., 150
Feyerabend, Paul, 76
Fissell, Mary, 49
Fleck, Ludwik, 64, 76
Flexner Report, 61
Foucault, Michel, 22, 81–82
Fox, Renée, 75
France, 58–59
Frank, Arthur, 117
Frankel, Charles, 34
Franklin, Benjamin, 54
Freeden, Michael, 63
freedom, 31, 53, 104–9, 111–31, 134–35, 138–41, 170
   negative, 105–6, 110, 114, 120
   positive, 105, 109, 115, 117, 135, 138, 158
   ringers (*Freiheitstrychler*), 130
   terminology of, 105, 142
Fuller, Steve, 79

Galen, 29, 40, 44–45
Galenism, 43
Garland-Thomson, Rosemarie, 139
Gaudillière, Jean-Paul, 169
Gawande, Atul, 17
Gawdat, Mo, 98

Gay, Peter, 46, 51
genomic, 1, 161
  enhancement, 137
  medicine, 31, 136
  research, 134
  technologies, 136
germ theory, 71–72, 107
Germany, 58–59
Gluckman, Peter, 58
Goodman, Melody, 136
Google, 98, 135
Gracia, Diego, 111
Great Depression, 61
Green, Stefanie, 124
Griffiths, Simon, 144
Gunter, Jen, 91
Guyatt, Gordon, 93–94
Guzzella, Lino, 136

Haller, Albrecht von, 55
Hanson, Mark, 12
Harding, Sandra, 83
Harris, John, 138
Harvey, William, 48
health
  biopsychosocial, 3, 9, 14, 16, 33, 71, 146
  determinants of, 144, 152–53, 156, 162
  ecological, 175, 178
  'health for all', 142, 147, 151
  inequalities, 6, 32, 100, 142, 145–46, 156, 164, 169
  justice, 32, 142–43, 147–48, 150–51, 153–54, 156, 158, 162–64, 166
  mental, 14, 60, 108, 125, 128, 180
  perfect, 39
  progress, 30, 70, 142, 151, 154, 156, 159, 162
healthcare
  access, 147–49, 164, 169
  costs, 6, 160, 164, 186
  green, 175, 183
  primary, 147, 150–51
  public, 59, 147
  unsustainable, 175
Herder, Johann Gottfried von, 54
Hesiod, 37
Hinton, Geoffrey, 99

Hippocrates, 29, 37, 48, 60
  English, 48
Hippocratic–Galenic tradition, 40, 180
Hippocratism, 37–40, 48–49, 61, 180
history
  philosophy of, 40, 51, 64
  progressive, 44
  Whig, 2
Hobhouse, L. T., 63
Hobson, J. A., 63
Hodgkin, Paul, 87, 93
Honneth, Axel, 25, 157
Horton, Richard, 102
Huber, Jakob, 25
Hughes, Stuart, 101
human universals, 13
Hutchins, Robert M., 70

iatrophysicists, 48
ibn Sina (Avicenna), 43
Illich, Ivan, 80–81
injustice, social, 140, 143, 149, 156–57, 160
intensive care units, 19, 122, 166
Intergovernmental Panel on Climate Change (IPCC), 179
Iran, 166
Islam, 43
Italy, 128
Izambert, Caroline, 169

Jameton, Andrew, 174
Jaspers, Karl, 65
Jenner, Edward, 183
Jonas, Hans, 120
justice, 139, 142, 147, 158–59, 161
  and freedom, 138–39, 141
  and medical ethics, 105, 114
  Rawlsian, 148
  social, 32, 143–44, 148, 157, 161, 163, 170
  sufficientarian, 147
Juven, Pierre-André, 169

Kalanithi, Paul, 91
Kamm, Frances, 163
Kant, Immanuel, 52–53, 105, 109–10, 113
Kaplan, Abraham, 109
Kelvin, William, 99

Kickbusch, Ilona, 178
Klee, Paul, 64
knowledge
   biomedical, 17, 66–67, 74, 79, 85, 87, 102, 140, 153–54
   exploding, 97–98
   integrated, 100
   moral, 109
   probabilistic, 95, 136
   progress of, 64, 66–67, 76, 87, 97, 106
Koch, Robert, 60
Koselleck, Reinhart, 34
Kuhn, Thomas, 76–78

Lasch, Christopher, 2, 54, 171
Latin, 41, 43
Latour, Bruno, 169
Laudan, Larry, 76
Le Clerc, Daniel, 51
Leibniz, Gottfried Wilhelm, 49
liberalism, 62, 78, 107, 172, 177
life expectancy, 123, 153–55, 159, 170
limits
   environmental, 32, 175, 177
   to knowledge, 72
Lister, Joseph, 29, 60
Lomasky, Loren, 148
Lyotard, Jean-François, 79

MacGregor, Gordon, 146
Macklin, Ruth, 6
Magalhães, Susana, 118
Mahler, Halfdan, 151
Malinowski, Bronisław, 76
Marmot, Michael, 157, 167, 169
Martin, Adrienne, 18
Marx, Karl, 144, 171
Marya, Rupa, 161
McGill University, 104
McKeown, Thomas, 152–53
McKibben, Bill, 171
McKinlay, John B., 152
medical education, 14, 89–90, 105
medical ethics, 105–6, 108, 118, 131
medical humanities, 27
medical nihilism, 60, 80
medicina, 43

medicine
   alternative, 6, 89, 129
   atomic, 70
   Chinese, 7
   commodification of, 80, 186
   digital, 105, 133, 141
   equitable, 20, 136
   goals of, 2–4, 6–7, 13, 20, 88, 161, 170, 183
   historians of, 8, 26, 29, 116
   history of, 26, 28, 35, 48, 62, 67, 71, 98, 113, 145
   humoral, 38, 48, 180
   narrative, 117
   neonatal, 19
   personalized, 133–37, 161, 177
   postmodern, 89
   preventative, 81, 135
   socialized, 62, 145, 164
   sustainable, 174, 178, 183–84
   Western, 1, 7, 17, 30, 69, 74, 85, 99, 105, 125
Meier, Christian, 50
Middle Ages, 40, 43–44, 47
molecular revolution, 133
Mondeville, Henri de, 44–45
Montréal, 133, 165, 168
multi-dimensionality, 13, 30, 105, 170, 186
Murray, Stuart J., 94

narrative ethics, 15, 116
Nash, Linda, 174
nature, 47–48, 106, 175–76, 181, 183–85
   ambivalence of, 119
   constructed, 179, 183
   end of, 171
   and health, 32, 55, 176, 179–80
   imitation of, 39
   mastery over, 51, 54, 65, 175
   and progress, 180–81
   progressive, 51–53, 57
   representation of, 77
   therapy, 180
nazism, 107
negative eugenics, 58
new optimists, 24
New Zealand, 148
Newell, Kenneth, 16

Newton, Isaac, 45
Newton, Warren, 95
Nietzsche, Friedrich, 60, 81
Nisbet, Robert, 5, 19, 34, 49, 61
Noll, Peter, 124
nuclear era, 70, 108
Nuremberg Code, 107
Nussbaum, Martha, 139, 158

Obama, Barack, 134
Oreskes, Naomi, 23
Organisation for Economic Cooperation and Development (OECD), 3, 6, 168
Osler, William, 26
Osterhausen, Johann Karl, 53

palliative care, 18, 122–24
Paracelsus, 48
Parsons, Talcott, 75–76
Pasteur, Louis, 60
Patel, Raj, 161
patient
  autonomy. *See* autonomy, of patients
  consumer, 135, 137
  digitally engaged, 132
  empowered, 31
  patient-centred history, 128
  and personhood, 10, 60, 114
PatientsLikeMe, 132
Peabody, Francis, 63
penicillin, 5, 19, 62, 69
personhood, 9–10, 12–13, 16, 30, 63, 65, 104–6, 110–11, 174–76, 186
  dimensions of, 10, 65
  and health, 13, 16
  holistic, 63, 104, 110
  integrated approach to, 12–13, 111
  and progress, 30, 106
physica, 44
Pickett, Kate, 160
Pierce, Jessica, 174–75, 178
Pinker, Steven, 24, 104
Plumwood, Val, 175
population health, 86, 149, 153, 164, 170
Porter, Dorothy, 115
Porter, Roy, 28, 115
postmodernism, 22, 66, 79

Potter, Van Rensselaer, 109
Precision Medicine Initiative, 134
profectus, 41, 49
progress
  access to, 144
  biomedical, 116, 124, 138, 164
  challenges to, 76, 80, 104, 108–9, 161
  dimensions of, 165, 179, 183, 186. *See also* multi-dimensionality
  economic, 4, 171
  epistemological, 66, 77, 82, 92
  first-order, 5
  green medical, 174–76
  of health, 32, 151
  historical, 49, 52, 56, 59, 171
  historiography of, 22
  human, 37, 46, 69, 132, 145, 160, 173
  inflationary, 186
  as justice, 142, 159, 165
  and liberation, 120, 137, 140
  linear, 7, 26–27, 169, 174
  meaningful, 9, 116, 118, 153
  measuring, 20–21, 82
  moral, 6, 25, 158
  non-linear, 185
  open-ended, 4, 32, 51, 56, 71, 120, 175, 177
  political, 25, 59
  rhetoric, 2, 9, 30–31, 35, 153, 166
  scientific, 54, 57, 62, 64–65, 68, 75–76, 78, 80–83, 85–86, 96, 102–4, 108–9, 165–66
  scientific and human, 102
  scientific and medical, 82, 85–86, 126
  scientific and problem-solving, 96
  scientific displaced, 80
  scientific knowledge, 71, 75, 86
  second-order, 18
  social, 58, 62–63, 144–47, 164–65
  sustainable, 32, 173
  technological, 4–6, 12, 25, 31, 63, 105, 117–22, 124–25, 141, 148, 166
  terminology of, 4, 16, 25, 35–36, 142, 172. *See also profectus; progressus*
  trap, 177

Index

progressivism, 144
  neo-, 25
progressus, 36, 41, 50
Protestantism, 48
public health, 15, 151, 166
  global, 129, 179

racism, 14, 58, 142, 155, 161–62
Ramsey, Paul, 110
randomized controlled trials (RCTs), 94–96
Rawls, John, 148
relationship, patient–physician, 107, 110, 115, 135, 137
relativism, 22, 28, 71, 78, 87, 93
Ritchie, D. G., 63
Rogoff, Ken, 159
Roman Empire, 40, 171
Romantic thinkers, 54, 180
Roosevelt, Franklin D., 67
Rose, Nikolas, 113
Rosenberg, Charles, 28
Rosenberg, Lawrence, 133
Rosenkrantz, Barbara, 169
Rousseau, Jean-Jacques, 55, 180
Russia, 166

Sackett, David, 94
Saint Victor's, Hugh of, 43
Saint-Pierre, Abbé de, 50
Sand, René, 145–46
Sarton, Georges, 64
Satel, Sally, 163
Saunders, Cicely, 123
Schwab, Aurore, 173
science
  philosophy of, 23, 76
  progressive, 26
Seigel, Jerrold, 10
self-determination, 11, 53, 104–5, 109, 114, 127, 141
selfhood, 10–11, 36, 141.
  See also personhood
self-mastery, 106–7
Sen, Amartya, 158
Seneca, 123
Sève, Lucien, 121
Shapin, Steven, 29
Siegler, Mark, 114
Sigerist, Henry, 62, 145

Simon, Jeremy, 88
Smith, Adam, 54
Smith, Christian, 12
smoking, 84, 92, 162–63
Social Darwinism, 57–58
socialism, 62, 144, 159
Solomon, Miriam, 9
Sorel, Georges, 64
Spencer, Herbert, 57, 61
Štampar, Andrija, 145
Starr, Paul, 69
Stehr, Nico, 86
sustainability, 173–74, 176, 181–83
  and democracy, 185
  development toward, 172–73, 178
  discourse around, 174
  and justice, 157, 169
  power of, 173
  problems of, 174, 185
  and progress, 171, 173–74, 178, 183
Sweeney, Peter, 97–98
Switzerland, 6, 124, 130, 145, 166
Sydenham, Thomas, 48, 59
Szreter, Simon, 153

Teggart, F. J., 37
Thailand, 167
thought styles, 64
Topol Review, 132
Trump, Donald, 168
truth
  competing visions of, 78
  medical, 83, 93
  objective, 22, 64, 77
  and science, 76, 95
  universalizable, 88
Turgot, Anne Robert Jacques, 50

uncertainty, 75–76
  new, 20
  pervasive, 87, 89
United Nations, 3, 70, 173
United States, 61, 68, 76, 134, 168
Unzicker, Rae, 128

vaccines, 5, 57, 80, 128–31, 144, 153, 165
  campaigns for, 131
  compulsory, 129
  hesitancy toward, 129–30

van Doren, Charles, 34
Varga, Somogy, 131
Veatch, Robert, 113
Venkatapuram, Sridhar, 158
Vesalius, Andreas, 48
Vietnam, 167
Virchow, Rudolf, 59, 144
Voltaire, 56
von Braun, Wernher, 68

Walter, Hubert, Archbishop of Canterbury, 42
war, 2, 64, 67–69, 88, 92
Warner, John Harley, 28
Weber, Max, 63
WebMD, 132
Weinberg, Robert, 92

Whitehead, Cynthia, 98
Wilkinson, Richard, 155, 160
Williams, Bernard, 148
Wissensgeschichte, 66
Wootton, David, 29
World Health Organization (WHO), 3, 15–16, 70, 145–46, 150–52, 156
World War I, 61
World War II, 67, 107
Wright, Ronald, 176–77
Wu, John, 96

Xenophanes, 37

Zuckerberg, Mark, 4
Zusammenhangwissen, 100

For EU product safety concerns, contact us at Calle de José Abascal, 56–1°,
28003 Madrid, Spain or eugpsr@cambridge.org.

www.ingramcontent.com/pod-product-compliance
Ingram Content Group UK Ltd.
Pitfield, Milton Keynes, MK11 3LW, UK
UKHW020451050226
467579UK00035B/466